1·85

# Aromatherapy

## *A Practical Approach*

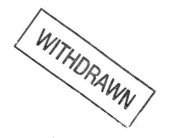

D0988326

Vicki Pitman

Published in 2004 by:
Nelson Thornes Ltd
Delta Place
27 Bath Road
CHELTENHAM
GL53 7TH
United Kingdom

04 05 06 07 08 / 10 9 8 7 6 5 4 3 2 1

A catalogue record for this book is available from the British Library.

ISBN 0 7487 7346 0

Illustrations by Oxford Designers and Illustrators
Page make-up by Florence Production Ltd, Stoodleigh, Devon

Printed in Great Britain by Scotprint

# CONTENTS

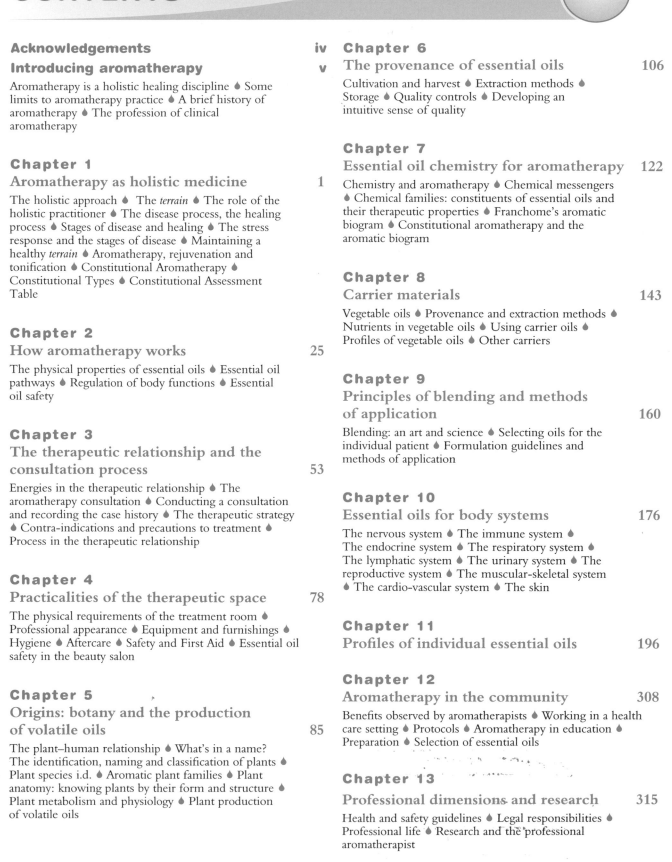

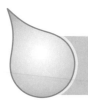

# ACKNOWLEDGEMENTS

This book makes no claim to originality. It is only intended to draw together as much relevant information as is practicable and will be useful for the modern student who is training to be a professional aromatherapist. Aromatherapy is a complex and wide ranging subject and the book cannot cover every aspect. By presenting the basic information in one volume I hope the book will also be of help to training schools and tutors of aromatherapy who can then augment it from their own considerable experience and expertise.

It would not have been possible without the work of previous aromatherapists and in particular those who have pioneered the development of the profession in the UK. This includes but is not limited to Robert Tisserand, Patricia Davis, Valerie Anne Worwood, Julia Lawless, Jan Kusmerik, Shirley Price, Len Price, Pierre Franchomme, Daniel Penoel, Bernie Hephrun, and Teddy Fearnhamm. There are many others. I am deeply grateful to their years of dedication, practice and experience which they have shared so generously with the rest of us.

My thanks go to Dr. Jeremy Ellston and Janet Anders who graciously answered my botanical questions. I am also very grateful to the teachers who so inspired me in my aromatherapy training: Shirley Price, Lieve Vandersloten, Jan Kusmirek, Daniel Penoel, and Lynn Bartholomew Orchard.

Finally, I am very grateful to Clare Hart, Carolyn Lee, Helen Kerindi and the folks at Nelson Thornes for bringing this book to fruition.

## Photo credits:

The author and publishers are grateful to the following for permission to reproduce material:

Steven Foster Group Inc. for the photographs on pp. 216, 222, 226, 232, 234, 240, 242, 270, 280, 284.

Martin Wall Photography for the photographs on pp. 198, 200, 206, 208, 210, 212, 214, 216, 230, 232, 234, 236, 246, 248, 250, 252, 254, 258, 262, 264, 276, 278, 286, 294, 298, 300, 302, 304, 306.

Garden World Images/Harry Smith Collection for the photographs on pp. 218, 220, 228, 256, 260, 282.

McOnegal Botanical for the photograph on p. 292.

The Bridgman Art Library p. viii; An ancient Egyptian Herbal by Lise Manniche/ The British Museum Press p. 160); © The Trustees of the British Museum Press p. 168; C.M. Dixon Photo Library p. 168; Fragrant Earth pp. 109, 171; Hitchin Museum Collection Ref. 10090/281 pp. xvi, 107; Dr. Kazuo Yamasaki p. 200; Microscopix Photo library p. 103; Science Photo Library p. 107; Traceability testing laboratory www.traceability.co.uk p. 118; Salamander Books Ltd pp. 170, 171.

Every effort has been made to contact copyright holders and we apologise if any have been overlooked. Should copyright have been unwittingly infringed in this book, the owners should contact the publishers, who will make corrections at reprint.

Picture research by Rosie Williams and Sue Sharp.

# INTRODUCING AROMATHERAPY

Until the late 1970s, the term 'aromatherapy' was little known outside France. This term, perhaps for the first time linking aroma (the scent or smell of a substance) with healing, is believed to have been first coined by a French chemist working in perfumery in the 1920s, René Gattefossé. He wished to distinguish the use of specific plant extracts – essences – for therapeutic or medicinal aims from their use merely as source materials for perfume manufacture. Actually, however, the use of aromatic plants for a therapeutic, healing or health promoting purpose is as old as the use of plants in general as medicines – i.e. probably as old as human life itself. So there has probably never been a time without 'aroma therapy', never a time when humans have not used aromatic plant materials for health and healing.

Soon after its more widespread introduction into the UK for healing, came its widespread introduction into the marketplace. Essential oils, as opposed to synthetic scents, became ingredients featured in toiletry, beauty and other commercial products to enhance their image as being more 'natural', luxurious and beneficial. As a result, to a certain extent there exists confusion in the mind of the general public as to the value of authentic clinical aromatherapy. As students-in-training it is important that you understand clearly the nature and value of aromatherapy as a healing art and science. It is equally important to understand its limitations.

## Aromatherapy is a holistic healing discipline

When used in its therapeutic sense, aromatherapy is the holistic art and science of choosing, blending and applying essential oils extracted from plants to heal conditions of disharmony and imbalance in an individual patient after a duly conducted consultation and assessment.

*Holos* is the ancient Greek concept of a divine wholeness inherent in the natural world and in each individual. Holistic aromatherapy recognises that the various aspects of a person – physical, mental, emotional, spiritual and social – cannot be understood in isolation from each other, nor from the environment. Rather, each must be understood within the context of the others, of the whole person, for a meaningful assessment leading to appropriate treatment and for relevant advice on health-enhancing life habits to be given.

Furthermore, holistic aromatherapy recognises the importance of wholeness with regard to its materials. For example, it is important to use the whole essence extracted from the plant, not an essence that has been adulterated or a substance that is an approximate copy of an essence.

### Aromatherapy uses essential oils as healing agents

Essential oils are the volatile substances extracted from aromatic plants by steam distillation, expression, maceration or solvent extraction. The subject of essential oils will be discussed in Chapters 2, 5, 6, 7 and 11.

### Aromatherapy is a special branch of herbal medicine

Because it makes use of substances extracted from plants, aromatherapy is a form of herbal medicine. It offers a *materia medica* specialising in aromatic plants and their extracts that is highly dynamic and vibrant.

### Aromatherapy is part of the naturopathic tradition in healing

Naturopathy is the healing system that places the study and following of nature at the heart of any healing treatment. It has its roots in pre-history, but was first developed as a methodical system by Greek physicians such as Hippocrates. In naturopathy, only substances readily found in or easily extracted from those occurring in nature are used. Healing methods also aim to follow natural processes. So, in addition to herbs and their essences, naturopathy employs the four elements of water (e.g. hydrotherapy), earth (e.g. clay), fire (e.g. sunlight or heat) and air, as well as foods and dietary regimens, and also vegetable oils, colour, heat and cold. Aromatherapy makes use of such naturopathic treatments as mediums through which the essences are introduced into the patient and by means of which their properties are enhanced.

### Aromatherapy is energetic medicine

Central to European naturopathic tradition has always been the concept of the vital force, vibrating through and giving life to our universe (see below). Today, through the science of physics, it is also understood that beneath the biochemical level there is an energetic level at which substances exist and interact with each other. The molecules and atoms of which essences are made are literally vibrating with electromagnetic energy and this energy carries information which influences human cells towards healthy functioning.

### Aromatherapy is a complementary medicine discipline

Aromatherapy, particularly as pioneered in the UK, US and Australia, is a healing modality in itself but it also takes its place within the wider health care system, truly complementing or 'completing' the care of the patient. Aromatherapists work alongside orthodox medical practitioners in GP surgeries, hospitals and hospices to enhance, augment or support any medical treatment prescribed.

## Some limits to aromatherapy practice

In France aromatherapy has been almost exclusively researched, developed and practised by chemists and medical doctors. There a prescription is given by the doctor, most often as an internal treatment for infection, prepared by the chemist and taken by the patient. As practised in the UK by appropriately qualified practitioners aromatherapy does not undertake to diagnose or cure specific disease conditions, but rather to so support and enhance the body's own healing mechanisms that conditions of imbalance are resolved as far as possible. Currently in the UK aromatherapists undertake not to advise or prescribe the oral ingestion of essential oils, but to restrict the methods of application to external pathways, unless they have undertaken the necessary additional specialised training.

## A brief history of aromatherapy

### Ancient usage *per fumare*

Plant medicine has probably always been used by humans, but it is only with the beginnings of recorded history – about 5000 BC – that we have direct evidence for this. From the archaeological discoveries of tombs engravings, papyri, stone and clay tablets and palm leaf texts of ancient Egypt, Mesopotamia (Assyria and Babylonia) and India we know that aromatic plant materials were very important not only in magico-religious rituals but also in practical life (cooking and bathing) and in medicine. These ancient cultures seem to have conducted themselves in an holistic way: all aspects of life were implicitly understood as interconnected. Hence, for example in healing, the spiritual aspects of the patient were attended with as much care as the physical, bodily suffering. Many aromatic plants were part of the ancient recipes and formulae prescribed by priest-physicians, as well as part of folk medicine. These include fennel, garlic, spikenard and cumin. We know how highly valued were myrrh and frankincense as they were chosen along with gold as gifts from the Magi to the Christ child. The Bible speaks of anointing (massage) with scented oils such as spikenard. Specific fragrant plants were associated with deities and spiritual purification.

Aromatic plants were particularly valued because of their unique property: scent, which is of course borne through air. And air and breath were considered particular manifestations of the Divine. Hence aromas could be used as vehicles between humankind and the divine, communicating prayers and creating the right spiritual atmosphere for communion. This is the probable origin of the use of censers and of aromatic woods in temple construction. Our word perfume comes from two Latin words: *per*, through, by means of, and *fumus*, smoke or rising air. This suggests that ancient uses of aromatic substances in incense, libations, anointing and ablutions were intended to carry the prayers and meditations of the supplicant to the gods above.

From around 600 BC a gradual shift occurred in several ancient cultures in people's understanding of the nature of both the human condition and of the divine. Before this time people tended to see themselves as completely subject to the whims of incomprehensible gods and goddesses. Gradually, people began to recognise that the human capacity for reasoning was in fact an attribute humans derived from a divine power, which had created the world along rational lines. Some intangible aspect of humanity is divine or spiritual and it resonates with the divine or spiritual within nature. With regard to health and disease, this attribute enables humans to understand what may bring on illness, rather than seeing it as a punishment, and thus take reasoned steps to return to health. Studying and then following nature's divine model, trying to live in harmony with it, is the surest way to as healthy a life as possible. This is the view found in the medical writings of the Hippocratic physicians (5th century BC) and Galen (2nd century AD), who taught the wisdom of *vis medicatrix nature*, the 'healing power of nature'.

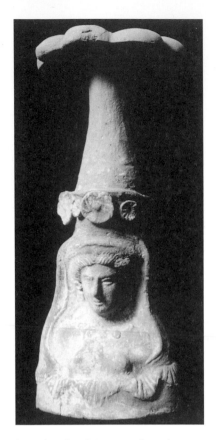

**Fig. I.1a** *Greek incenser from the temple of Hera, Paestum, Italy*

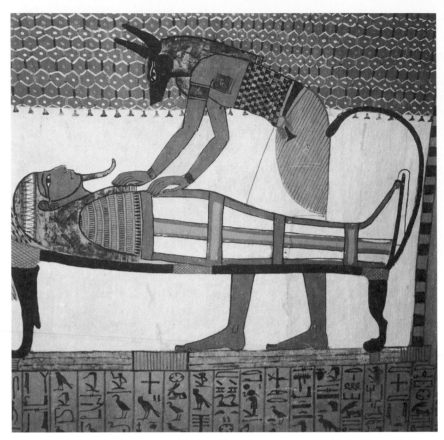

**Fig. I.1b** *Anubis, Egyptian god of the dead and patron of embalmers, embalms a mummy, 1320–1200 BC. Aromatic plants were used in mummification and helped preserve the corpses from decay. From* An Ancient Egyptian Herbal, *Lise Manniche*

Health was viewed as a balance among the natural elements – earth, water, fire, air and the *quintessence* or fifth element, ether (*aither* in Greek), and among the corresponding *humours* or fluids that constitute the human body. Disease arises from a fundamental disorder or imbalance among these elements or in the balanced flow of *pneuma*, the vital breath. Similar views are found in ancient medical texts of India and China. Ayurvedic medicine speaks of balance among the *dosas* (vata, pitta, kapha) and in the flow of *prana*. Chinese medicine speaks of balance in the flow of *chi* or *qi* through the meridians and among the five elements of earth, water, metal, wood and fire.

In each of these ancient medical systems, aromatic plants are used to great effect primarily in the form of fresh juices, infusions, decoctions, alcoholic macerations, poultices, enemas, pessaries, dietary modulators, and notably fumigation and oil massage. These methods are still in use in herbal medicine and naturopathy.

In addition to their use in medicine, ancient peoples used aromas in celebrations and religious practice – either fresh, as in the millions of rose petals lavished on his guests by the Roman emperor Nero, or extracted into fats and oils to form unguents, perfumes, toiletries and embalming agents. An example of how aromatic preparations featured in many ways in everyday life is the renowned Egyptian remedy *kyphi*. Made of 16 different ingredients, it became a panacea of the ancient world used as medicine, incense, perfume, poison antidote and tranquilliser.

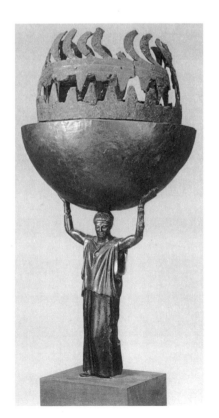

**Fig. I.1c** *Incenser from Delphi, Greece, abode of Apollo, god of medicine*

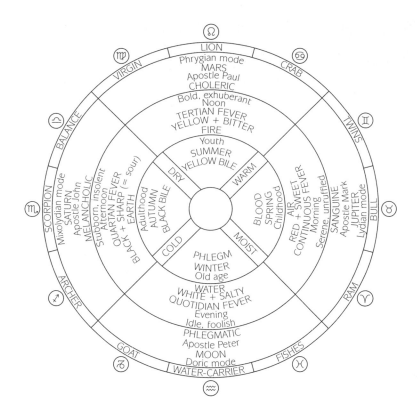

**Fig. I.2a** *Hippocratic scheme of the four humours (innermost ring) and its development in European tradition. Galen added some correlations: imbalanced humour is related to types of fevers and patient temperament is indicated (second inner ring). Others accrued later with the influences of Christianity and astrology (see Culpeper's herbal). Man as microcosm is placed within the macrocosm of Nature including: daily and seasonal cycles, the elements, energetic qualities, planets, tastes, stages of life, vital organs and even musical modes.*

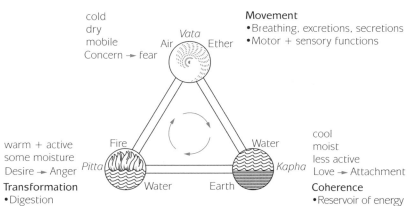

**Fig. I.2b** *Tridosa model of Ayurvedic medicine. The dosas represent biological aspects of the five elements and the primal energy* prana

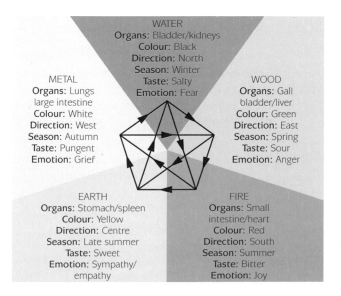

**Fig. I.2c** *Model of the five phases of transformation in Chinese medicine. Qi flows through each phase at different times of the day. Each element and organ either nourishes or controls another*

## 171. OKIMON. **Ocymum basilicum**
### Basil

Ocimum is commonly knowne, being eaten much it dulls the eyesight, but it is a softner of ye belly, a mouer of flatulencies, vreticall,
and calling out of milke. It is hard of digestion. Being applyed
with the flour of Polenta, & Rosaceum, & vinegar, it doth help
inflammations, & ye stroke of ye Sea dragon, and of ye Scorpion.
Of itself with Chian wine (it is good) for ye griefs of the eyes. But
ye iuyce of it, doth take away the dimnesse that is in the eyes, and
drie vp the rhumes. But the seed being dranck is good for such
as breed melancholy, & for ye Dysureticall and for the Flatulent.
It causeth also many sneesings, being drawn vp by the smell, &
the herb doth the like. But the eyes must be shut whilst ye
sneesing holds. Somme also doe avoyd it and doe not eate it,
because that being chewed, and set in the Sunne, it breeds little
wormes. But the Africans haue entertained it, because they which
eate it & are smitten of a Scorpion, yet remaine without paine.

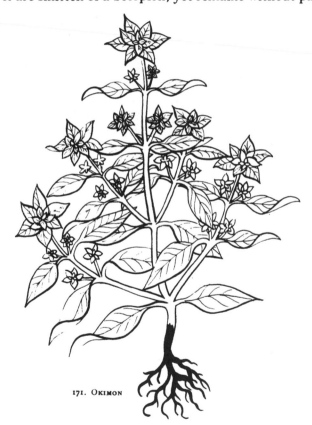

171. OKIMON

**Fig. I.3** *A page from Dioscorides' herbal* De Materia Medica, *the oldest surviving
Greek herbal dating to the 1st century* AD. *Each herb had its own page and this set the
pattern for future herbals. Here basil is recommended for flatulence, as a lactagogue and
diuretic. A basil poultice with flour helps inflammations and insect and 'sea dragon'
bites. The seeds are to be used for melancholy. This translation in 17th-century English
was by John Goodyer in 1640. The ancient text (Vienna Codex), first printed in
1478, inspired a renaissance in herbals by herbalists such as Fuchs, Brunfels, Gerard
and Culpeper*

## Distillation and the appearance of 'essential oils'

As far as we know ancient peoples extracted aromatic substances in fats and oils, water and clays for the most part. Distilled extracts from plants were not in common use. However, there is evidence that suggests stills may have been used. At Taxila, an ancient city at the crossroads of many cultures and empires (now in modern Pakistan), a clay distillation unit has been found.

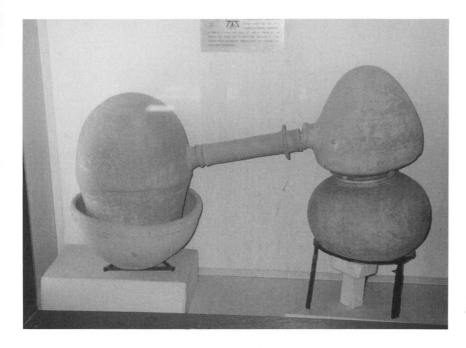

**Fig. I.4** *A terracotta still from early civilisations at the ancient city of Taxila (near Rawalpindi, Pakistan)*

The invention of the still and the refinement of the distillation process did not occur until the medieval period, the 11th century. It is traditionally attributed to Ibn Sena, known to us by his latinised name Avicenna. He was one of the most renowned and influential physicians, scholars and scientists of the Islamic-Arab Empire. Physicians like Ibn Sena practised Unani Tibb, a medical system that preserved and built on the ancient system of Hippocrates and Galen. Unani Tibb in effect saved Greco-Roman medical texts from disappearing during the fall of the Roman Empire, in around AD 400. It still flourishes in many Muslim countries today.

Ibn Sena is credited with the invention of the refrigerated coil, which condenses the aromatic vapours. With the perfection of the distillation process, essences, or as we now call them 'essential oils', were more available and perfumes could be more easily produced and preserved. The Arabs, Persians and Turks became adept at creating wonderful perfumes, eagerly desired by Europeans.

## The Renaissance, a rebirth of pan-European culture

With the fall of the Roman Empire, European peoples suffered wars, isolation, and the fragmentation and loss of much of their cultural inheritance. The Crusades, a bloody and ultimately futile attack on the Arab empire, stimulated contact with a sophisticated and learned culture and ironically with their own Greco-Roman heritage again. During the 14th, 15th and 16th centuries, Europeans experienced a rebirth of connection to their ancient past and a renewed passion for learning,

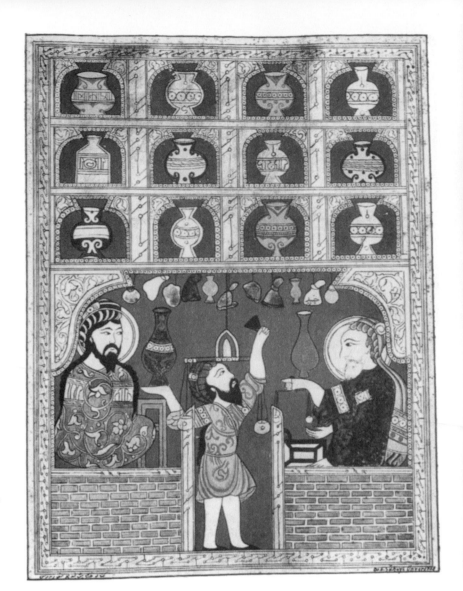

**Fig. I.5** *A Baghdad pharmacy in 1224, illustrated in an Arabic copy of Dioscorides'* Materia Medica. The Western Medical Tradition, *The Wellcome Centre for the History of Medicine, London*

philosophy, art, music, science and medicine. Ancient texts were translated from Arabic back into Latin; works of art from ancient Greece and Rome were rediscovered. With the invention of printing, books of medicine and alchemical works could be produced and circulated widely, using ancient knowledge in the service of present day concerns. Important in England were Gerard's *Herbal* and Culpeper's *The English Physician*. Also during this time the profession of the apothecary became clearly distinct from that of the physician, who previously would have made many of his own medicines.

One feature of the Renaissance, which combined reverence for ancient knowledge with interest in practical discovery, was alchemy. Alchemy is seen as both forerunner of modern chemistry and pharmacy, and a mystical quest for true knowledge. Inspired by ancient hermetical writings, its practitioners were trying to discover a method of transforming base metals such as mercury and lead into pure gold. Distillation was an important laboratory method. By their studies they discovered many chemical properties of their materials. But alchemy was

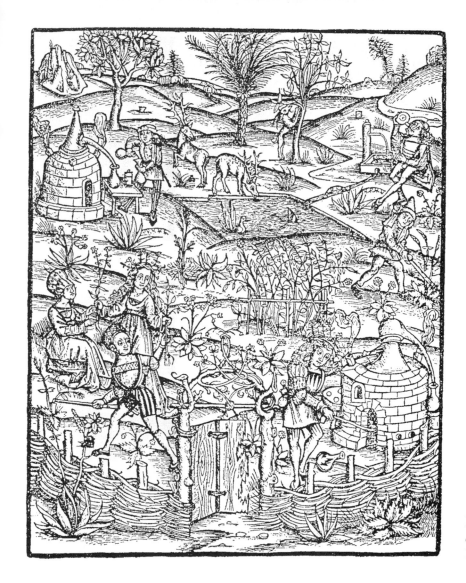

**Fig. I.6** *A scene of herb culture and distillation, Hieronymus Branschweig's* Liber de Arte Distillandi, *1527*

also a philosophical discipline: the work in the laboratory was intended to be paralleled by the inner change in the alchemist, whose soul was purified from its mixture with base emotions into its quintessence or spiritual nature. Distillation was both a practical method of working with substances and a metaphor for this inner transformation and concentration of the pure essence of the soul.

With distillation essential oils entered the *materia medica* of herbalists and apothecaries and also became more available to the general public. Many Renaissance households had their 'still room' where the women prepared domestic medicines including medicinal vinegars, wines, and distilled spirits from herbs and spices. This was known as the art of simpling. The famous Four Thieves Vinegar was an aromatic blend used to protect those who had to bury plague victims, and who availed themselves of the chance to plunder their pockets. Similarly, dried aromatic herbs were strewn on the floors of a household and hung in the rooms to cleanse and purify them. Without being aware how, the people knew very definitely by empirical experience that essential oils protect against infection.

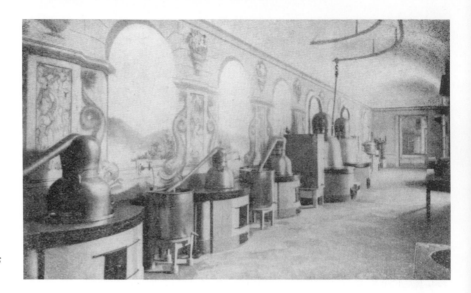

**Fig. I.7a** *The still room of the Profumo-Farmacia. The pharmacy dates from the 13th century*

## A new scientific paradigm

Beginning in the 16th and 17th centuries another shift gradually occurred in how we understand ourselves and the natural world around us, culminating in what is called the scientific revolution. Great advances in science and technology were made in the 18th, 19th and 20th centuries and continue today. Important discoveries in the very *physical* sciences – physics, chemistry and biology – encouraged the view that humans could now control and manipulate the natural forces – gravity, electricity, water

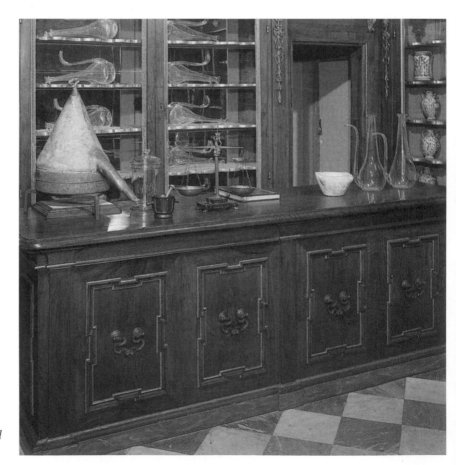

**Fig. I.7b** *Sales table of the Profumo-Farmacia de Santa Maria Novella in Florence showing a small tin and copper still and glass distillation vessels, 16th and 17th century*

power, and the chemical properties of minerals, metals and plants – to enhance our comfort and convenience, and to 'conquer' disease. Unfortunately, this was at the expense of a sense of the oneness and harmony within nature. The scientific discoveries also challenged the Church's control over knowledge, with the result that the Church at first tried to oppose the new scientific theories. This opposition provoked many scientists to repudiate anything that smacked of the spiritual, 'superstitious' or the subjective in favour of the objectivity and reason perceived to be available only to science. One result was a fragmentation of the understanding of what human life consists of, which one might call the loss of a sense of *holos*. Medicine has since become increasingly more scientific and technological and less of an art, tending to concentrate – until only recently – exclusively on disease as a physical entity. This trend was accelerated with the discovery of germs as agents of infectious diseases by Pasteur in the 19th century.

The tendency of concentrating on the disease was at the expense of the patient as a whole person, the one who was experiencing the disease. Disease was seen increasingly as something coming from without, rather than as something occurring because of the state within the body. Any type of healing practice outside the new scientific norm was considered outdated, superstitious and ridiculous and was discouraged or made illegal.

Fortunately, healers from the various naturopathic traditions continued to practise and defy medical convention. In the latter part of the 20th century, science itself 'rediscovered' realms of psychology and consciousness so that today, *holism* is accepted as fundamental once again. Today the two approaches are striving to work together for the patient's benefit. Many physicians and scientists of course never lost sight of the vital and spiritual aspects of their subjects and had always continued to put science at the service of a holistic understanding.

## The birth of aroma therapy

One of these scientists was René Gattefossé. In the early 19th century, plant distillates were still very much used in perfumes and much scientific work was done on their properties. Gattefosse discovered that lavender essential oil had powerful healing properties after an accident occurred in his labaratory. He was burned and he treated himself with the lavender oil near to hand. He was so impressed with the result that from this point he began researching the healing potential of pure essential oils. One thing he learned was that the whole oil was more effective in healing than any single, so-called 'active' component. He also found synthetic imitations much less effective. In his 1928 book, he coined the term *aromathérapie*. In 1923 two Italians, Giovanni Gatti and Ranto Cayola, published their researches into the psychological effects of essential oils, *The Action of Essences on the Nervous System*. They discussed how odours influence mood and emotions; via respiration they affect the functioning of the central nervous system – i.e. that part which is not under our conscious control. They identified sedative and stimulating essential oils. Paolo Rovesti, also of Italy, has also contributed to this field of psycho-aromatherapy, working with patients with psychiatric disorders.

In the middle 20th century, another Frenchman, a physician Dr Jean Valnet, began using pure essential oils and researching how they can be such effective healing agents against infectious pathogens. As an army doctor he successfully treated the wounds of soldiers with essential oils, and continued to use them in his medical practice. In 1964 he published his work, *Aromatherapie*. Many others in France and Italy were also publishing research on essential oils as healing agents. In Australia, work on the properties of native trees, tea tree and eucalyptus, was also being published.

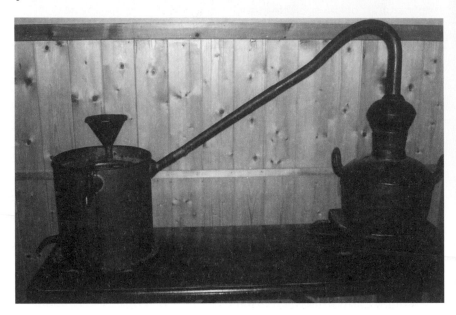

**Fig. I.7c** *Home made still dating from the late 18th century*

In the 1950s Margaret Maury, a biochemist and cosmetologist, learned about the work of Valnet and other French researchers of aromatherapy. Mme Maury believed deeply that beauty came from the person's inner vitality and health. This led her to study the great healing traditions of Tibet, India and China. Combining this deep holistic sense with her intuition about essential oils, she began to use this knowledge to create individual aromatic complexes for each client, based on their individual constitution or temperament and its imbalances. Maury tried to interest many doctors in using essential oils in their practice, but to no avail. Like herbalists, she knew that substances could be absorbed into the bloodstream through the skin, so she introduced the concept of the aromatherapy massage. Fifty years before medical science fully appreciated the permeability of the skin, Maury had promoted the advantages of percutaneous application of medicinal substances and a holistic approach, which blended complexes to match the needs of each individual patient. She began to train beauty and massage therapists in her 'art of aromatherapy'. She was the mentor of Micheline Arcier and Danielle Ryman. Her work began to be taken up and developed by more people in the late 1970s and early 1980s. Robert Tisserand, Patricia Davis, Shirley Price, Valerie Ann Worwood, Bernie Hephrun and Jan Kusmerik and many others contributed significantly to the development of aromatherapy in the UK, and abroad.

## The profession of clinical aromatherapy

As this brief history shows, 'aromatherapy' has meant different things in different times and places. In France, it is practised as an aspect of

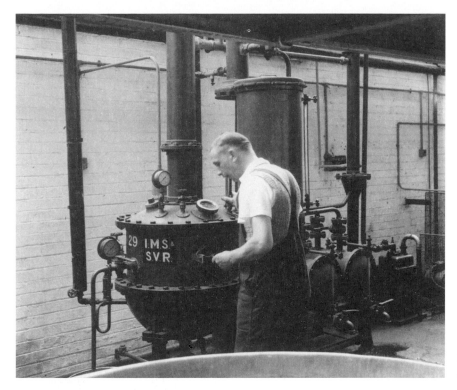

**Fig. I.7d** *Commercial still in the factory of William Ransom and Son Ltd., 1958*

orthodox medicine by doctors, in a rather allopathic way; this is sometimes called medical aromatherapy. French aromatherapists use essential oils internally. Some such as Dr Daniel Penoel and Pierre Franchome combine detailed knowledge of the chemistry of the essential oils with a holistic approach based on naturopathic, constitutional principles. In the UK, US and Australia (and countries that follow their model) the profession of clinical aromatherapy has traditionally been based on naturopathic and holistic principles and a thorough training in the *materia medica* of essential oils, but has limited their use to external applications formulated individually for each patient. As such it requires training in massage therapy. Many nurses and other orthodox health care professionals have become trained in aromatherapy and have been able to introduce its use to hospitals and other health service settings.

Some practitioners in the UK, US and Australia have taken further training in the internal administration of essential oils based on Franchome's work. Professional herbalists are also qualified in their internal use. Many beauty therapists also undertake aromatherapy training to a professional standard beyond the introductory training in the use of pre-formulated aromatherapy blends.

Today, the training of practitioners is of a high clinical standard and aromatherapy well deserves to be regarded as an autonomous profession. It embodies the fundamental hallmarks of a profession:

- a specialist knowledge base
- a distinctive service to the client or patient
- independence in professional decision making
- a defined and widely owned ethical framework for practice.
  (from *Developing Professionalism: A case study of Chinese medicine in the UK*, Catherine O'Sullivan, unpublished doctoral thesis, 2000, Leeds Metropolitan University.)

# AROMATHERAPY AS HOLISTIC MEDICINE

'. . . to do away with that which causes pain, and by taking away
the cause of his suffering to make him sound [healthy]. Nature
of herself knows how to do these things.'
                Hippocrates, *Regimen I*, XV (translated by W. H. S. Jones)

After working through this chapter you will be able to:

- understand the distinctive approach of holistic medicine to health
  and disease
- understand the holistic concept of stages of disease
- understand the mechanism of the stress response and how stress
  contributes to disease
- appreciate the role of diet, exercise, recreation, rest and cleansing
  in a holistic aromatherapy practice
- use your knowledge of aromatherapy as rejuvenation and
  tonification to extend your practice
- understand the concept of the constitutional type or *terrain*
- understand the importance of practising within the limits of your
  training.

Hippocratic physicians realised that in the healing arts 'it is necessary to
know what man is, by what causes he is made and . . . what [he] is in
relation to food and drinks, and to habits generally and what will be the
effects of each on each individual' (Hippocrates, *Ancient Medicine*,
translated by W. H. S. Jones). These words reflect the Greek emphasis
on *holos* – literally the divine Whole, revealed in nature – as central to any
understanding of ourselves and our purpose in life. Health is founded on
*isonomia* or balance, and *harmonia* or harmony among the various aspects
of ourselves and between ourselves and our external surroundings.

The **holistic** tradition has experienced a renaissance since the latter
part of the 20th century. Once invoked only by those on the 'fringe',
those engaged in 'alternative' medicine – which of course means
aromatherapists – the holistic approach is now familiar to the wider
public and even accepted in orthodox medical circles. As aromatherapy
takes its place within mainstream health care let us not forget the
inheritance and traditions that have formed aromatherapy and within
which we practise.

## The holistic approach

### The vital force

Holistic medicine is first and foremost vitalistic. There is a *vis vitalis* or
life force, the source of vital energy within each of us, and within all
beings, the energy that initiates and sustains life. Its nature is to ever
seek a state of health and positive well-being. In other cultures this

universal principle of energy goes by different names. It is called *chi* or *qi* in China, *prana* in India. Western traditional medicine based on Hippocratic concepts has sometimes called it *pneuma*, vital breath or air, sometimes simply *phusis*, nature. *Phusis* gives us our word 'physician', originally one who heals through the power of nature. The Latin phrase *vis medicatrix naturae* sums up these ideas in the credo of Western traditional, naturopathic and herbal medicine: 'the healing power of nature'.

This **vital force** exists at a subtle level and permeates the whole creation with its life-giving energy, which is why we sense a relationship with other creatures and with the very elements of nature. Being subtle, the vital force is not always perceived directly by our five senses, which are there to give us information about the physical world within and around us. So it cannot be measured or quantified. But it does have an effect on our physical bodies. It is present within every living cell and makes life possible. It is rather like electricity: we can't see electricity, though it is always present about us, but we can observe it with the right equipment and we can harness its power for our benefit.

The vital force manifests gradually from a subtle level of higher consciousness to first the mental, then the emotional and finally the physical level, which is why these three levels affect each other so profoundly, and are so inter-related. Holistic medicine recognises this force and seeks to work with it. This is why we say that holistic medicine works with the mind, body, emotions and spirit.

## Disease is imbalance of the whole organism

Disease, even a short-term, minor ailment, doesn't just happen at the physical level, or to a single body part, for example, the throat. The psychological, emotional, mental and even spiritual aspects of the person are always involved in the disease process and likewise the recovery of well-being – the healing process. When any specific part of the body is diseased the whole body is recognised as being involved and affected, whether this is detectable at the physical level or not. This has important implications for treatment. Orthodox medicine may treat repeated

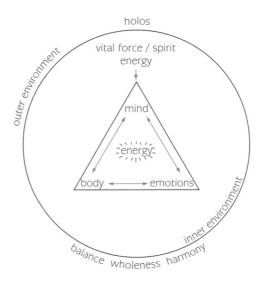

**Fig. 1.1** *The flow of the vital force and the relationships of body, mind and spirit*

tonsillitis with surgery or, as is more preferred now, with antibiotics. When the inflammation has gone, the problem is considered solved. However, from a holistic point of view the inflamed tonsils are in reality a signal that the entire body is in some way experiencing ill health and other aspects in addition to the inflammation in the tonsils must be addressed. When this is done, not only are the symptoms relieved, but also the person as a whole becomes well, and returns to positive health.

## Health is positive well-being not just absence of disease

Typically, medical science measures things to determine if we have disease, for example a blood test is taken to determine levels of enzymes, hormones, or the presence of bacteria or viruses. This approach does not necessarily take into account that the person may feel significantly unwell, yet have no measurable symptoms from a clinical point of view. If there are no measurable symptoms or signs, then it is considered no disease is present. Health and disease are thus defined exclusively in terms of quantitative measurements.

Holistic medicine takes a comprehensive view of the patient from the beginning and recognises that mind, body and spirit are all parts of one living being. It maintains and promotes the **synergy** of the body, the combined healthy functioning of all its parts. It aims at a positive state of health and wellness, a harmonious balance among many aspects, and not only the removal of disease symptoms, important though this certainly is. While recognising the value of all that medical science has achieved, holistic medicine has long emphasised that the patient's experience of illness and the state of his or her mind and emotions actually has a significant influence on the physical symptoms, the measurable disease. It does this because it has a fundamentally different philosophy about the nature of the human body and the causes of disease. Orthodox medicine has recently become more interested in these mind–body relationships (it excludes spirit). This is evident in its new discipline of 'psycho-neuro-immunology'.

The nature of the vital force is to flow in a free and balanced way, energising every cell and tissue and promoting the flow of blood, lymph and nerve energy. If this flow becomes congested, blocked, excessive or deficient in any particular place – be it at a subtle or a physical level – the stage is set or a predisposition has developed for disease. Keeping our organism in an open, freely flowing state is keeping it in health.

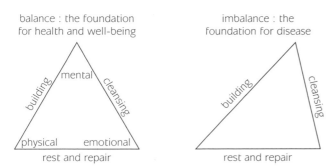

**Fig. 1.2** *A comparison of balanced with imbalanced functions*

## Homeostasis

The traditional concept of balance in the vital force corresponds to the medical concept of **homeostasis**: the body's condition of relative stability in its internal environment. This favourable internal environment, which the body strives to maintain, consists of:

- optimum concentration of gases, nutrients, ions and water
- optimum temperature
- optimum pressure in the fluid surrounding its cells.

For health the different aspects of our selves need to work together in a harmonious balance of activity. If any one aspect becomes either too excessive or too deficient, hyperactive or hypoactive, it gradually affects all the others and a negative imbalance is created. This gradually depletes the vitality of the body's energy, leaving it more susceptible to disease.

Health is a dynamic process, like a dance, not a fixed state of perfection. Our healthy state of well-being is constantly being challenged by different aspects of and experiences in our lives. The key to health is to understand ourselves, our particular balance of the different aspects involved, so we can order and live our lives accordingly, meeting challenges without becoming too out of balance. Knowing ourselves, we enhance our strengths while minimising our weaknesses rather than living in ways that weaken us, block the flow or drain our innate energy, our vital force. Becoming more attuned to when our individual healthy balance becomes weakened and taking appropriate measures to restore balance before serious disease takes hold, we live to a greater potential of harmony whatever our individual circumstances.

## The body has its wisdom: the self-healing energy

According to naturopathic, holistic principles the vital force is intelligent and so is the body through which it manifests. The life principle naturally always strives for survival, health and well-being. Therefore, even though the body may give us symptoms of illness, such as headaches and fevers – and we call these 'dis ease' and wish to rid ourselves of them – such symptoms also represent the body's best method of dealing with an imbalanced state through its self-healing mechanisms. Through manifesting such symptoms it is doing two things:

- trying to re-establish its equilibrium or homeostasis. Given its present circumstances, it creates the symptoms in order to restore the balance. Uncomfortable symptoms are the most intelligent means to do this.
- signalling to us that there is a serious imbalanced state present, which should be attended to. When we feel the symptoms we have to stop and take care of ourselves.

Symptoms, though unpleasant, even painful, can now be understood in a positive light as the body trying to grab our attention, to communicate that it is imbalanced in some way and needs attending to. We all know that feeling run-down is often the prelude to the onset of a really bad cold, fever or flu, which literally makes us take to our beds – at last! We may blame it on a 'bug' but really we have been ignoring the state of the body, letting its vitality become so low or depleted that the infection has been able to take hold.

This is why it's not a good idea to suppress minor ailments with drug medications. This makes us feel a little better temporarily, but prevents us from addressing the imbalance that caused the ailment and, in the longer term, weakens our health. Feeling symptom free, we do not pause to adjust the way we are living that made us get ill in the first place. This allows the imbalance to continue, become worse or 'go underground', displaced to deeper tissues and systems. A long-term imbalance begins to drain the body's vital energy and immunity and fosters a state in which a more serious disease can occur. It is such repeated suppression of the body's healing efforts, such ignoring of the body's signals that can set the stage for chronic disease. Being naturopathy-based, complementary medicine does not block but works with the body's natural healing intentions to restore positive health or optimum function.

## The unity behind diseases

Holistically, any disease, at its fundamental level, is perceived to result from a disharmony in the flow of the vital force – the flow is blocked, congested, hyperactive or hypoactive. Disharmony, in turn, creates congestions or imbalanced activity in the physical body. Such disharmony becomes the context in which it is possible for disease to develop. It is the real disease, of which the many diagnosed conditions – migraine, depression, flu, fever and so on – are the manifestation. The causes of disharmony can come from any area of our lives: spiritual, mental, emotional, social or environmental, physical – often a combination of two or more of these. We cannot always avoid these disruptions – life is meant to challenge us – but we can deal positively with the situation, trying to re-establish our best balance. Whether the individual disease manifested is a cancer, a bout of infection or the result of an accident, while relieving the symptoms we need to address the imbalance and restore harmony.

> **REMEMBER**
>
> Given the present circumstances, symptoms are the body's best, most intelligent response to an imbalanced situation. Holistic medicine, while relieving symptoms, goes further and seeks to restore balance, by working with nature's innate healing force. Emphasis is placed on re-establishing normal optimal functioning as the key to resolving conditions in the long term.

## *The Terrain*

In 19th-century France, the state of the organism began to be referred to as the **terrain**. The term indicates the background condition of the organism, which determines if disease can take hold or allows for healing to take place. Today we would see it as the inherent homeostasis the body strives to maintain. It is also the mind–body–spirit complex, the sum of all the factors in the organism, which predispose it either towards health or disease. In assessing a patient we can ask: What is the terrain of this patient? What adjustment to the terrain does the patient need to make to become well or to remain well? The terrain is closely related to the concept of **constitutional type**, which we find in traditional medical systems.

**Progress Check**

1. What is the origin of the term holistic?
2. What is one important distinction between holistic medicine and conventional medicine?
3. In what ways does holistic medicine offer a multi-dimensional approach to health care?

**ACTIVITY**

1   Start a health journal. Consider your own health: what are your typical illnesses or aches and pains, the things you are most prone to, if any? List these on a piece of paper.
2   Now think about what aspects of your life give you most cause for worry, strain or stress. These could be relatively straightforward things, such as the environment at the workplace is bad for you because your desk is too low or high, causing back ache. They may be more complex: you've never completely got over a childhood shock. List any such aspects. If you feel one of these may be creating an upset of the natural energy balance within yourself, put a star by it.
3   Finally, think about little ways in which you might begin to balance yourself and who might help you in this. Note these down.

**GOOD PRACTICE**

When assessing a patient, seek to understand his or her particular symptoms within the larger, holistic context of his or her life and situation.

## The role of the holistic practitioner

**REMEMBER**

Aromatherapy is 'complementary' to orthodox medicine. In other words it 'completes' the health care, which otherwise would be incomplete because it does not address the whole person and the optimum balance within the person.

The holistic approach respects the patient as the most important part of the healing process. This may seem obvious but experience shows that often the patient gets lost in the focus on the disease. With treatments and advice based on holistic concepts, this is less likely because from the start it is crucial that the patient play a part in the recovery. For example, the patient learns about which factors in his or her life may have laid the foundation for the disease and works with the practitioner to avoid these and to establish habits of health and a frame of mind that fosters health. Responsibility for healing rests ultimately with the patient. The practitioner's role is to support the patient's own healing mechanisms and help create the right conditions for recovery.

### Support and rebalance the body: the triad of treatment

This positive approach to maintaining health and resolving disease is one that may seem difficult at first, but which brings long-term results. It supports the body in its natural activities of nourishing, cleansing and maintaining and in its healing efforts. It attends to the symptoms in a way that both relieves them *and* clears the underlying cause of the imbalances, optimising the patient's health. These are the ultimate aims of aromatherapy.

A basic approach is threefold:

1   Energise and support the body to remove blockages by activating the cleansing of tissues.
2   Bring about deep relaxation, which also frees blockages and removes tensions. Through relaxation the patient feels more at ease, secure, can become open to positive change.
3   Strengthen any weak tissues, organs or functions and tonify the vital energy.

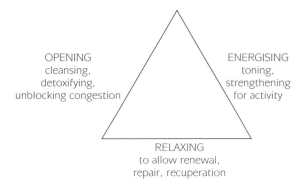

OPENING
cleansing,
detoxifying,
unblocking congestion

ENERGISING
toning,
strengthening
for activity

RELAXING
to allow renewal,
repair, recuperation

**Fig. 1.3** *The triad of treatment*

**ACTIVITY**

Breath awareness: get in touch with your own vital force through breath awareness. For just five minutes a day, sit calmly or lie down in a quiet place and observe your own breath. Breath is the vehicle for the vital force. Just allow your mind to pay attention only to your breath as it flows smoothly and rhythmically in and out. If the mind wanders to other thoughts, as it will naturally want to do, just keep returning it to the breathing. Feel the breath as it enters your nostrils and consciously follow its path through the nasal passages, into the lungs and out again. Allow your breathing to gradually become slower and deeper. Next, feel that you are relaxing a little more with each breath out, letting any cares and tension flow out with the out-breath. Feel that the out-breath is carrying these out of the body with it. Feel that the in-breath is bringing in vitality and energy along with oxyen, recharging your batteries. Feel yourself balanced and calm, at ease yet poised for activity.

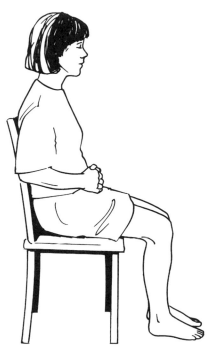

**Fig. 1.4** *Relaxation with deep abdominal breathing*

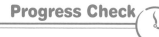
**Progress Check**

1   What is meant by the term vital force?
2   What are some possible consequences of the vital force being blocked or congested?
3   What do symptoms indicate from a holistic point of view?
4   What is the approach of holistic medicine in treating symptoms?

**GOOD PRACTICE**

Fundamentally, treat the person not the disease or symptoms. Seek to restore balance and harmony.

## The disease process, the healing process

Disease does not really manifest 'out of the blue', nor can it even be attributed solely to a pathogenic organism. We do not simply catch flu from someone else. The pathogen is part of the cause but not the whole story. We have many pathogens in our bodies all the time and our immune system usually destroys them before they take hold and provoke symptoms. But if this immunity becomes weak for any reason – whether a sudden shock or trauma, or a long-term unhealthy lifestyle – then we have altered the healthy *terrain* to one in which pathogens can thrive. Inevitably the symptoms of disease occur as the body deals with the situation. Unhealthy living includes mental–emotional aspects as well as the physical ones. Stress may be caused by the loss of a loved one as well the exhaustion of overworking. Both have been found to lower immunity. Sometimes a small event can be the trigger that finally tips the scales when there has been a long period of imbalance building up almost unnoticed; suddenly a disease is manifested.

## Stages of disease and healing

Naturopathy provides a very useful model for understanding the disease process. It recognises that there are acute, sub-acute, chronic and degenerative **stages of disease** – stages of dis-harmony.

Disease or the imbalances leading to disease pass through these recognisable stages and the healing process also passes through these stages as the body returns to health.

### Acute stage
First the imbalance is at a relatively superficial and minor stage. The body's basic immunity has not been able to deal with a pathogen or an imbalance in the normal course of its activity, so it mounts a more active, acute defence, which produces symptoms such as fever or inflammation (a local fever) with accompanying pain and swelling. Such fevers are part of the body's method of cure – heat itself kills many pathogenic organisms. In the process the body may create phlegm or catarrh, or may produce sweating, or diarrhoea, depending on the nature of the pathogen or area of imbalance. Notice that such symptoms are located at the sites of elimination – the nasal and respiratory passages, the skin, the colon, sometimes the kidney-bladder, as in a case of cystitis. The body is in effect striving to eliminate the toxic matter through the nearest or most appropriate eliminative channel and prevent it going deeper.

If the body is successful and its self-healing reaction is not suppressed, the body recovers and is in a healthier state. Often such an acute, self-limiting illness appears when the body has become toxic to an excess, so

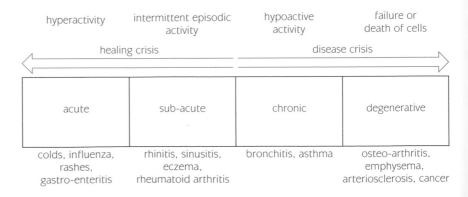

**Fig. 1.5** *The stages of disease and healing and some examples of disease conditions*

| hyperactivity | intermittent episodic activity | hypoactive activity | failure or death of cells |
|---|---|---|---|
| healing crisis | | disease crisis | |
| acute | sub-acute | chronic | degenerative |
| colds, influenza, rashes, gastro-enteritis | rhinitis, sinusitis, eczema, rheumatoid arthritis | bronchitis, asthma | osteo-arthritis, emphysema, arteriosclerosis, cancer |

much so that the normal **elimination channels** – the respiratory system, kidneys, colon and skin aided by the lymph – are not able to remove toxins in their normal course of activity. Toxin excess can be created by factors such as poor diet or eating too much of the wrong types of food, lack of exercise, a weakly functioning organ not able to perform its role, or even by negative thoughts and emotions. For example, constipation can actually be caused by a frame of mind that is obsessed with 'holding on' or with controlling everything; the tension in the mind influences the muscles of the intestines. Long-term constipation allows fermentation to occur in the bowel, creating toxins that accumulate and eventually become the breeding ground for pathogens, which can weaken and then permeate the bowel wall. This state, which is known as **dysbiosis** or intestinal wall permeability, can cause inflammation.

If the body is not at first successful in ridding itself of toxicity and rebalancing itself, or if its efforts are suppressed, it will try once more to mount an acute eliminative process and we experience disease again. Such acute eliminative episodes are thus best seen as a healthy body rebalancing itself and treatments are aimed at supporting the body through this process.

If the body is not strong enough to eliminate the pathogen or the pathogen is too strong for a particular body then a simple acute fever can become a life-threatening illness. For example, a disease such as measles, which is now usually mild in Western countries, is life threatening in areas where the overall health of the population is lower due to factors related to poverty and poor diet. Also in conditions such as meningitis, the pathogen is so strong that the disease quickly becomes life threatening and urgent medical attention is required. Acute stages can occur also as complications to chronic diseases. Extremely high fevers or inflammation can destroy tissues of vital organs and in these situations there is need for medical intervention.

## Sub-acute stage

If the acute state is not successful, and particularly if acute stages are repeatedly suppressed, the person may recover to some extent but the body will be left weaker, with the imbalance or toxicity not resolved. The disease then passes to a deeper level in the body. The body has adapted to an imbalanced state and carries on, but its efficiency is compromised. If it is a question of toxic material – anything that the body cannot use – that cannot be eliminated, the body may localise it in, for example, a joint, or encapsulate it in the form of a polyp or cyst. This mildly impaired state of less than optimum function is the sub-acute stage.

In this stage, symptoms may not manifest, or they may manifest only at a sub-clinical or low-grade level. The person can function well enough, does not feel ill, but also reports several mild or vague symptoms that don't seem to add up to any one recognised condition. The person in fact does not feel really well. The body can carry on in this stage for a very long time. However, the effect of long-term imbalance is that major organs are gradually weakened as their functions become impaired. Within the sub-acute state there may be some acute eliminative activity, localised in the area where the body has isolated the toxicity or where toxins have gathered because the tissues are weak: the body is trying again to resolve the situation. There may be periodic local inflammation of an area, for example, the joints, but it does not truly heal.

### The chronic stage

In this stage of disease, weakness and toxicity have continued so long that major organ functions have become compromised. Often one eliminative organ has had to work harder because another organ has been weak. It can carry on for quite a while but eventually it too becomes weaker due to the stress of overwork. Thus the chronic stage shows that the imbalance in the body has become more complex, and more organs and systems are involved. For example, if the blood is not properly cleansed through the action of the liver, plaque and atherosclerosis can accumulate in the walls of the arteries. This state can be in existence for a long time, unknown to the sufferer. All the while the heart muscle is working harder to pump blood through arteries that are getting smaller and smaller. Reduced blood supply to the heart itself means that this vital muscle is not receiving the nutrition it needs. Gradually the heart becomes weak and a chronic diseased state exists.

### Degenerative stage

Tissues that do not receive the right amount of both nutrition and cleansing through proper blood and lymphatic circulation, or the right amount of nerve stimulation, eventually degenerate. When organs and systems are in the chronic stage for long enough, such blood, nerve and lymph supply is diminished and the tissues eventually degenerate to the point where they cannot function enough to support life. Degeneration can be restricted to a local area, which causes loss of function, as we see in the degenerative stages of arthritis. Cancer causes the gradual degeneration of tissues and organs, preventing proper nutrition to healthy cells. If systemic degeneration continues unreversed, death ensues.

### The healing process and healing crisis

From the above discussion, we can see that many acute reactions, while uncomfortable or even painful to experience, are the sign of a healthy body throwing off its diseased state. Holistic medicine seeks to work with this process. Acute phases of eliminative or inflammatory activity as part of healthy function are what has been called the '**healing crisis**'. We have come to consider a crisis as always being something bad, but really the word just means a *turning point*, and indicates here the point at which the body turns itself from disease to health. Actually it is a healing 'achievement' because it means the body's healing, vital force is strong enough to mount a successful healing process.

### Stages of healing

Just as disease is a process involving many factors, so too is healing. The 'Law of Cure' identified by the homeopath Hering states that healing occurs:

- from inside to outside
- from the top down
- in the reverse order.

The first statement tells us that healing must come from within. There needs to be real inner change towards the positive in the person's emotional and mental state, as well as physically among the organs and systems. This doesn't have to be dramatic, or instantaneous, though it can be. Just deciding to come for aromatherapy treatments itself indicates that the person is motivated and engaged in the process of getting well.

Often a person begins to feel better emotionally before the physical symptoms are resolved.

The second statement tells us that if the important organs and systems have been compromised, they need to return to healthy function first before healing can be effected throughout the system. The third statement explains that symptoms of diseases or conditions we have experienced in the past will occur again as the body throws the factors that created them out of the system and in the reverse order in which they occurred. The deepest imbalance will be the last to be resolved. Since this is now a process of healing, the symptoms will be of shorter duration, less severe and the person will feel not worse, but better, more vital after such crises.

Not every patient experiences a healing crisis, but understanding this Law of Cure, we will not be surprised if patients sometimes seem to get a little worse before they get better, or if they report the reoccurrence of a condition they had years before, or we see a skin condition that improves slowly at first and continues to improve until the last traces disappear from the hands or feet. If occurring as part of a recovery process, these 'healing crises' are to be welcomed. A patient naturally will be concerned about such apparent setbacks, but we will be able to reassure them that as long as the momentum is one of changing from negative to positive, and in which they are feeling better in themselves, such episodes are normal and are part of the healing process. If old conditions or symptoms reappear, this time they are on the way out as the body has the positive energy to eliminate their causes completely. When the symptoms pass, the patient will report feeling better and having more energy than previously.

**Progress Check**

1 What are the four stages of disease?
2 What is the purpose of the acute state?
3 What is going on during the sub-acute stage?
4 What does the term chronic denote?
5 How would you explain a healing crisis to your client?

## The stress response and the stages of disease

In *Naturopathy* (1990), Roger Newman-Turner draws attention to the fact that this understanding of the stages of the disease process in fact corresponds closely to Hans Seyle's stages of the adaptive **stress response**. An endocrinologist, Seyle pioneered the research into the body's response to stress and explained his ideas to the general public in his book *The Stress of Life* (1990). His work shows a profound awareness for the deeper issues involved in discussions of health and disease. Seyle emphasised that it is each individual's ability to cope with stressors, with threatening events or challenging demands that matters, not the quality or intensity of these stressors. It's 'not what happens but how we take it'. He distinguished between the 'eustress' or good kinds of stress that challenge us in positive ways, causing us to grow and develop, and the 'distress' or negative kinds of stress that wear us down. We need a certain amount of stress to grow and develop into our full potential. Exercise is a form of stress that strengthens our muscles and general health. Working

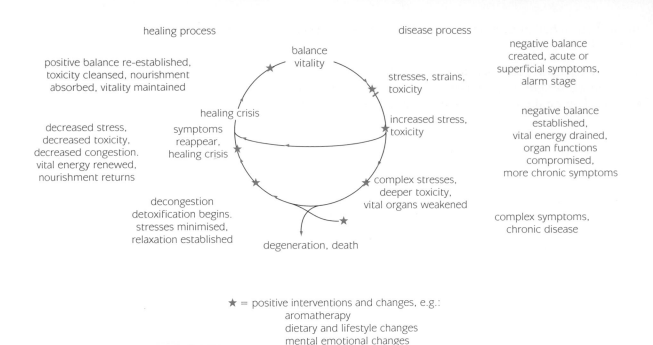

healing process       disease process

balance
vitality

positive balance re-established,
toxicity cleansed, nourishment
absorbed, vitality maintained

negative balance
created, acute or
superficial symptoms,
alarm stage

stresses, strains,
toxicity

healing crisis

increased stress,
toxicity

decreased stress,
decreased toxicity,
decreased congestion.
vital energy renewed,
nourishment returns

symptoms
reappear,
healing crisis

negative balance
established,
vital energy drained,
organ functions
compromised,
more chronic symptoms

complex stresses,
deeper toxicity,
vital organs weakened

decongestion
detoxification begins.
stresses minimised,
relaxation established

complex symptoms,
chronic disease

degeneration, death

★ = positive interventions and changes, e.g.:
      aromatherapy
      dietary and lifestyle changes
      mental emotional changes

**Fig. 1.6** *A flow chart of the disease process and the healing process, illustrating how positive changes can affect the course of the process*

hard to complete a task and learning to speak up for yourself in order to change a negative situation are other forms of positive stress. When stress is – or is perceived to be – a challenge that encourages or prompts us to raise our level of performance, when it stimulates us to adopt better habits it is a very positive thing.

## The stress response

Seyle discovered that the body has certain unconscious mechanisms, which are triggered when a dangerous or potentially harmful situation is perceived. This response is controlled by the nervous system and by the endocrine system. The sympathetic nerves initiate certain changes while other changes are initiated by hormones – the chemical substances secreted by glands to control and integrate metabolism and co-ordinate the response to certain stimuli. Hormones carry messages like nerves but their messages act more slowly and over a longer period of time. Nerves can be seen as the body's e-mail system, hormones as its postal service. Together they govern the stress response. These responses happen in a certain sequence:

1   An alarm stage (corresponds to the acute stage): The body mounts its defences.
2   A resistance stage (corresponds to the sub-acute and chronic stage after a sustained period of imbalance): The body adjusts to a sustained situation and manages to cope and to survive.
3   An exhaustion stage (corresponds to the weakest level of chronic stage moving towards degeneration): Major organ functions begin to fail, cells to die. If the resistance phase does not resolve the situation and return the body to homeostasis, a chronic stage ensues, which gradually uses up body energy in maintaining an inherently imbalanced condition. Finally there is degeneration, ageing and death of cells or the entire organism.

Aromatherapy aims to help the body be able to mount a successful stress response by:

- supporting the immune system
- helping restore homeostasis after the alarm and resistance phases
- helping the body recover as much as possible from the exhaustion stage.

It aids the body's recovery from the negative effects of stress.

## Stressors

Things that may generate the stress response vary greatly. Stressors include anything that challenges us in a way that triggers the nerves and hormones to respond. Seyle called them non-specific. Even a seemingly small stressor – if repeatedly encountered and perceived to be threatening or even just worrying – may eventually cause damage because the body is repeatedly being thrown into a stress response. Repeated smaller local stress responses can eventually develop into a general **adaptation** syndrome.

Stressors include such things as:

- loud noises, e.g. constant telephone ringing, noise of machinery, tension of a production line
- threats (real or imagined), e.g. job insecurity, wounds or the potential for a wound (i.e. a car accident just avoided)
- pathogens or poisons, including those released inside the body as a by-product of infection
- fear, or prolonged anxiety or worry of any kind, any emotional upset.

## The stresses of life

Seyle discovered important things about the stress response.

- It is *non-specific* – many different stressors can initiate the stress response and also, most importantly, the changes initiated by the stressor will affect the *whole* body, not just a part.
- It is a *syndrome* – i.e. the body responds with not just one change but a number of changes and their effects accumulate over time. Several episodes of stress or repeated stressful events can create a syndrome or group of changes. Seyle called it the **general adaptation** syndrome.
- Effects of stress can occur both locally, in specific areas and generally, affecting the entire system. An example of a local stress response is how the immune system responds to infection introduced by a cut or wound. We get swelling, heat and pain as the body sends in its defensive army of immune cells to fight and contain the infection.
- A general adaptation response is typified by what happens, for example, when we experience a sudden threat. Its first stage has been called the fight or flight response and is mediated through the sympathetic nervous system and the adrenal glands.

## The mechanism of stress: the general adaptation syndrome

### Stage one: alarm reaction, the sympathetic response

When threatened, your body prepares for fight or flight. The sympathetic nerves signal the adrenal glands to release hormones: adrenaline and corticosteroids. These enter the bloodstream and initiate changes to the metabolism:

- more blood is directed away to the large muscles and brain
- the heart beats faster and heart muscle contracts more frequently and more strongly
- perspiration (the cooling system) is activated
- the liver releases sugar into the blood to be the fuel for the muscles to stand and fight or flee
- the spleen contracts to make more blood available; red blood cell production and clotting ability increases
- digestive, urinary and reproductive activities are inhibited.

The body is effectively in a state of red alert.

All this is well and good, the body copes and responds and when the threat is over it returns to its homeostasis. The body has used the energy provided, the sugar is burned up with exertion, the muscles work and the danger having been successfully met, the body returns to a recuperating state for repair and renewal of energy.

However, the problem for our health comes when this recuperation and restoration of homeostasis does not happen. If we are overworking at a challenging job and we do not take time for adequate rest, we may encounter so many repeated stressful situations that the body is not allowed to recuperate adequately afterwards. It is important to remind ourselves here that stressors can be emotional and mental as well as physical. Our thoughts and emotions can initiate the alarm reaction. For example, we can be so anxious about our job security, or a sick loved one that our body responds with a stress adaptation. So how we perceive ourselves and the world around us is important in this regard.

### Some symptoms of alarm reactions

Repeated alarm reactions can lead to many minor symptoms and ailments associated with the physiological changes initiated by the alarm phase of the stress response such as:

| | |
|---|---|
| Churning stomach | Aching or stiff neck |
| Sweating | Diarrhoea |
| Nausea or even vomiting | Clenched jaw or fists |
| Breathlessness | Dry mouth |
| Racing heart or palpitations | Dizziness |
| Aching head | Confused thoughts |
| Trembling | |

Although the immediate threat of a stressor may have been met, if stress becomes chronic the body still senses all is not well. At this point the stress response passes to the resistance stage.

### Stage two: resistance
In this stage the response is initiated by regulating factors of the endocrine system. Hormones continue to circulate in the bloodstream.

They allow the body to continue to fight the perceived stressor long after the effects of the alarm reaction have died down. In the resistance stage, the rate at which life processes occur is significantly increased – you could say that we are ageing faster – and although blood chemistry returns to normal, blood pressure levels and water retention remained raised. The continuing circulation of hormones in the resistance stage, if continued long term, puts a heavy demand on the body, especially the circulatory system and the adrenal glands. Continued release of adrenal cortisone is especially harmful; a high level in the blood is associated with diabetes, ulcers and heart attacks, and it has been found to suppress the immune system, leaving the body's resistance to disease weaker. This lowered state of the resistance phase is perhaps typified by the experience of chronically feeling low on energy.

What in fact is happening is that the body is now having to maintain a state of 'balanced imbalance'. An imbalance exists, which it can't resolve, so it adapts and makes the best of that state of continuing stress. An imbalanced state causes an eventual draining of energy, under-nourishment of cells and under-functioning of organs. Such a state, unrelieved by adequate recuperation, eventually leads to symptoms of disease. These will manifest differently in different people, but they may all be to a significant extent related to chronic stress.

---

**Symptoms and ailments associated with the resistance stage**

| | |
|---|---|
| Chest pains | Wheezing |
| Colds and flu | Accidents |
| High blood pressure | Dermatitis or eczema |
| Overeating | Alcoholism |
| Abdominal pain | Pre-menstrual syndrome |
| Loss of libido | Excessive smoking |
| Migraine | Loss of appetite |
| Phobias or obsessions | Low back pain |
| Insomnia and/or tiredness | Indigestion |
| Depression | Persistent anxiety |

---

### Stage three: exhaustion

If the resistance stage continues long enough without let up, major organs are becoming more and more weakened and their functions compromised. In the exhaustion stage, the internal environment around cells cannot be maintained, and cells begin to die. The adaptation has become chronic and finally degenerative.

## The stress factor in disease and health

Having shown how repeated or sustained states of stress can so profoundly affect the body's internal organs and tissues, literally causing energy to be used up and the body's functions to work harder to maintain 'balanced imbalance', Seyle demonstrated how stress is an important factor in many chronic diseases. The resistance and exhaustion stages are in fact what naturopaths saw as the chronic and degenerative stages. Seyle's work in effect proved that disease comes from within, a consequence of the body's eventual inability to respond to repeated stress unrelieved by periods of recuperation. Seyle came to realise that each of us has a reservoir of 'adaptative energy' and that this is depleted by chronic stress. In effect, when this adaptative energy is drained or exhausted, chronic diseases result. Seyle calls such chronic diseases the diseases of adaptation. They include such conditions as hypertension, diabetes, migraines and obesity.

Seyle was careful to emphasise that it is not so much the stressor agent that is important but our response to it. This is an extremely important point to remember. It means that rather than being passive victims of stress, of disease, we in fact have the ability to minimise its effects on our bodies according to how we choose to live. We can protect, nurture and extend the life of our adaptive energy by the thoughts we entertain, by the way we respond to challenges, by emotions we enjoy, by the lifestyle we lead and many other means. Many other thinkers have come to the same conclusions and they teach that it is not what happens to us in life that matters so much as how we respond to it, learn and grow through our challenges.

Seyle's approach allows us to see that stress can be positive and is not necessarily always negative. But if we perceive life events as stressful, or allow temporary acute stresses to become chronic and the dominating factor in our lives, we can allow stress to set the stage for many diseases. It has been said that stress is a factor in at least 75 per cent of diseases. Thus learning methods of dealing with stress in our lives is one of the most health enhancing things we can do. Following nature, a holistic

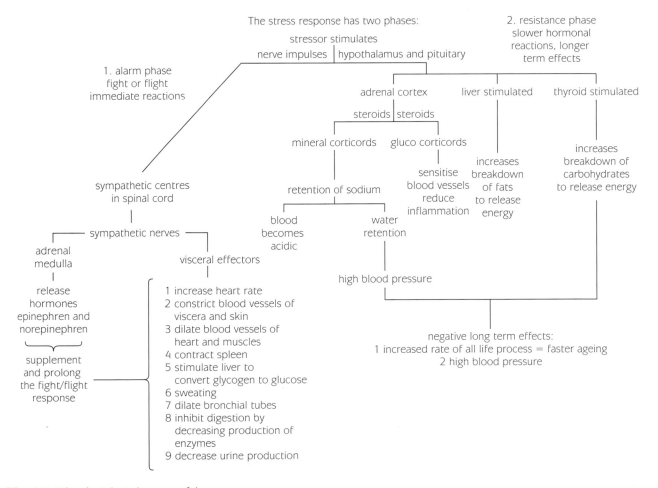

**Fig. 1.7** *The physiological process of the stress response*

approach aims to restore normal functioning of the body systems and provide for adequate rest, relaxation and recreation – the keys to recovering from stress.

## Maintaining a healthy *terrain*: breathing, diet, exercise, recreation, rest, cleansing

From the above discussion of stages of disease and healing, we can see that the body's overall health lies in the health and vitality of each cell and tissue, and of psychological factors – a healthy *terrain*. Every cell, every tissue, every organ needs energy to do its work, regular cleansing to remove the waste products from cell metabolism and open channels of communication to the body-whole. These factors are supplied by our breathing, diet and activities.

### Respiration
In addition to clean air, adequate respiration of our cells involves the way we breathe. Factors that impair breathing include: poor posture, breathing that is too shallow, 'overbreathing' (taking in more air than we can actually process) and mouth breathing.

### Nutrition, digestion, absorption
To maintain health or revitalise an ailing body, these of course need attention. As regards diet, not only is the quality of the food important, to ensure vital nutrients like vitamins, minerals and enzymes but also the quality of the digestion itself. Emotional factors, a happy atmosphere and regularity in eating habits all affect the digestion and absorption of nutrients, which in turn feed our cells.

### Cleansing
Cells and tissues need to have the by-products of their metabolism removed regularly. In our homes we cannot allow waste to build up in our kitchens or toilets or they would soon become a breeding ground for germs and disease, and places where space is clogged up and activity compromised. In our bodies also, regular cleansing is vital. The five eliminative channels and the liver need to be active and well functioning so that cell waste and food by-products are regularly excreted. The five eliminative channels are: the lungs and respiratory system; the colon; the kidneys; the skin; and the lymph system. In addition, the liver, in company with the lungs and the kidneys, is responsible for keeping the blood healthy so that it can carry nutrients to the cells. The liver neutralises toxins in the blood. At the mental–emotional level too each of us could use a little house cleaning from time to time, examining which attitudes and habitual emotional responses may be blocking our clarity of thought and motivation.

### Exercise, rest and recreation
A healthy body needs both regular exercise and regular periods of rest and relaxation. Exercise tones muscles, increases circulation to cells and aids elimination through sweating. It also helps maintain good co-ordination between mind and body. Rest and relaxation allow the body time for self-repair and recovery from stress; and for release of the tensions that can build up and block the circulation and other body functions. Recreation is providing ample space in one's life for creativity and self-expression. This, too, is important for our inner sense of well-being.

# Aromatherapy, rejuvenation and tonification

Margarite Maury believed that optimum health was linked to **rejuvenation**. This term does not really mean a futile search for eternal youth. Rather it describes the body's own capacity for regeneration and its impetus towards well-being. Today medical science itself is beginning to recognise the importance of this area of health care. It has begun to speak of 'inhibiting the ageing process'. Traditional healing systems, such as that of Hippocrates and Galen, and of Ayurvedic and Chinese medicine, have always emphasised that curing disease is not the only function of medicine. Medicine should also strengthen the body's health so as to prevent disease and promote longevity. In traditional healing systems special practices and herbal combinations were developed to tonify and rejuvenate the body's organs and tissues and the body as a whole. Maury implanted this same concern into aromatherapy when she emphasised that the dynamism of essential oils plays a major role not only in curing disease but also in rejuvenation therapy. Aromatherapy uses the properties of essential oils such as astringent, tonifying, digestive, relaxing and stimulating to rejuvenate the organism so that the patient can live life to the full.

## REMEMBER

The basics of healing and health apply as much to the mind and emotions as to the physical body.

Passionately interested by works dealing with the essential oils, perfumes and aromatics we have discovered their vast possibilities – particularly with regard to the problem of regeneration.

Margarite Maury (1989) *Margarite Maury's Guide to Aromatherapy*, p. 51

## ACTIVITY

In your health journal, reflect on one of your own past diseases or ailments, whether minor or more serious. Consider what factors in your life as a whole may have been involved in the experience for you. Study the next section on constitutional aromatherapy. Having learned about your constitutional type, consider what aspects of your nature may have been imbalanced before the illness. What steps would you take today to bring yourself into balance as much as possible following such an illness?

## GOOD PRACTICE

Aromatherapy respects the person's whole being: body, mind and spirit.
- Its fundamental aim is to restore a positive, dynamic balance of these factors to bring about healing.
- It realises the patient's feelings and sensibilities are important factors in assessing the condition.
- By creating individual blends of essential oils for each patient, the aromatherapist is treating the whole person.

1   What are stressors? Give **four** examples.
2   What are the three stages of the general adaptation syndrome or the stress response?
3   What effects does the continued circulation of hormones in the resistance stage have on the body?
4   How do the stages of disease and the stages of the stress response correspond?
5   What are some important aspects of the body's functioning, which are important for health?
6   Think further about 'rejuvenation', then explain its meaning in your own words.

# Constitutional aromatherapy

Knowledge of aromatic plants has been used successfully for thousands of years in traditional medical systems like the Hippocratic-Galenic medicine of Europe, Chinese medicine and Ayurvedic medicine of India. As well as knowing the actions of medicines, these systems evaluate the energy and qualities of medicinal substances and these are seen to correspond to and influence similar qualities within human beings. In healing two principles are applied:

♦   Like attracts like. A healing substance of like quality enhances that quality in the body. The many properties and qualities in nature can be conveniently grouped into the following categories: stimulating-calming (sometimes a substance can combine the two, acting on different systems); warming-cooling, moistening-drying. Substances that promote good quality of vital heat and moisture in the body are those that are warming (for example, pepper, ginger) and moistening (for example, water, oils or foods with a high water content or gels that retain water).
♦   Opposites counteract. Cooling lowers heat, moistening lessens dryness, warming relieves cold, drying reduces excess moisture.

Essential oils, like other medicinal or food substances, can be grouped according to their warming, moistening, cooling, drying, stimulating and calming effects. In constitutional aromatherapy these qualities are used to help balance the constitutional predispositions and imbalances of the patient.

## Constitutional types

Humans can be grouped according to certain characteristic tendencies. Psychologists recognise certain personality types: type A, B and so forth. Geno-type or bio-type is another term used to describe this phenomenon. Traditional medical systems call them constitutional types, temperaments or humoural types. Each type exhibits a particular pattern of characteristics and qualities both physically and psychologically. The characteristic qualities are inherent from birth and give a predisposition for types of behaviour, thoughts, feelings and types of health issues. They are common to all of us; it is just that each of us tends to exhibit a greater proportion of certain characteristics. In this book we will describe the constitutional types of traditional Western medicine based on Hippocrates and Galen. This model was also used by Avicenna and Culpeper. Many of the terms are actually quite familiar to us through words in general use, such as **phlegmatic**, **choleric,** **bilious, melancholic**, **sanguine**, even-tempered, warm or cold 'natured', hot-headed or cool-headed.

The idea of constitutional types has many similarities to the idea of the *terrain* discussed above. The terms are effectively interchangeable.

For the aromatherapist, assessing a patient's constitutional type helps by:

- giving a structure within which to process all the information we gather about the patient in the therapeutic context.
- helping explain why each person may react differently to the same set of circumstances, for example the degree of touch, helping our approach to be adapted accordingly
- guiding the planning of treatments and in judging the likely process an imbalance may go through as it returns to harmony, for example, a 'hot' person may have cleansing symptoms of a hotter nature, perhaps a mild infection or inflammation, than one who is temperamentally 'colder'. It helps if we can anticipate this and advise our patients accordingly
- enhancing our self-awareness as practitioners in order to approach the patient with more clarity, knowing that our understanding of them is influenced by our own nature.

> **REMEMBER**
>
> Selecting essential oils to harmonise with the patient's inherent constitutional pattern helps restore balance to the whole.

In the Western traditional model, the four constitutional types are based on the four humours or bodily fluids, which themselves were derived from the five elements that, in Greek thought, constitute the world: earth, water, fire, air and ether. Each element has certain qualities, which it contributes to the humours. Earth is cold and dry, for example, water moist and cool, fire hot and dry, air moist and warm.

| Humour | Temperament/constitutional type |
|---|---|
| Blood | Sanguine |
| Bile | Choleric or bilious |
| Phlegm | Phlegmatic |
| Black bile/melancholy | Melancholic |

In modern times, the terms phlegmatic and melancholic have sometimes been called **lymphatic** and **neurogenic** (nervous-type). The qualities of each humoural type are described below.

If a humour tends to be dominant in a person, then that person will have mostly those characteristics. We all have a bit of each humour in us, for we are all made of the same elements that comprise the world. It's only a question of degree and tendency. A person can certainly show at different times and in different circumstances any of the characteristics. But usually one or two humours (group of characteristics) will be stronger from birth. Some people are strongly of one humour, some are more of a mixed type and have strong tendencies from two humours.

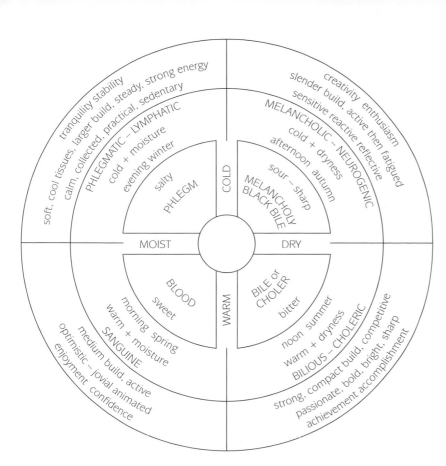

**Fig. 1.8** *The Hippocratic temperament model*

## The Hippocratic constitutional types or temperaments

These can be supported or balanced by corresponding types of food, exercise, colours, climates and, most importantly, essential oils. In Chapter 7 there is a more detailed discussion of the chemistry of essential oils that relates them to constitutional types.

### Sanguine

- Warm and moist: a higher proportion of water and fire elements; corresponds to the blood, to springtime and morning.
- Physically of a medium, strong build and have an abundance of warmth and energy. Usually enjoy excellent health, unless overindulge.
- Psychologically of a sunny, optimistic nature; usually serene and unruffled; outgoing, enjoy other's company, bringing people together; enjoy their food and other sensual stimulations.

- Prone to imbalances of: congestion due to over-indulgence; heart/circulatory problems; over-stimulation leading to exhaustion.
- Benefits from esters, sesquiterpenes to relax; terpenes if too damp (e.g. excess mucous or fluid retention); ketones and aldehydes if hyperactive or catarrhal.

## Bilious

- Warm and dry, reflecting a higher proportion of fire and air elements typified by bile and summer.
- Physically of a strong, compact, slender or wiry build with good energy; tendency to dryness.
- Psychologically of a hot, passionate, ambitious, bold or exhuberant nature; competitive, enjoy excitement, workaholic, independent thinkers, mentally quick with a tendency to more easily become irritable, angry.
- Prone to imbalances of the liver, and heat and dryness; gall or kidney stones; enjoy stimulation, are used to having energy, so may turn to drugs, such as caffeine to boost levels, and perhaps alcohol to relax.
- Benefits from small amounts of ketones or aldehydes to cool, moisten and relax.

## Phlegmatic/lymphatic

- Cool and moist, reflecting a higher proportion of water and earth elements, typified by mucus, lymph fluid and winter, evening.
- Physically of a softer but large-boned build with a steady energy. Skin will feel cool and soft.
- Psychologically of a prudent, calm nature; tendency to sedentary habits, even idleness; slower to accept the need for/ initiate change.
- Prone to accumulate water or damp or have moist-type inflammations, swellings, water retention; to gain weight more easily.
- Benefits from warm and dry: terpenes for fluid retention, congestion of phlegm; ethers for antispasmodic action on physical level.

## Melancholic/neurogenic

- Cold and dry, reflecting a higher proportion of air and earth elements typified by nerves, autumn and afternoon.
- Physically of more slender build; more lacking reserves of energy; tendency to dryness; enjoys or benefits from movement.
- Psychologically sensitive, which can manifest either as quiet, reserve or erratic, ungrounded or overenthusiastic behaviour; when imbalanced can be prone to discouragement/self-pity, or to fear, anxiety or nervousness or to react to situations by being stubborn or insolent.
- Prone to reactions: may have more infections, allergic reactions; or cope less well with stress and suffer spasms, tension or stiffness (earlier onset of osteo-arthritis).
- Benefits from warm and moist, centring or grounding; use oils rich in molecules close to centre of biogram: small amounts of ketones if patient has phlegm or aldehydes, especially for inflammatory reactions; ethers for antispasmodic action; alcohols and small amounts of phenols for infections.
- To correct coldness, oxides such as cineol are helpful; terpenes for short-term use.

## ACTIVITY

Determine your own constitutional type using the table below. With greater awareness of your own constitutional balance, you will better understand patients. Then use the table to understand the basic constitutional type and assess imbalances of each patient. Combine it with a knowledge of chemical constituents (Chapter 7) to choose essential oils for patients.

### Constitutional assessment table

The table is a shortened form of one used by traditional healers to assess constitutional type and *terrain*. Other factors and aspects can be added to the classifications.

Method:

1 Make several photocopies of the table.
2 Tick which quality of a temperament applies to you the most. Add up all the numbers under each temperament and see what your basic predominant tendency is. When assessing, consider your overall predisposition from birth; don't be misled by temporary short-term situations. Remember that we all have some of each quality to a certain extent; it's a question of degree. Also each quality is relative to the others; there are no absolutes. Those of African racial origin will find that the skin colours may not apply to them. Become aware of what factors aggravate an imbalance in your life and what factors, therapies, strategies you can use to balance this.
3 Add up the number of ticks in each column. Their proportion shows the predominance of characteristics of the subject.
4 Using the table assess your own constitutional type. Then assess the constitutional type of three fellow students and discuss your results.

Note: persons of African origin may fall into any of the four categories regardless of colour indications given under 'Complexion'. Such colouring may apply to them, but if not, they can be assessed according to the other factors. In particular, skin can be assessed in the Skin/touch category.

| Temperament | Sanguine | Phlegmatic | Bilious | Neurogenic/melancholic | |
|---|---|---|---|---|---|
| Complexion | Ruddy, reddish-brown | Creamy, pale, moist | Yellowish | Darker, drier | |
| Build | Muscular, ample | Large-boned, thicker | Muscular, lean | Slender, delicate | |
| Skin, touch | Warm, soft | Cool, soft | Warm, dry | Cold, dry | |
| Energy, movement | Active | Sedentary | Very active/hyperactive | Active, but can become 'stuck' | |
| Sleep | Normal | Enjoys long sleep | Thrives on less sleep | Light, can be poor | |
| Pulse | Normal, 70–80/min, normal volume | Slower, 60–70/min, fuller | Rapid 80–100/min, normal volume | Slower, 60–70/min, less volume | |
| Emotional tendency | Sunny, positive disposition, likes company | Calm, quiet, enjoys solitude | Quick reacting, irritable, angry, enjoys competition | Variable, nervous, uncertain, enthused, depressive | |
| | | | | | Totals |

## Key Terms

You need to know what these words mean. Go back through the chapter or check in the glossary to find out.

- ◊ adaptation
- ◊ choleric/bilious
- ◊ constitutional type
- ◊ dysbiosis
- ◊ elimination channels
- ◊ healing crisis
- ◊ holistic
- ◊ homeostasis
- ◊ lymphatic
- ◊ melancholic/neurogenic
- ◊ phlegmatic
- ◊ rejuvenation
- ◊ sanguine
- ◊ stages of disease
- ◊ stress response
- ◊ synergy
- ◊ *terrain*
- ◊ vital force

# HOW AROMATHERAPY WORKS

'. . . when we are dealing with an essential oil and its odoriferance, we are dealing directly with a vital force. . . . By inserting this energy force into our body, we can therefore expect an efficacious and selective action on its part. The body will thus have at its disposal a vital and living element. It will use its energy for its own ends.'

*Margarite Maury's Guide to Aromatherapy,* pp. 80–1

After working through this chapter you will be able to:

- recognise the important physical characteristics of essential oils
- understand the three pathways by which essential oils interface with the body
- understand the influence of hormones on the body's functions and mental–emotional states
- appreciate the oral pathway of interface
- recognise the range of odours that characterise essential oils
- understand the safety considerations relevant to the use of essential oils
- reinforce your understanding of practising within the limits of your training
- exercise appropriate cautions and contra-indications for aromatherapy treatment.

Chapter 7 discusses the chemistry and energy of essential oils that makes them such potent healing agents. This is known as pharmacology, the study of biologically active substances, their composition, uses and effects.

In this chapter we examine the physical characteristics of essential oils, their therapeutic effects and to some extent their 'pharma-kinetics' (from two Greek words for 'drug' and 'movement') or how they can enter, circulate and leave the body, including the possible effects the body may have on the essential oils. The therapeutic effects or actions of essential oils are described in the Therapeutic Index at the end of this chapter.

Like our bodies, plants and their extracts are complex and dynamic, two qualities that make them so effective for human health. The aromatic molecules are considerably bio-active even in small amounts. Their chemical components have known therapeutic actions. Put another way, it can be said that they communicate biological information, which 'signals' the body to initiate changes that in turn help restore normal functions and homeostasis. Ultimately, the effects we find in aromatherapy rest on the communication between one complex form of life and another.

**REMEMBER**

As distinct from the single 'magic bullet', drug approach of orthodox medicine, aromatherapy values the complexity of essential oils as ideal for positively influencing the complexity of the human body.

# The physical properties of essential oils

Essential oils are composed of different types of molecules, all based on carbon (see Chapter 7). As a group, these molecules have certain physical properties.

- Essential oil molecules are volatile, which makes them unstable, i.e not 'fixed'. They evaporate readily on exposure to air, transforming to a gaseous state. Evaporation is a form of osmosis.
- Essential oils have consistency varying from very fluid (lavender, German chamomile, cypress) through fluid (Roman chamomile, ylang ylang) and viscous – of a thick, adhesive consistency resistant to flow (patchouli, sandalwood, vetiver) – to semi-solid (myrrh). Ambient temperature and pressure can affect the consistency.
- Essential oil molecules are **lipophilic** and they are **lipid** soluble, i.e. they are attracted to and are soluble in oils, fats and lipids (from the Greek *philia,* love).
- Essential oil molecules are alcohol soluble.
- Essential oil molecules are only slightly water soluble or **hydrophilic**.
- Essential oils are concentrated; only a small amount is needed to stimulate a healing effect.
- Essential oils are odoriferous: compounds of molecules with highly complex scents.
- Essential oils are flammable. They must be stored and handled with due care and safety.
- Essential oils are dynamic and bio-active; their molecules are of small molecular weight and size, with active components, which allow them to penetrate and react with our tissues.
- Essential oils are complex; their complexity of molecular structure allows for a varied range of applications.

In the discussion that follows you will see how these characteristics contribute to the effectiveness of aromatherapy.

# Essential oil pathways

Essential oils interface or contact with the body via three important pathways. Each pathway is discussed individually but in reality each pathway interacts with and influences the others since the body is an integrated *holos*. It is by means of these routes that the properties of essential oils can interact with the body. The pathways are:

- through the skin mantle – the cutaneous pathway
- through the respiratory membrane – the respiratory pathway
- through the neuro-endocrine system – the olfactory pathway.

In addition there is the oral pathway, which is used in aromatic medicine as practised in the UK only by qualified clinical herbalists or by specially trained practitioners, and as practised in France by medical doctors.

Once in the body, essential oils act both systemically and locally.

**1** What is the technical meaning of 'volatile'?
**2** What does viscous mean?
**3** What are the three main pathways by which essential oils interact with the body?

## The cutaneous pathway

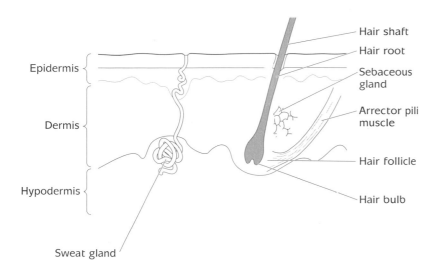

Epidermis
Dermis
Hypodermis
Sweat gland

Hair shaft
Hair root
Sebaceous gland
Arrector pili muscle
Hair follicle
Hair bulb

**Fig. 2.1a** *The zones of the skin. The transit time of a cell from the deepest layer to the surface is 15–30 days*

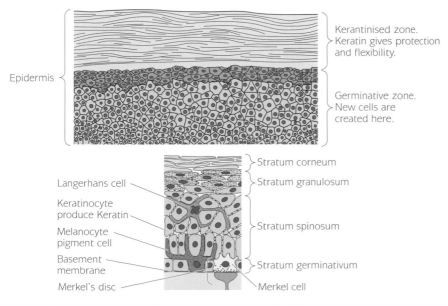

Epidermis

Kerantinised zone. Keratin gives protection and flexibility.

Germinative zone. New cells are created here.

Langerhans cell
Keratinocyte produce Keratin
Melanocyte pigment cell
Basement membrane
Merkel's disc

Stratum corneum
Stratum granulosum
Stratum spinosum
Stratum germinativum
Merkel cell

**Fig. 2.1b** *Detail of the epidermis, showing its types of cells. Langerhans cells are macrophages, part of the immune system. Merkel's cells react to pressure on the skin*

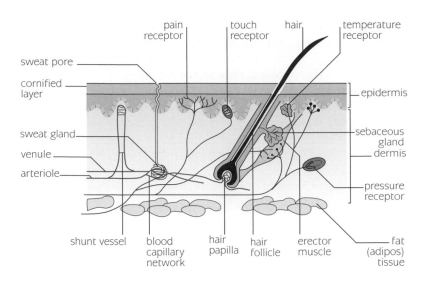

**Fig. 2.1c** *Detail of the skin showing its nerve supply, glands, muscles and hair follicles. Touch receptors react to light pressure and low frequency vibrations; pressure receptors react to deep pressure and high frequency vibrations*

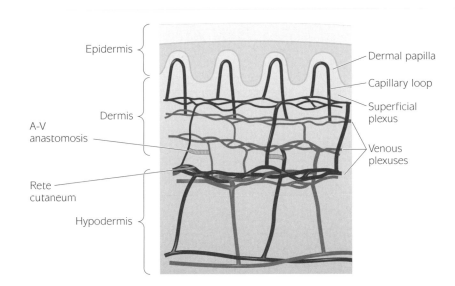

**Fig. 2.1d** *Details of skin, showing its blood supply*

## The skin

As Madame Maury realised massage is an ideal mode of application for essential oils.

The skin is not an impenetrable barrier, as was once believed, but a dermal mantle permeable to water and lipid-based substances. These include essential oils, vegetable oils and many other substances that can dissolve in fats, including even pesticides (Price and Price, 1999, p. 96). It is the largest body organ, averaging about 2 m in size in the adult. One square centimetre of skin contains 3.5 m of nerves and 1 m of blood vessels by which it interacts with other organs and systems of the body.

*The skin is part of the neuro-immune system:*
1    Its surface is a specialised micro-environment containing acids, protective bacteria and enzymes. This mantle helps protect against infection by foreign bacteria. It is thought that a small portion of an applied essential oil will react with the skin's mantle and be

changed before entering the blood circulation. The skin also contains immune cells: Langerhan's cells, which communicate information about the surface environment to the immune system; neutrophil and phagocyte cells to protect against pathogen penetration.

2   The skin interfaces with the lymph system's first line of defence. It is notable that major lymph nodes are located close to the skin surface.

3   Pressure sensitive nerve endings mean that caring touch is relayed to the brain where it influences the sense of well-being and function of vital organs (Montague). The skin also reflexes to body organs via the spinal cord synapses called dermatomes. Touch stimulation can beneficially affect internal organs. (See Figure 2.2 below.)

4   Heat-sensitive nerve endings relay temperature information so the body can adjust itself to extremes of temperature.

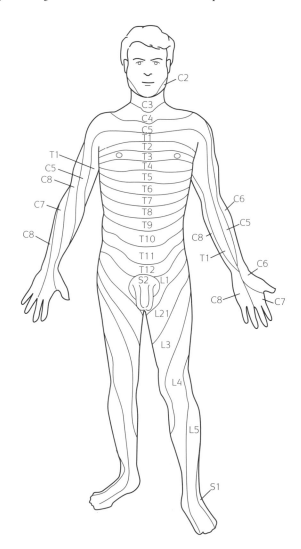

**Fig. 2.2** *Dermatomes*

*The skin interacts with the muscle–skeletal system:*
1   Pressure-sensitive nerves make possible proprioception, our sense of the body's placement in space, which helps us balance and move.

**REMEMBER**

The skin is a protective organ of the immune system. Its surface has a natural acidity, pH 5.5, which deters growth of infectious microbes and is home to beneficial bacteria, which keep infectious bacteria in check. Essential oils are also slightly acidic, and work with natural immunity and skin metabolism to inhibit infection.

2   Its cells interface with the connective tissue and muscle tissue. Essential oil molecules influence local connective tissue, and muscle–skeletal tissue (See Figure 2.3).

*The skin is an organ of excretion:*
1   The skin helps remove wastes from the body through diaphoresis or sweating.
2   It interacts with the kidneys and respiratory excretion pathways. When excretion by these organs is impaired, the skin often takes up the burden. This is why many skin eruptions are improved when the kidney and respiratory blood-cleansing functions are improved.

*The skin is an organ of absorption, of nourishment:*
The skin is composed of layers of different types of cells, together with sebum glands, hair follicles, collagen, elastin, nerves, capillaries of lymph and blood vessels. (See figures on pages 27 and 28.) Beyond the thick, external keratin layer (epidermis), all cell membranes contain lipids, to which essential oil molecules are attracted. This is the same mechanism by which oestrogen patches and other drug patches work. This pathway avoids the entero-hepatic circulation by which substances taken orally are broken down by the liver.

1   The small size of the molecules of essential oils and their bio-activity allows them to penetrate the epidermis. Travelling both through the fatty substance between other cells and across the lipids of the cells themselves, they enter the lymphatic and blood circulation. From there they can be carried to the entire body, even crossing the blood–brain barrier via their lipid solubility.
2   Essential oil molecules are absorbed by sebum (a lipid substance) and also via hair shafts; they enter local micro-circulation of the skin's lymph and blood vessels.
3   Molecules of nourishing substances such as vitamins and proteins can also be absorbed through the skin, by-passing the liver metabolism.

## REMEMBER

Aromatherapy and herbal medicine pioneered the percutaneous application of medicinal substances.

## REMEMBER

The rate of absorption varies depending on the circumstances of application, the nature of the skin and also the essential oil itself. Eucalyptus and thyme have been shown to take 20–40 minutes, bergamot and lemon from 40–60 minutes, pine from 60–80 minutes and peppermint from 100–120 minutes.

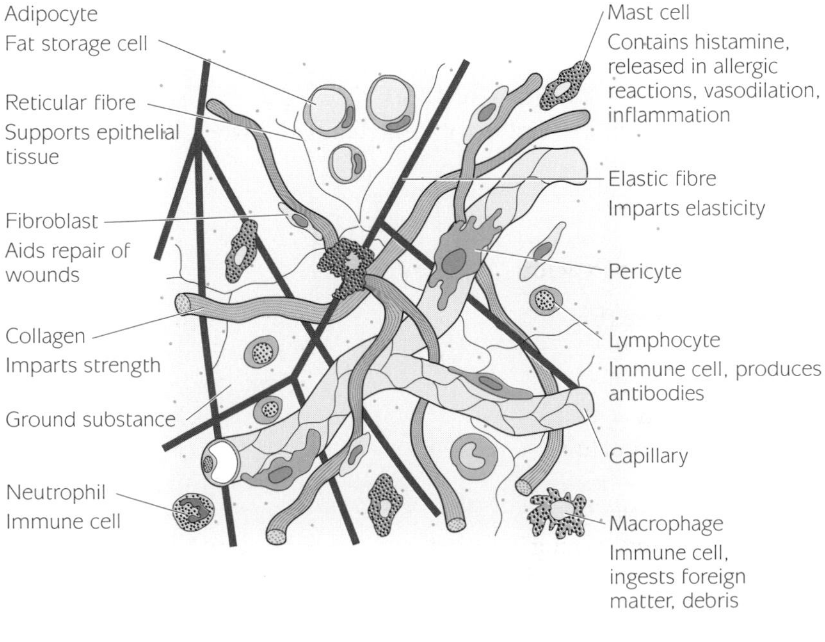

Adipocyte
Fat storage cell

Reticular fibre
Supports epithelial tissue

Fibroblast
Aids repair of wounds

Collagen
Imparts strength

Ground substance

Neutrophil
Immune cell

Mast cell
Contains histamine, released in allergic reactions, vasodilation, inflammation

Elastic fibre
Imparts elasticity

Pericyte

Lymphocyte
Immune cell, produces antibodies

Capillary

Macrophage
Immune cell, ingests foreign matter, debris

**Fig. 2.3** *Loose connective tissue (areolar), a matrix of different types of cells, which supports the skin. Note: adipocytes or fat cells are found in this tissue*

Always use the best quality vegetal oils, creams and lotions to help the essential oils penetrate the skin. These will also have a local nourishing effect on the skin.

*Skin types*

The skin of individuals varies in several ways. The chart below outlines the basic skin types.

**Chart of skin type**

**By genetic or ethnic type:**

Oriental – well lubricated, more sebum but without being oily

Dark/African skin – with more pigmentation, well lubricated without being oily

Mediterranean/olive – well lubricated without being oily

Northern European – the 'peaches and cream' complexion, transparent/less pigment; prone to thread veins after age 30 and sensitive to sunlight

Celtic – thinner, often with freckles, sensitive to sunlight

**By general type (within the genetic types, the following ranges are found):**

Normal – balanced without dryness or excess oiliness; with a bright tone; evenly textured and supple. 'Normal' indicates what is normal for an individual

Dry/sensitive/dehydrated – more finely textured, with tendency to dryness, flaking off of cells; dry skin is more sensitive, reacts easily to weather extremes (roughness, chapping); ages early

Oily – more coarsely textured, shiny, prone to blemishes; ages more slowly; oiliness can make it feel grubby by afternoon, but gives it greater resilience

Combination – having a mixture of areas of dryness and oiliness

*Skin permeability*

The skin of different body regions has slightly differing structure. This gives a different permeability in different areas. In areas of thinner skin, or in more exposed areas or in those with thinner muscle layers beneath, it is more permeable. Permeability is a way of saying the skin 'breathes', taking in and letting out, mediating between the inner and outer environments.

**Permeability of various body regions**

| More permeable | Less permeable |
| --- | --- |
| the inside of the arm, wrist or leg | the back |
| behind the ears | the abdomen |
| the forehead | the buttocks |
| the soles and palms | the chest |
| the scalp | outer thighs, lower legs |
| shoulder areas | outer arms |
| skin of infants, young children, the elderly, if thinned, injured | dry skin |

### Advantages of massage application

During massage the warmth of the room and of the practitioner's hands, and the rubbing itself, warm the patient's body and increase peripheral blood circulation. This enhances the penetration and absorption of essential oils. Although the quantity of essential oil used is small in comparison to the size of the body, the effect is still potent. This is because of the highly active nature of the essential oils: a minute proportion has a major effect.

Essential oil molecules vary in size, so their absorption rate varies: Linalool and linalyl acteate (molecules present in lavender e.o.) have been detected in blood samples taken 5 minutes after application (Price and Price, 1999). Others may take anywhere from 20 to 120 minutes.

The shape and structure of essential oil molecules also plays a role (Chapter 7). Their complexity and molecular structure give them great flexibility. This helps them pass through the layers of skin cells.

### Other percutaneous applications

In addition to massage, essential oils can enter the skin through the use of other methods such as pessaries, compresses, liniments and baths (Chapter 9). In baths, penetration is facilitated by the fact that water is absorbed also and water increases skin permeability up to 100 times. The property of essential oils to be slightly water soluble facilitates absorption also.

### Metabolism, distribution and excretion of essential oils in percutaneous application

While the metabolism of essential oils is not completely understood at present, the following reflects current understanding.

After permeating the skin, essential oil molecules have four possible outcomes:

1   They may be metabolised (broken down, changed) by cutaneous enzymes.
2   Some of them may remain in the cutaneous fat cells as a reservoir from which they are slowly released to the capillary circulation.
3   Some may be completely absorbed in the local skin tissue and micro-circulation.
4   Most pass into the general arterial–venous circulation for systemic distribution.

From empirical experience, it is found that a significant number of essential oil molecules applied by aromatherapy do pass into the general blood circulation. Unlike substances taken into the body orally, essential oils entering via the skin do not have to pass through the liver (enterohepatic circulation), where they would be extensively changed. The liver aims to convert lipid-soluble substances into water-soluble ones, which are more easily distributed, used and excreted by the body. With cutaneous application, after passing into the arterial circulation (blood and lymph) a portion of an essential oil's molecules are distributed in their original state throughout the body. With the blood and lymph fluid, they will pass into and out of internal organs and structures, all of which are nourished and cleansed by the circulation.

*Factors affecting distribution*
The type of skin in the area of application has some effect on their distribution. Some areas are relatively more conducive to permeation than others (see above). Some essential oils demonstrate an affinity for certain organs, fennel and juniper for the kidneys, for example. Herbal–naturopathic tradition has found that essential oils will be particularly taken up by the weak organs, which need their effects.

According to the extent of the blood passing through an organ or tissue, called **perfusion**, cells will receive more or less of the essential oils, and hence of their effects. The endocrine glands, heart, lungs, brain, liver and kidneys receive the most blood circulation, followed by lean muscle and skin, then fat tissue and finally the ligaments, tendons, teeth and bone. Any adipose tissue deposits will inhibit essential oil penetration.

**GOOD PRACTICE**

After the warmth of a bath, sauna or exercise, the skin is actively eliminating and slightly less receptive to absorption of essential oils. Ideally wait until the body has cooled down before applications. Massage and passive warmth (e.g. hot water bottle) increase the circulation to the skin and enhance penetration and absorption of essential oils.

*Excretion*
Entering the venous circulation, the molecules are carried to the lungs, kidneys and skin to be excreted along with other body wastes in the form of breath, urine and perspiration. About 95 per cent of excretion is via the kidney–urine pathway. A certain amount of lipid-soluble molecules will diffuse back into the blood from the tubule walls of the kidneys. Once applied to the body, analysis of breath, blood, urine and sweat samples will show traces of the molecules. (See Battaglia, 1995, pp. 115–19 and Price and Price, 1999, pp. 96–9 for further discussion.)

Cautions:

♦   Some components of essential oils are capable of binding to the body's protein plasma albumin. It is advisable to reduce dosage for patients with a history of kidney or liver disease. Their plasma protein levels may be low making the essential oils more available in the blood, and these patients may be more vulnerable to their normal presence in the blood.

- Essential oils may have an effect on drug metabolism, influencing their absorption, for example, or inhibiting their action. While no conclusive studies on drug-essential oil interaction have been done, patients on drug medication should be advised to ask their physician to monitor them for such effects, so that their medication can be adjusted accordingly. It happens that after an aromatherapy treatment programme, a person may need less medication than previously.

## ACTIVITY

Rub a clove of raw garlic or some raw onion on to the soles of your feet. Time yourself to see how long it takes before its odour is present on your breath, your sweat and your urine.

Follow this by eating some raw garlic or onion and next a big bunch of fresh parsley, or some cumin, cardamom or fennel seeds. Compare the two procedures and discuss your results with colleagues.

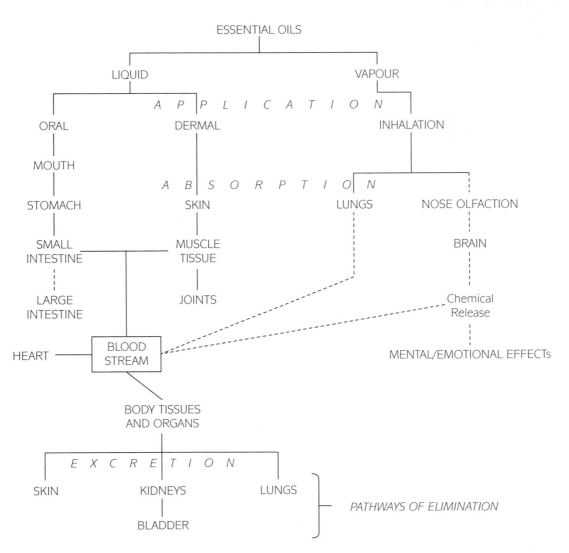

**Fig. 2.4** *Flow chart of essential oils' interface, absorption, circulation and excretion in the body. See Fig. 2.8 for details of olfaction.*

1. What are the functions of the skin?
2. How does the size of essential oil molecules affect their activity when applied to the skin?
3. What does lipophilic mean?
4. Name three factors that aid the penetration of essential oils through the skin.
5. Describe what happens to an aromatic molecule after it enters the bloodstream.

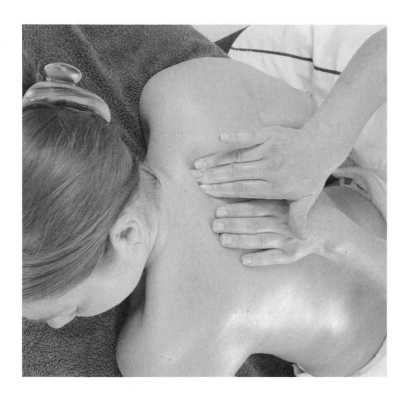

**Fig. 2.5** *Giving and receiving massage: for optimum health, our bodies are designed to receive loving or therapeutic touch – a gesture of comfort, a stroke of tenderness, a massage (Montague, 1986). In an aromatherapy massage, the nerves in the skin detect the healing or care intended by the giver and communicate this to the brain. This stimulates* **endorphin** *release and a sense of well-being, relaxation and calm within the body. The receiver's consciousness comes to a still point of inner balance. The body recovers its essential integrity*

## The respiratory pathway

Breath is next to life itself for it nourishes the body with oxygen-rich air. The lungs are responsible for our primary respiration and our most immediate interaction with our environment. We can live only a few minutes without air, whereas we can go for days without water and weeks without food. Imbalances and blockages in the respiratory system or in breathing mechanism as well as the quality of the air have profound affects on other body functions, both physical and psychological. Both the quality of the air we breathe and the way we breathe affect our bodies and our consciousness.

### Respiratory physiology

In a way the lungs are a type of skin membrane, but one which is on the inside. In this sense some of the above characteristics of the skin apply to the nature of respiratory membranes, lymph and blood circulation. All respiratory tissues (nasal, larynx, bronchial) are constantly exposed to air, which has a drying effect. To counterbalance this, the membranes lining the tract secrete a moistening mucus. The mucous membrane is also full of cilia, which help catch and deter micro-pathogens and other particles from entering and damaging the lungs or body. The mucous lining also

> **REMEMBER**
> 'Volatile' comes from the Latin *volare*, meaning to fly away, move quickly. In chemistry it indicates the capability of entering a gaseous state. As organs of respiration, the lungs are naturally receptive to the airborne aromatic molecules of essential oils.

acts as a moisture-rich environment, which facilitates the absorption of oxygen. Air moves to alveoli at the end of each bronchial tube. The wall of each alveolus has the thinnest membranes of the body. Here gaseous exchange occurs via the lymph–blood capillaries. (Oxygen comes in, carbon dioxide and wastes pass out.) Absorption by inhalation is even faster than by dermal or oral application.

The bronchial tubes are also lined with smooth muscles, which can contract to help expel excess mucus via expectoration.

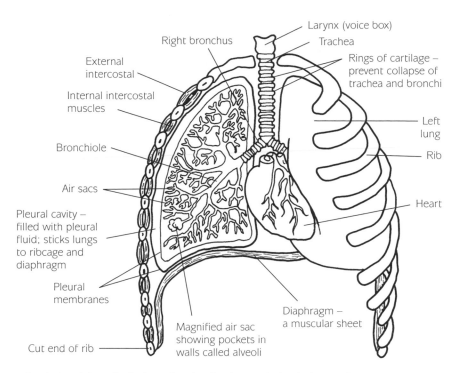

**Fig. 2.6a** *A bronchiole, bronchi, alveolar duct and alveoli (air sacs)*

## REMEMBER

On inhalation essential oils are taken with air into the bronchial tubes. They stimulate increased bronchial secretion, thus having a moistening effect locally. This is of benefit in nose, throat and lung infections. Essential oils with antispasmodic effects can benefit excess bronchial contraction by their action on smooth muscle.

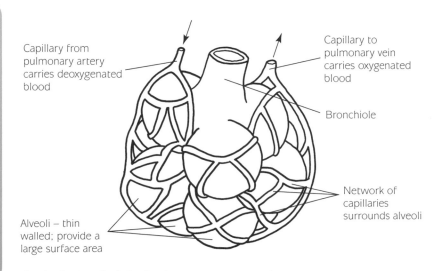

**Fig. 2.6b** *Detail of alveolar sac*

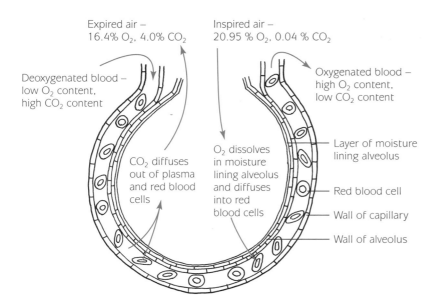

Expired air –
16.4% $O_2$, 4.0% $CO_2$

Inspired air –
20.95 % $O_2$, 0.04 % $CO_2$

Deoxygenated blood –
low $O_2$ content,
high $CO_2$ content

Oxygenated blood –
high $O_2$ content,
low $CO_2$ content

$CO_2$ diffuses
out of plasma
and red blood
cells

$O_2$ dissolves
in moisture
lining alveolus
and diffuses
into red
blood cells

Layer of moisture
lining alveolus

Red blood cell

Wall of capillary

Wall of alveolus

**Fig. 2.6c** *Detail of $O^2$–$CO^2$ exchange with capillaries*

### Distribution, metabolism and excretion of essential oils via the respiratory pathway

Essential oil molecules penetrate the mucous membranes of the lungs and affect the local tissues according to their therapeutic actions (pages 53ff). They also enter the local lymph and blood capillaries. In the lungs they facilitate the nutritious and gaseous exchange between the blood and lung cells, and assist elimination of wastes. They then pass on via the blood to circulate throughout the system, passing into organs and tissues by means of the arterial circulation, having effects by means of perfusion through the tissues. The venous circulation takes them back to the lungs, kidneys and sudoriferous glands for elimination by breath, urine and sweat.

**ACTIVITY**

Practise a visualisation of the respiratory pathway. Sitting quietly, imagine a molecule of essential oil attached to an oxygen molecule in the air. Imagine its circular journey as it passes into the respiratory tract and trace the journey through the gaseous exchange there and on to the systemic distribution until it reaches excretion by the lungs (now with carbon dioxide) and kidneys.

1 Which structures or tissues of the lungs facilitate the penetration of essential oils into the body by this pathway?
2 How can essential oils affect the local environment and tissues in the lungs?
3 What happens to essential oils when they enter the blood circulation from the lungs?

### The olfactory or neuro-endocrine pathway

Maury noted that essential oils affect directly our consciousness and consciousness affects behaviour: 'the powers of perception become clearer and more acute, we can see things and events in their true perspective. The conscious mind is alerted and one feels great enrichment. They induce true sentimental and mental liberation' (Maury, 1989, p. 82). Recently science has learned more about the physiological mechanisms by which these effects occur.

### *Olfaction and the sense of smell*

The human sense of smell, olfaction, is both primitive and sophisticated. It is fundamental to our survival, to our identity and contributes to our health and sense of well-being – our *euphoria*.

Olfaction is more important than we tend to think. Olfactory nerve cells are the only ones capable of regeneration, indicating the priority the body places on olfaction. Our reaction to smells is quicker than our reaction to pain or sound – 0.5 seconds versus 0.9 or 0.15 seconds, respectively. This suggests olfaction may be the primary defence mechanism and the prime importance of smell to preserving life.

The sense of smell can be classified into two categories: primary, or instinctive, and secondary, or learned by experience. The secondary sense of smell will always be influenced by the primary one.

*Primary*

The instinct of smell is part of our survival kit. Infants quickly learn to recognise the scent of their parents or carers. It is an aspect of bonding. They know the scent of the mother's skin and automatically turn towards her for nourishment and affection. Simultaneously, the infant's scent attracts the mother and stimulates her care. The sense of smell allows us to discriminate between wholesome and unhealthy foods and environments. As we reach puberty, we become (unconsciously) sensitive to the pheremones of potential sexual partners.

*Secondary*

From the moment of birth our sense of smell is growing and developing. As we are exposed to more and more odours we learn to recognise them and also our minds are automatically associating them with either pleasant or unpleasant experiences. Thus smell is closely related to memory and the recording of experiences. If strong emotions are associated with a particular odour, then the sensations of that experience will be recalled – if only unconsciously – when we detect the odour again. The range of odours to which we are sensitive varies with the individual. Some of us are highly sensitive and others less so. It may be that as humans have become more civilised and technology oriented we have lost our conscious awareness of smells, but parts of our brain still can respond to them. Ordinarily, we don't usually live up to our smell potential, but we can increase it with practice.

With training, humans can detect up to 3,000 different scents. (It is thought we recognise tens of thousands unconsciously.) This ability is the foundation of the perfumers' art, and highly developed in the so-called 'noses' who create perfumes. Some illness can be detected by the odorants emitted by the diseased organism, for example, the breath of schizophrenics is known to have a particular odour. The sense of smell is also strongly connected to important brain functions such as cognition, concentration, learning and, again, memory.

Anyone who enjoys the scent of a flower or a perfume or a good meal in preparation is aware that aromas have profound psychological effects. They are capable of strongly influencing our moods by stimulating the production-release of hormones, neurotransmitters and neuropeptides. Biochemists in the perfume industry have long studied the psychological effects of odours. More recently psychiatrists, psychologists and neuroscientists have also begun to study their effects on behaviour, memory and concentration. Medical doctors have used fragrances in treating some conditions.

In epilepsy, for example, if the person can develop the ability to sense an oncoming seizure, and then practise using a fragrance that induces a relaxed, positive mood, the two skills can be combined to beneficial effect. When an oncoming seizure is detected, the person smells the chosen essential oil, and triggers a more positive, less stressful state, which can lessen or even prevent the seizure. Some essential oils can also act via the nervous system as anticonvulsants.

In recent years science has gained greater knowledge of how the brain functions, particularly the **limbic system** and its production of hormones and neurotransmitters. This has helped explain the mechanisms of the mood effects of aromas that people experience. It has in fact helped science come to a more holistic understanding of human behaviour.

> **REMEMBER**
> Because of their mind–body effects through scent, essential oils can help in psychological, stress-related and even psychiatric disorders.

## Olfactory physiology

In their volatile state, essential oils are gaseous, air-borne molecules. Indeed their association with air and breath, the body's primary physiological function, may be the key to their profound effects. A substance must be gaseous and capable of dissolving into mucus to affect our olfactory nerves. As can be seen from Figure 2.7a the nose itself is not, strictly speaking, the organ of smell but a structure that contains the olfactory nerve receptors or cilia (hairs) and about 20 million nerve cells, 10 million above each nostril.

Passing through the mucous membranes of the nostrils, essential oils stimulate the nerve cilia, which in turn generate a nerve impulse to the two olfactory bulbs at the top of the nostrils, one on each side of the brain. This is an electro-chemically generated stimulation. It is thought that the olfactory cells here are extensions of the first cranial nerves.

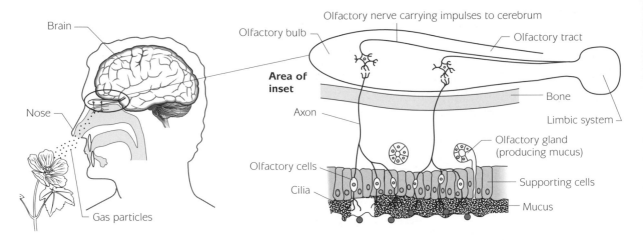

**Fig. 2.7a** *Organs of olfaction in the nasal cavity. Odorants dissolve in the mucus covering the epithelium and stimulate nerve receptor cells, which conduct electro-chemical information along the olfactory nerve to the limbic centre*

The first cranial nerves conduct the stimuli of the odorant along the olfactory tract, which branches to several sites in the brain, primarily the olfactory cortex of the temporal lobes and the amygdala in the limbic area of the brain.

The olfactory part of the cerebral cortex in the temporal lobes enables us to interpret impulses as odours and be aware of the sensation of smell. The olfactory area recognises and distinguishes between different odours. For example, it allows us to identify an odorant very specifically – distinguishing a rose from a violet, for example, or even identifying different types of roses.

### The limbic system

The limbic system (Latin *limbus*, a threshold or border) or limbic area (see Figure 2.7b) comprises the thalamus (Greek, 'inner chamber'), hypothalamus, pituitary and pineal glands, the hippocampus (Greek, 'sea horse') and amygdala (Greek, 'almond'). These structures are linked by a nerve tract called the fornix. The limbic system is part of what has been called the old or primitive brain, sometimes the emotional brain. It is located in the middle of the brain, above the brain stem, below the cerebrum. Its activities affect the cerebrum (cortex) which performs higher brain functions as well as the cerebellum and its functions.

The area is only beginning to be understood. From what we know, this area is responsible for survival senses such as hunger and thirst, the stress response, and basic emotions like fear, pain, pleasure, joy, anger, affection, sexual arousal along with the subsequent behaviours that they prompt. It also plays a part in memory. Learning from experience is necessary for survival so the organism can distinguish between what aids survival and health, and what doesn't. People who have sustained damage to the limbic system suffer from memory impairment. Odours help with memory.

Olfactory impulses stimulate the amygdala, an organ comprised of two almond-shaped structures lying either side of the frontal cortex (about an inch into the brain from the ears). When stimulated, the amygdala releases emotions, particularly pleasure, pain, anger, contentment, fear,

**REMEMBER**

Damage to the hypothalmus may result in a range of effects such as:

● diabetes insipidus
● sleepiness
● disturbed autonomic functions.

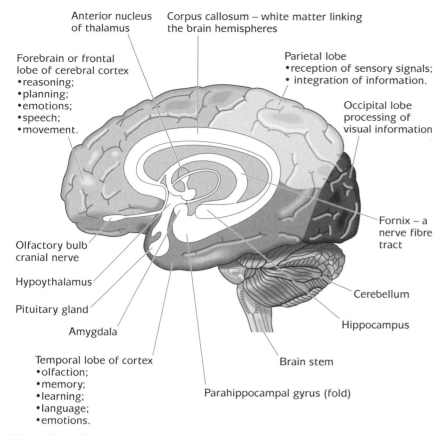

Anterior nucleus of thalamus

Corpus callosum – white matter linking the brain hemispheres

Forebrain or frontal lobe of cerebral cortex
•reasoning;
•planning;
•emotions;
•speech;
•movement.

Parietal lobe
•reception of sensory signals;
• integration of information.

Occipital lobe processing of visual information

Fornix – a nerve fibre tract

Olfactory bulb cranial nerve

Hypoythalamus

Pituitary gland

Amygdala

Cerebellum

Hippocampus

Temporal lobe of cortex
•olfaction;
•memory;
•learning;
•language;
•emotions.

Brain stem

Parahippocampal gyrus (fold)

**Fig. 2.7b** *Olfactory organs connect to the limbic system which influences moods and mental processes and helps regulate functions of many body organs and systems*

sorrow and sexual feelings. It also plays a role in memory. In both emotions and memory it influences the body sensations and movements that accompany these experiences. It controls the overall pattern of our behaviour. The amygdala also shares many interconnections with the frontal cortex, the cognitive part of the brain and the area of learning and mental activity.

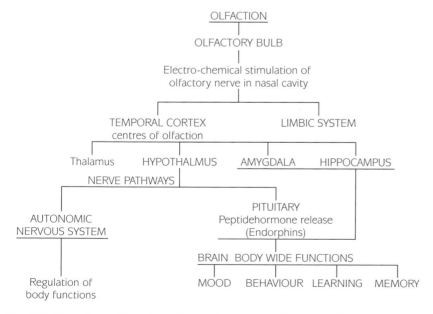

OLFACTION

OLFACTORY BULB

Electro-chemical stimulation of olfactory nerve in nasal cavity

TEMPORAL CORTEX
centres of olfaction

LIMBIC SYSTEM

Thalamus    HYPOTHALMUS    AMYGDALA    HIPPOCAMPUS

NERVE PATHWAYS

AUTONOMIC NERVOUS SYSTEM

PITUITARY
Peptidehormone release
(Endorphins)

BRAIN  BODY WIDE FUNCTIONS

Regulation of body functions

MOOD    BEHAVIOUR    LEARNING    MEMORY

**Fig. 2.8** *Flow chart of the effects of electrochemical stimulation of olfactory nerve in nasal cavity*

The hippocampus, a structure with a seahorse-like shape, also plays a part in memory formation, and helps identify sensory information worth saving, such as smells. It interprets odorants. If it is damaged, memory may be impaired.

The hypothalamus is connected to and influences the thalamus and thus the cerebral cortex and it receives messages from these. Part of the role of the thalamus is concerned with memory and emotions. It also influences the pituitary gland via chemical messengers called regulating factors. It receives information from outside the body via the sensory pathways, including smell. It receives information about the internal state of the body from internal viscera via nerve impulses. It can thus help control many body activities, most of which relate to homeostasis. It also helps control emotions, heart rate, blood pressure and secretions of the pituitary, which in turn influence the adrenal glands.

## Regulation of body functions

**Essential oils and 'molecules of emotion'**
The hypothalamus, by a complex system of nerve pathways, blood vessels and electro-chemical exchanges, is linked to:

- the central nervous system, with its two autonomic branches: sympathetic and parasympathetic
- the endocrine system
- the body-wide network of information exchange available to cells

Odorant stimulation of the hypothalamus – such as occurs during an aromatherapy treatment – stimulates the anterior pituitary gland to secrete substances called **peptides**. Peptides are a type of hormone and made of amino acid protein molecules. One hormone of particular interest in aromatherapy is the endorphin. It has also been discovered that nerve cells or neurons also secrete neuro-peptides, in addition to the neurotransmitters such as noradrenalin involved in the stress response (Chapter 1).

*Endorphins*
Endorphins, first discovered in the pituitary gland, were some of the first peptides to be found. Scientists determined that their release produces pleasurable sensations and even have opium and morphine-like effects, capable of overcoming or reducing sensations of pain.

Later scientists discovered that these natural opiate peptide-hormones can be produced not only in the brain by the pituitary gland but are also found throughout the body, such as cells of the digestive tract, the circulatory system, the skin, the kidneys and the lungs.

When released either from the limbic system or other cells in other body tissues, endorphin molecules travel through the blood stream or by means of nerves. They find and bind to receptor sites on the walls of cells all over the body. This 'binding' allows the information to be conveyed into the cells and the cells are stimulated to perform certain functions.

The discovery that this information exchange between cells takes place by means of peptide-hormone molecules has changed the way we understand the body-mind interaction to occur. We have learned that:

- Rather than being a totally brain-directed central command system, information-exchange is a feedback loop system. The brain and the rest of the body communicate in a two-way exchange.
- In addition to regulation by the autonomic nervous system, many body functions are now know to be regulated and coordinated by the circulation of peptide-hormones like endorphins.

### Essential oils and body-mind communication

Essential oil odorant molecules can stimulate the release of these peptides and thus affect the regulation of body functions. If those peptides, which initiate positive sensations, can be induced to flow, they can overcome or ease pain sensations. They can be harnessed in the treatment of disorders caused by chronic stress or depression. Just as the hormonal–nerve pathways orchestrate a stress response to pain, trauma or threat, so the peptide–hormonal network can orchestrate a pleasure response.

Dr Candace Pert discovered the opiate receptor and went on to discover how peptides affect us. She called peptides 'molecules of emotions'. In her book *Molecules of Emotion* she explains that our emotions can now be understood in a biochemical, i.e. physical way, as the flow and reception of peptide molecules creating mood states and prompting behaviours.

According to Dr Pert's research, it is not only the classic brain areas of emotional response – the hippocampus, the hypothalamus and the amygdala – that are responsible for generating emotion in response to stimuli. Because receptors for peptides exist throughout the body, feelings can be both generated or expressed not only in the brain but also in other parts of the body. This helps explain the expression 'gut feeling'. Pert says that when we have a particularly strong, memorable experience – whether positive or negative – peptides are released, inducing either positive or negative moods. At the same time body-wide tissues are also flooded with the peptides, setting up feedback systems of either positivity or negativity, depending on the nature of the experience. In this way the emotion or mood connected to the experience can be 'stored' in body tissues as well as being present in the brain. This release of hormones also influences learning and memory centres in the forebrain.

Since scent is one of the experiences that can trigger the release of morphine-like peptide endorphins, via the hypothalamus–pituitary hormonal information pathways, we find an explanation in very precise physical terms for how essential oils can affect our mood and help induce healing in the organism. Dr Pert's work helps explain what Margarite Maury and aromatherapists have found through empirical experience: the pleasurable sensations of scenting essential oils can profoundly affect our moods, our mental functioning and the health of every cell. Scenting of a pleasurable essential oil can stimulate the release of these peptides and initiate a cascade of beneficial activities in the body–mind whole.

**REMEMBER**

Peptide-hormones, like endorphins, have been called 'informational substances' because they carry signals to the cells which then trigger certain functions. These include:
- regulation of body temperature
- insulin production or inhibition
- regulation of heartbeat
- involuntary muscle contraction
- regulation of sleep cycles
- inducement of moods and emotions
- regulation of appetite and thirst
- regulation of calorific levels
- digestive functions
- sexual arousal and sexual satisfaction
- the stress response.

**REMEMBER**

This peptide-cell network, through projections from the limbic system into the cerebral cortex or forebrain, can affect the cognitive centres where higher learning, discernment and cognition take place.

To sum up, essential oils can affect the body via olfaction and the limbic system by a stimulation of the hypothalamus, which in turn stimulates the following:

- The autonomic nervous system, i.e. parasympathetic and sympathetic functions
  - via the sympathetic nervous system an odorant can initiate the calming of hyperactive sympathetic functions
  - via the parasympathetic nervous system an odour can initiate the stimulation of hypoactive parasympathetic functions.
- The limbic–pituitary and the peptide-cell receptor network; the release of endorphin peptides induces a state of euphoria or inner sense of well-being at an emotional and body-wide cellular level. Aroused emotions such as anger, fear or anxiety are calmed. Body functions are beneficially regulated.

**THE AUTONOMIC NERVOUS SYSTEM**

| parts affected | para-sympathetic | sympathetic | general result |
|---|---|---|---|
| **pupils** | contracted | dilated | controls the amount of light entering the eyes |
| **cilary muscles** | contracted | relaxed | controls accommodation of the eye |
| **blood vessels** | arterioles of glands and viscera dilated | arterioles of alimentary canal and skin con-stricted; those of skeletal muscles dilated or constricted by different fibres; tone raised in walls of larger vessels | adjusts the blood pressure and the distribution of the blood |
| **spleen** | dilated | constricted | adjusts the quality and quantity of blood in circulation |
| **heart beat** | slowed and weakened | hastened and strengthened | adjusts the rate of the heart according to the blood pressure and varying muscle activity |
| **bronchioles** | constricted | dilated | adjusts ease of breathing to requirements |
| **sweat glands** | | activity increased | produces extra sweat in anticipation of heat production during activity |
| **adrenal medulla** | | activity increased | reinforces direct effects mentioned above |
| **peristalsis of the alimen-tary canal** | increased | decreased | controls the speed of passage of food and the rate of digestion |
| **sphincters** | relaxed | contracted | |
| **digestive glands** | activity increased | activity decreased | *note*: digestion is slow when body activity is great and vice versa |

**Fig. 2.9** *The autonomic nervous system*

## Brainwaves and odour

Experiments measuring brain waves, the alpha, beta and gamma electrical vibrations emitted by the brain, also show a response to essential oil fragrance. An electroencephalogram, EEG, has revealed that inhaling essential oils promotes coordination between the activity of both left and right brain hemispheres. This promotes a feeling of harmony, calm and well-being within the self and alertness and clarity of mind (from Batagglia, 1995). This is yet another way essential oils can benefit the mind-body-spirit whole.

| Essential oil | Biorhythm affected | Sensation |
|---|---|---|
| jasmine, neroli, rose | alpha delta | calm, harmony reverie, sleep |
| black pepper, rosemary basil, and cardamom | beta | alertness, clarity, arousal |

**GOOD PRACTICE**

Avoid scenting essential oils straight from the bottle or holding a sample too close to the nose. They are very concentrated and this practice is not needed or helpful. If the nose is blocked, you may pinch it closed for 30 seconds while you shake your head; this relieves congestion. Repeat if necessary at intervals until passages are clearer.

**Progress Check**

1  What is the mechanism by which an odorant stimulates olfaction?
2  Which cranial nerve conducts olfactory stimuli to the brain?
3  What is the limbic area of the brain? Where is it located?
4  How are peptide-hormones, such as endorphins, which are released from the limbic system (hypothalamus–pituitary pathway), able to trigger changes in mood, affect body sensations and regulate cell activities?

## The oral pathway

It is possible to take essential oils into the body by the digestive route, the oral pathway. This has traditionally been done by mixing a very small amount of essential oil with honey, oil or a sugar cube. This pathway is not used by aromatherapists unless they are also trained clinical herbalists or have undergone further special training in the use of essential oils internally. It is a practice used by medical doctors in France primarily for infectious diseases. Essential oils are potent agents for overcoming infections (see Chapter 7). In France doctors usually obtain a swab with infected tissue on it, which is sent to a laboratory for **aromatogram** analysis.

**REMEMBER**

While internal use of essential oils has advantages, effective results can also be obtained by correct and thoughtful use of the external pathways.

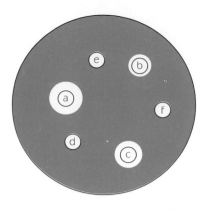

**Fig. 2.10** *An aromatogram. In this example, essential oils a and c produce a larger zone, so are having most effect on the bacteria and would be chosen for treatment*

An aromatogram determines which essential oil is best suited to kill or inhibit the particular pathogen. The swabbed pathogens are cultured (multiplied) in a Petri dish. Several different essential oils are added to the culture, which is placed in an incubator. The culture is observed periodically for several hours or days to see which essential oil(s) slows or stops the pathogen's growth as indicated by the formation of a visible zone around the culture – the 'zone of inhibition'. Thus the selection of essential oils can be highly tuned to the individual patient and specific pathogen. The doctor then writes a prescription, which is filled by the chemist, who dispenses the essential oils in a carrier called an exipient. The exipient facilitates absorption while protecting the digestive membranes from harmful effects of contact with the essential oil.

## GOOD PRACTICE

Aromatherapists do not prescribe or advise the internal use of essential oils, unless they have undertaken specialised training.

## ACTIVITY:
## DEVELOPING YOUR SENSE OF SMELL

One of the best ways to learn about essential oils and how they affect us through olfaction is to begin to keep a smell database of your own experience. Gradually, with time and patient practice, you can distinguish such things as the character, originality and authenticity of a good quality essential oil.

You may structure your database in any way you or your tutor wish, but here is one way to do it.

Take one to three essential oils a week. Create a record chart or use the example given on page 48. Smell each essential oil at regular intervals, noting the time and any relevant circumstances (perhaps physical, perhaps psychological) and record your response. To describe the character of the scent, use the vocabulary of perfumers as given.

Preparation:

Obtain some good quality essential oils and some of inferior quality. Obtain two chemotypes of one or more oils. You learn from comparing them. Obtain some smell strips or blotting paper strips. Place some coffee grounds in a closed jar. Open and smell at intervals if you feel fatigued. This refreshes your senses. Place yourself in a quiet setting without interruptions.

Method:

1   Add a drop of essential oil to the smell strip. (Sometimes it is enough to just wipe it across the tip of the bottle. It depends on the oil.)

2   Move the strip slowly back and forth below your nose. It is not necessary to have it very close as the oils are so concentrated. As you move the strip, take a few short, small sniffs, inhaling.

3   Pause and become aware of your response, and concentrate. How would you describe the odour?

4   Record your response. The main point is to do exactly the same thing each time you practise. Some people may be more visual than verbal, and may prefer to record their response with colours or shapes, not words.

Here are some of the qualities you might consider:

◊   Strength: assertive, aggressive, mild, soft, subtle.
◊   Type: the character of odour – fruity, spicy, pungent, sharp, musty, floral, sweet, green or herbal, woody, balsamic, medicinal; other? Does the odour remind you of something? Does it remind you of a past experience?
◊   Depth: light, powdery, i.e. indistinct or vanishing in about 60 seconds; or rich, complex, i.e. as you continue to smell the essential oil, you detect more nuances of its fragrance.
◊   Effect: How does the essential oil affect you? Can you name a mood, state or emotion, or a state of mental or physical awareness that it triggers? Describe in words, colours, shapes or other quality that is meaningful to you.

To help you, some fragrance vocabulary used by perfumers includes the following:

| | |
|---|---|
| Aldehydic | presence of the long-chain fatty aldehydes, e.g. the scent of ironed laundry or sea water |
| Balsamic | presence of heavy, sweet, odour as in vanilla or cinnamon |
| Camphorous | presence of camphor, medicinal-like |
| Citrus | presence of citrus odour |
| Earthy | reminiscent of humus-rich or moist earth |
| Floral, flowery | presence of various sweet, floral odours |
| Fruity | presence of various fruit odours |
| Green | reminiscent of cut grass and fresh leaves |
| Herbaceous | a complex odour, reminiscent of mint, eucaplytus or other plants |
| Medicinal | reminiscent of disinfectants, phenol, salicylate |
| Metallic | odour found near metals, particularly when wet |
| Minty | like peppermint |
| Mossy | like moss |
| Resinous | presence of resins, e.g. myrrh, pine |
| Spicy | presence of various spice odours: pepper, clove, etc. |
| Woody | reminiscent of trees, wood |

5   Repeat the exercise using essential oils of lower quality or essential oil scented toiletry products. Compare your reactions.

**Developing your sense of smell: record sheet**

| Essential oil | | | | | | | | | | | | |
|---|---|---|---|---|---|---|---|---|---|---|---|---|

**Quality of Odour**

Strength
- Aggressive
- Assertive
- Mild
- Soft
- Subtle

Depth
- Light
- Powdery
- Rich, complex
- Heavy, deep

Aldehydic

Balsamic

Camphorous

Citrus

Earth

Floral, flowery, sweet

Fruity

Green

Herbaceous

Medicinal

Metalic

Minty

Mossy

Resinous

Spicy

Woody

Other

Effect
- Uplift
- Calm
- Invigorate, etc.

# Essential oil safety

Experience teaches that what has the potential for good can also harm if given in the wrong way, the wrong circumstances or the wrong place. However, when used by trained aromatherapists, the possible risks that could occur in using essential oils are extremely low.

Issues of safety and essential oils may be grouped under the following categories.

1 Risks by route:
   - oral ingestion
   - external application.
2 Risks by site of effect:
   - whole body – by ingestion causing death
   - skin reaction
   - **neurotoxicity** – damaging to the nerve tissue
   - **hepatotoxicity** – damaging to the liver
   - hazards during pregnancy
   - carcinogenesis – cancer causing.

Aromatherapy as professionally practised in the UK and several other countries does not make use of the oral ingestion of essential oils. Nevertheless, it is important that aromatherapists are aware of the potential dangers of taking them internally. There are cases on record in which individuals have taken essential oils orally and caused great harm.

## Lethal dose evaluation

In science and industry, the method for establishing the toxicity of a substance is called the lethal dose evaluation. Test animals are given a range of doses for a substance and the dose at which the substance is lethal for 50 per cent of the animals is called the $LD_{50.}$ It is given in grams per kilogram of body weight of the animal. Thus, an $LD_{50}$ of 1 means that 1 g of essential oil per kilogram of body weight of the test animal induces death in 50 per cent of the animals tested.

When this toxicity data is applied to humans we assume an average body weight of 70 kg (11 stone). So, for example, for a $LD_{50}$ value of 2.6 g per kg of a substance, it would take 170 ml of actual oral dose to cause death in someone weighing 60 kg (9½ stone). That's much more than anyone is likely to take.

Leaving aside the ethical issues, it is questionable whether test results from animals such as rats and rabbits are transferable to humans because of differences in our skin and metabolism.

Essential oils that have been recorded as causing considerable toxicity if orally ingested in higher than therapeutic quantities include: wintergreen, camphor, eucalyptus and pennyroyal, clove, hyssop, nutmeg, sage, sassafras, cinnamon, thuja (Battaglia, 1995).

## Skin reactions

Skin and mucous membrane reactions to essential oils include: irritation, **sensitisation** and **phototoxicity**.

### Irritation

People can have skin reactions to many substances, including essential oils, even when these are administered in small doses. An irritation is a local, inflammatory reaction on exposure to the essential oil: redness, possibly a rash.

Often people know that they have quite sensitive skin as they already react easily to a variety of substances. In this case, before giving an essential oil that is known to be possibly irritating, it is wise to perform a patch skin test.

*Giving a patch test*
Apply a small amount of diluted essential oil (2.5%) to a patch of skin, for example, on the inner forearm. Cover with cotton gauze and wait 12–24 hours. Observe for any signs of irritation.

Essential oils containing significant amounts of phenol molecules are the most common causes of skin irritation: these include clove, oregano, thyme.

## Sensitisation
This involves an allergic reaction. The body perceives the essential oil as a foreign body and mounts an immune reaction causing dermatitis: rash, inflammation, redness, possibly slight blistering. In sensitisation, once the dermatitis has been provoked, it is likely that the reaction will recur whenever the person is exposed to the chemical causing it, whether this is found in an essential oil or from some other source in the environment.

This is a highly individualised reaction. It may still be possible to use an essential oil that has caused a reaction if one first starts with a very high dilution and only gradually increases it.

Also, the potentially sensitising effects of a substance when used alone may be quenched, or rendered harmless, by the presence of other substances or constituents when it is combined with them.

## Photosensitivity
This is a skin reaction caused by exposure to ultraviolet light of the sun's rays. Some essential oil molecules – specifically, bergaptene and furocoumarin 5-MOP – can increase the skin's absorption of sunlight, and thus increase the chance of sunburn. It is recommended that if such essential oils are used, the client is advised not to expose the skin to sunlight, or UV lamps for at least 12 hours.

Photosensitising essential oils are some of the citrus group: bergamot, lime, bitter orange, and angelica.

## Hepatotoxicity
Some constituents of essential oils have been known to damage liver cells on oral ingestion. It is highly unlikely that damage could be caused by dermal absorption under normal, diluted use.

### Hepatotoxic essential oil molecules

| Constituent | Essential oil |
| --- | --- |
| trans-anethole | aniseed, fennel |
| cinnamaldehyde | cassia, cinnamon bark |
| methyl chavicol | basil (ct. tropical), tarragon |
| eugenol | bay, cinnamon leaf, clove |
| pulegone | buchu, pennyroyal |
| safrole | sassafras, camphor (brown and yellow) |

## Neurotoxicity

Since essential oil molecules are lipid-soluble, they can cross the blood–brain barrier and reach the brain tissue. Here they can potentially cause:

- convulsant effects – provoke epileptic seizures
  - fenchone in fennel
  - pinocamphone in hyssop
  - camphor in camphor, spike, lavender, rosemary, sage
- negative psychotrophic effects – alter mood and/or perception
  - thujone in sage (*Salvia officinalis*), wormwood
  - myristicin in nutmeg
  - elemicin in nutmeg.

## Carcinogenesis

This term means the stimulation, formation and/or growth of cancer cells. There is no real evidence that this has ever been caused by essential oils used in aromatherapy. The precaution is based on evidence that certain molecules of the volatile components of the herbs calamus, sassafras and camphor (beta asarone and safrole) have stimulated cancer either when these herbs have been ingested, or when their essential oils have been repeatedly applied in high doses.

## Hazards during pregnancy

It is a general rule among herbalists and naturopaths that no treatment should be given during pregnancy, unless for very minor ailments. Pregnancy is not the time to be engaging in active cleansing or tonification therapy.

The concern with using essential oils during pregnancy is due to the properties of some of their constituents. Please refer to the list at the end of the chapter for details.

- Hormone-like properties in some oils may disturb the natural balance of the hormones oestrogen and progesterone during the pregnancy.
- Emmenagogue properties become potentially abortifacient in the context of pregnancy, since emmengogues act on the uterine muscle causing contraction. They may trigger miscarriage if a foetus is not viable. If the woman has had previous experience of miscarriage any emmenagogue oil is avoided as potentially destablising to the pregnancy. Certain essential oils may be safely used in the last six weeks of a normal pregnancy to strengthen the uterus for the birth.
- Toxic properties (see above discussion) in some essential oils. These should be avoided during pregnancy because of the theoretical risk that even tiny amounts are capable of crossing the blood–brain barrier or affecting the liver or kidneys of the foetus.

### Essential oils to avoid in pregnancy

| Essential oil | Property |
|---|---|
| pennyroyal, sage, thuja, wormwood, tansy, mugwort, savin | abortifacient and toxic |
| mustard, wormseed, horseradish | toxic |
| aniseed, fennel, basil | oestrogenic |
| clove, hyssop, savory, thyme, wintergreen | moderately toxic |
| cedarwood, clary sage, jasmine, juniper, marjoram, myrrh, peppermint, rose, rosemary, lavender | emmenagogue* |

*\* Emmenagogue essential oils are also those that may help at the time of childbirth. They can be safe when used only at the time of labour and delivery*

## General safety precautions

- Keep to the correct therapeutic dose guidelines for the patient and circumstances.
- Abide by cautions, avoid using hazardous oils.
- Do not apply essential oils neat to the skin. Always dilute.
- Keep essential oils away from eyes and mucous membranes.
- Keep out of reach of children.
- Keep away from naked flame and heat.
- Label all blends and products clearly with name, date, quantity and instructions for use, i.e.:
  - Keep away from children.
  - Store in a cool place, away from sunlight.
  - Do not use internally.

## Safe doses and dilutions

Because essential oils vary in their viscosity, a drop of a viscous essential oil from a standard dispensing bottle will not be exactly equal to that of another, thinner essential oil. However, as a rough guide it is assumed that 20 drops of essential oil is equal to 1 ml in volume.

### Guidelines for dilutions

Infants, birth–12 months: 1 drop of appropriate essential oil in 10 ml carrier, a 0.5% dilution

Children, 1–5 years: 2–3 drops of appropriate safe essential oil, depending on weight, in 10 ml carrier

Children, 6–12 years: half the recommended adult dose, 1% dilution or 3 drops in 15–20ml carrier

Children, 12 years and above: use adult dose, 2.5% dilution or 6 drops in 12–20 ml carrier

Elderly: if frail, or with thinned skin, use half adult dose

See Appendix 2 for a full list of potentially hazardous essential oils and Appendix 3 for a list of the therapeutic properties of essential oils.

## Key Terms

You need to know what these words mean. Go back through the chapter or check in the glossary to find out.

- anosmia
- aromatogram
- endorphin
- hepatotoxicity
- hydrophilic
- lethal dose evaluation
- limbic system
- lipid
- lipophilic
- neurotoxicity
- peptide
- perfusion
- phototoxicity
- sensitisation
- smell fatigue

# THE THERAPEUTIC RELATIONSHIP AND THE CONSULTATION PROCESS

After reading this chapter you will be able to:

- understand the nature of the therapeutic relationship, the responsibilities and boundaries existing between practitioner and patient
- understand the aims, objectives and procedures of a consultation
- use active listening, reflecting and eliciting information when taking a case history
- make a clear record of the initial consultation and subsequent consultations and treatments
- observe for imbalances in the skin and posture
- give after care advice to your aromatherapy patient
- formulate a therapeutic strategy and manage treatment sessions
- be aware of precautions and contra-indications to aromatherapy treatment.

In addition to the essential oils themselves, one of the most important aspects of aromatherapy is the relationship between the practitioner and patient – the therapeutic relationship. The nature of the relationship has significant implications for the healing process. It is important that the practitioner assesses the patient using a consultation procedure in which a patient's information is recorded clearly and confidentially. This combined with a physical examination and the two assessments forms the basis of the **therapeutic strategy**: the selection of essential oils and of the appropriate method of application. Treatment is given as part of a holistic approach in which the practitioner aims to support or guide the patient's healing journey towards greater understanding of his or her own nature.

## Energies in the therapeutic relationship

As a practitioner you bring something of your own energy, state of mind and being to every treatment, so it is best to be aware of this and endeavour to keep your intentions clear and positive. In addition to the dynamics of the essential oils themselves (see Chapters 2 and 7), holistically we could say there are three more energies present in a therapeutic relationship:

- the energy of the patient
- the energy of the practitioner
- the energy of the healing power of the vital force underlying both.

### The patient's energy
The patient brings his or her own energy into the relationship. Usually, if he or she has come because of feeling unwell, the patient's energy is imbalanced in some way. Assessing the pattern or quality is an important

**REMEMBER**

An imbalance means the vital force of the person is caught in a negative pattern – a pattern that may eventually weaken the body and will provide conditions for illness.

first step to understanding the symptoms presented and the underlying causes for them. If his or her health or energy is weak the patient may be to some extent vulnerable and the practitioner takes care to respect the patient's **integrity** at all times.

### Variety among patients

Some patients may be already quite self-aware and just need a little support for their own growth and healing. Some may be very stuck and stagnant in the habits that have brought them to their present condition. Others may have suffered a trauma, which will take some time to resolve; more prolonged treatment, deeper work, may be required to change their pattern from a negative to a positive one. Some patients are very 'head oriented', want to participate actively in the process and respond best if given a lot of information along with treatment; they often bring a lot of information about themselves to treatment. Others respond best by just receiving the treatments and the deep relaxation that goes with it, without articulating what they feel. Still others, while initially enthusiastic, in practice may find it more difficult to commit to treatment or initiate changes that are indicated, beneficial though these may be. Some patients react quickly or strongly to the stimulation of the treatment; in others responses may take more time to be felt. These individual tendencies are part of the patient's inherent nature, *terrain* or constitutional type (Chapter 2). Some patients, especially those with several different areas of concern, may not be aware of how much progress they have made. If we ask them how they feel, verbally, the initial response may not indicate progress. This is one reason why during the first consultation and subsequent sessions, the practitioner uses follow-up questions to explore issues and get the patient to be as specific as possible. Recording the information means it can be later compared with information given at subsequent treatments. The 'before and after' record can help a patient realise that progress has been made. The record can also help the sceptical or discouraged patient be more open to the possibility of change, or renew his or her commitment to the healing process. Even if a condition is not fully resolved, because of the holistic treatments the patient will have gained new insights or the strength to tackle issues that were perhaps previously too daunting.

If the patient can engage in the processes of change and co-operate with the practitioner's recommendations that will enhance the effects of the essential oils. As the treatments continue, as changes occur, the practitioner will adapt the treatment and advice to new circumstances. A practitioner should not feel that he or she is either totally responsible for any progress or any apparent lack of progress in the patient.

### Patient in charge

Ultimately, the power for healing lies in the patient's own hands; aromatherapy's role is to be the catalyst for positive change. Sometimes a patient may not like to recognise this and will tend to look on the practitioner as the expert who will put things right or the patient transfers all his or her hopes on to the practitioner, much like a child trusts in a parent. As holistic practitioners we try to recognise if the **transference** is happening and we guide the patient to a more adult role of responsibility and acknowledgement of his or her own inner resources. To do this the practitioner responds as an adult from his or her place of inner calm (Chapter 1). In addition practitioners need to avoid exploiting, however unconsciously, the patient's vulnerability for the benefit of their own self-esteem. Equally they need not accept any undue share of responsibility. It is not practitioners who do the healing but the patient and his or her own vital force, engaged and energised by the application of essential oils.

### Respecting the patient's space
Being 'in charge' also means the patient is free to initiate changes in his or her own time. Our job is not to impose rigid ideas on the patient but to advise while the patient chooses what feels right for him or her to take on board at the time.

Progress Check

1 How might it help the healing process if the patient feels involved?
2 What does respecting the patient involve?
3 How might you use knowledge of a patient's energy pattern to help your work?

## The practitioner's energy
Since the practitioner is also a factor in the healing process, it is important for the quality of his or her energy to be as positive as possible. Developing self-awareness and the skill of working from a point of inner calm facilitates this capacity.

### Responding, not reacting
If the practitioner works from an inner point or fulcrum of balance, no matter what type of patient comes or the nature of the patient's imbalances the practitioner can respond positively. If we as practitioners do not know ourselves well first – are not aware of our own weaknesses and strengths – we may only react. Reacting means involving ourselves in that energy imbalance, whereas responding allows us to keep our balance without draining our own energy. The key here is self-awareness: if we are not clear in ourselves about who we are and where we are coming from – about our own issues, predispositions and habitual attitudes – we might unwittingly impose on the patient, or misunderstand what the patient is trying to communicate to us. Being clear in ourselves avoids this. Finally, it enhances the flow of healing energy.

### Protecting our space
Self-awareness and being centred also helps to protect us from absorbing any negativity of the patient. We are mindful not to take on the problems of the patient, not to take them too much to heart or to allow the patient to transfer any negativity. By creating and working from a place of balance within ourselves, we avoid this potential problem area.

To help create such a beneficial detachment different practitioners have different strategies. One of these is to ritualise the separation in some way. For example, as we wash our hands immediately after treatment, we consciously visualise that the water is clearing away the energy between us and the patient. Another is to take a minute or two for quiet meditation in between each patient, mentally clearing the mind and body (Fig. 3.1).

> **REMEMBER**
> - The responsibility of the patient: to give co-operation and participation.
> - The power of the patient: to be in charge of his or her own health; having access to his or her own healing power.
> - The vulnerability of the patient: needing respect and loving care.

## The practitioner's responsibility

To inspire others in healthy living the practitioner needs to take responsibility for his or her own health. Again different practitioners do this in different ways. For example, it is good to receive treatments from another practitioner or to engage in periods of peer supervision to identify and balance areas needing attention. Regular updating of skills and knowledge – called continuing professional development (Chapter 13) – keeps the practitioner open and competent. For some practitioners, practices such as meditation, yoga, t'ai chi, breathing techniques, relaxation, engaging in regular periods of inner reflection all help to foster self-awareness and access inner resources. The world is never perfectly harmonious and we all are affected by what goes on in and around us. A practitioner will try to counter the tendency for the world to spill over to the **therapeutic space**. For example, even if we are having a 'bad' day personally, we can still be present in a calm frame of mind for giving treatment. Or, if we sense this is not possible, we can make arrangements to give treatments at another time. Such self-awareness helps us offer our skills in a loving but detached manner, and we do not misuse the patient's trust or transfer to her our own imbalances. These intentions are aspects of integrity, of our being so connected to our true selves, so integrated within, that we naturally behave in a genuinely honest way towards others.

Essential oils are a powerful tool for health and healing but not a cure-all for every condition. Promising to cure every condition would be a breach of trust between practitioner and patient. Knowing this, aromatherapy practitioners work within certain guidelines:

- We never claim to 'cure' any disease or condition. Diagnosing and curing diseases is the province of the medical physician.
- We do not advise patients to stop taking medically prescribed medications. If done, it is only by the patient in consultation with his or her physician. However, with the patient's permission, we may contact the physician, to inform him or her about aromatherapy treatments.
- We do not give or advise on treatments for which we are not fully trained and qualified. When we feel our own expertise has come to a point where it is no longer helping a particular patient, bearing the patient's best interests in mind we refer the patient to some other form of treatment that we think will help.
- When we feel that understanding a condition or symptom is beyond our expertise or we suspect a serious medical condition, we do not hesitate to advise the patient to check with his or her GP.

> **REMEMBER**
>
> As practitioners we too are on a journey towards our wholeness: outwardly we develop and improve our skills; inwardly we develop our self-awareness.

> **REMEMBER**
>
> - The responsibility of the practitioner: to continue to develop his or her skills and self-awareness.
> - The power of the practitioner: expertise within his or her training, access to his or her inner resources.
> - The vulnerability of the practitioner: to any negativity of the patient.

> **ACTIVITY**
>
> With a fellow student or students, identify and discuss five conditions or situations in which you would refer a patient to another practitioner or medical physician.

> **GOOD PRACTICE**
>
> Between patients take a few moments to do five deep, relaxing breaths to clear the space. As you breathe in, repeat to yourself the word 'peace'. As you breathe out, say to yourself the word 'calm'.

## The healing energy of the vital force

The third energy in the therapeutic relationship is that of the vital force itself. With our knowledge of essential oils and methods of their application we try to release any blockages to the energy, create optimum conditions and promote its freer flow. We try to bring our patients in touch with the inner resource. This is the true healing power in the patient. Exactly why the positive energy begins to flow strongly and the healing begins is sometimes a mystery.

### ACTIVITY

Practise this centring exercise:

1  Place your hand on your abdomen just below the navel. Breathe five times into your lower abdomen, feeling that with each breath out you are releasing all the tension in your body, all discomfort – all that is flowing out with the out-breath. With the in-breath, you are renewing your energy. Feel the breath as it comes in through your nostrils and down into the deep lungs to your centre around the navel. From there it diffuses to every cell of your body, carrying oxygen and the energy of the vital force. Each in-breath renews the body with fresh oxygen and vitality. Each in-breath flows into your nostrils, down into your lungs to your navel area and, from there, diffuses throughout the body. Every organ, tissue and cell is revitalised and nourished with the healing breath. Through the breathing you can even increase the reservoir of energy within yourself as you nourish it with the conscious breathing awareness. After five breaths, rest a few moments in normal breathing, absorbing the feeling of relaxation and calm. Feel yourself connected to your inner core, a place of strength and calm, a place not of 'doing' but 'being'. This is your centre of gravity, your fulcrum of balance and poise.

2  Return to normal breathing again. Rest in this state, breathing calmly into your centre, feeling warm, heavy, relaxed. Be aware also that you feel renewed, vital and poised for whatever may come to you. Now that you have found the place of dynamic poise, know that you can return to it whenever you need – by using your breath and your awareness. Whenever you want to, using your breath, you can calm your mind and emotions and recharge your energy by returning to your centre of calmness, peace and strength. The more you practice this, the easier it becomes to access your inner strength and power, which is always there for you whenever you need it.

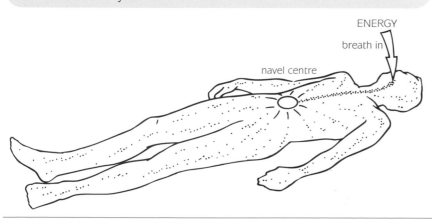

ENERGY

breath in

navel centre

**Fig. 3.1** *Relaxation with deep abdominal breathing while lying down. Visualise an inward flow of energy with the in-breath, energy radiating from navel throughout the body on the out-breath*

## Progress Check

1 In addition to the essential oils, what are the three energies that combine in the healing process?
2 What is the difference between reacting and responding?
3 How can the practitioner's self-awareness help protect both the practitioner and his or her patient?
4 Why is it important not to advise a patient to reduce any medication prescribed by his or her GP?
5 When might you advise a patient to have a check-up from his or her GP?

## Pitfalls and possibilities in the therapeutic relationship

### Pitfalls

- The practitioner becomes the 'expert' in the situation.
- The patient is merely the passive recipient of treatment without an active role.
- The gender of the practitioner or patient becomes an issue.
- The relationship becomes personal and does not remain professional.
- In talking with a patient, the practitioner may use language or terms, which, while meaningful to him or her, are not understood by the patient.
- The practitioner allows his or her own imbalances to interfere with the treatments, or allows negative energy of the patient to be transferred to him or herself.
- Either the practitioner or patient focuses too much on the physical aspects of the illness, measures improvement only on that basis, disregarding any healing taking place at other levels.

### Possibilities

- Positive communication. The practitioner actively listens to the patient's experience and explains his or her intentions in a way the patient can understand.
- Mutual respect, trust and care. The practitioner respects and genuinely cares for the integrity of the patient. The patient feels safe and in control. Compassion motivates the practitioner to foster the patient's own healing process. The practitioner takes care not to abuse his or her expertise at the patient's expense.
- Realistic and positive expectations. Confidence in the healing power of essential oils helps the patient be comfortable with the treatment process. Realising limitations allows the practitioner to refer the patient to other helpers when necessary.

## The aromatherapy consultation

Conducting a consultation on the patient's first visit and in briefer form on all subsequent visits is one of the most important aspects of a professional therapy. It forms the basis of the practitioner's assessment of the patient and the therapeutic strategy. Clear, continual record-keeping allows for reflecting on and evaluating the effectiveness of treatments and planning future treatments. It can provide the raw material for research.

The aims of a consultation are:

- to observe and record factors relevant to the patient's condition and to understand the whole person
- to allow the patient to express any concerns or experiences in a safe environment
- to allow the practitioner to explain the nature and efficacy of the treatment proposed and give supporting advice
- to foster a partnership based on mutual trust and respect.

### Confidentiality

In order to feel free to express even quite deep and personal feelings, the patient needs to know his or her information will be kept absolutely confidential. Reassure the patient of this at the first visit. As professionals we undertake not to pass on information to a third party without the patient's permission, although we are bound by law to report such things as instances of communicable diseases to the relevant health authorities.

---

**GOOD PRACTICE**

Patient records should be kept secure, under lock and key.

---

**Progress Check**

1. What are two advantages of recording the first and subsequent consultations?
2. What are three aims of a consultation?
3. Why is it important to assure the patient of confidentiality?

---

### Active listening

The term 'active listening' was coined to highlight the fact that often we really only pay partial attention to what people are saying. We may 'hear' the speaker, but we are not really taking it all in, not really paying attention nor being fully receptive. Active listening is a mark of respect because we give the speaker the gift of our full attention and show our acceptance of them. We do this by:

- not interrupting with comments
- not taking over the conversation with our own concerns or redirecting it towards ourselves
- not being judgemental
- not changing the subject
- not allowing our minds to wander as we listen to the speaker.

**GOOD PRACTICE**

During the consultation check that you are listening to your patient and not to yourself.

### Reflecting

When responding to our patients it helps if we show that we have understood them. One technique to help show this is to reflect back to the speaker the essence of what he or she has just said by paraphrasing it and saying it back to the speaker. The reflecting phase is important in allowing the speaker to know that we have understood what the speaker wanted to be understood, that the story has been communicated successfully; or, to know that it hasn't been and to give him or her the chance to explain again. Reflecting may be done by using such expressions as 'I understand you are saying that . . .', or 'I take you to mean that . . .', or 'So you feel that . . .' and then rephrasing the patient's main point(s).

### Eliciting information

Eliciting is another aspect of a consultation. It is used to bring out more details about a particular aspect of the case, more specific information than may have first been given. Eliciting uses open-ended questions instead of closed questions. An open-ended question invites an explanatory response; a closed question invites only a yes/no response. A practitioner employs follow-up questions to ensure relevant details are recorded.

For example, a patient says that she has headaches. But in order for the practitioner to understand the nature of the headaches and to relate it to the whole, to the *terrain*, the person's constitutional make-up, the practitioner needs to ask follow-up questions, such as the following:

- Which areas does the headache affect: the front/back/sides/sinuses/ and/or neck or shoulder area?
- When does it occur? – e.g. time of day, associated with an activity such as eating/exercise/work/other?
- Can you tell me about any particular event or experience, which may prompt a headache?

- What makes it better or worse – movement/rest/heat/cold/other?
- How do you usually cope with it or treat it?
- How long has it been happening? How long does it last?
- Does the condition irritate, frustrate, depress, worry or evoke other responses in you? How does it make you feel in yourself, in addition to the discomfort?

Such details are important for discovering any pattern to the symptoms and to give insight into the patient's mental–emotional make-up.

## ACTIVITY

1   With a partner, practise active listening and eliciting. In turn each of you relates a condition or experience you have had. It could be a journey, an illness or any memorable experience. The listener responds with reflecting techniques, with open-ended questions and follow-up questions to bring out more detail. Using the guidelines above, you each give feedback on how your partner performed. Did your partner wait to share comments until after you had finished? Did your partner reflect back your thoughts to you?

2   This activity is called 'Listening within'.
   (a) Find about 15 minutes when you can be uninterrupted.
   (b) Sit quietly and focus on your breathing for a couple of minutes, diverting your mind's attention from preoccupations with all external duties and activities and towards your inner state of being. Breathe normally but just observe your breath as it gently flows in and out in its own rhythmic cycle.
   (c) Allow yourself to attend to how you are feeling. Is there something between you and feeling fine? If so, can you identify it?
   (d) Pretend that your mind's eye is travelling around the different parts of your body – your face, shoulders, neck, stomach, legs. At each place you ask if that area is feeling OK. If you get a negative answer, such as 'neck feels really tense', acknowledge that, but put it aside for the moment as you move to another body part. As you find areas of tension, pain or excessive cold or heat, acknowledge each one and continue to check out your body until you have 'listened' and paid attention to all the parts that feel uncomfortable. If all of you is feeling well, be grateful and accept that too.
   (e) Choose one of your uncomfortable parts (or any part of you, if all are feeling well), think about that body part and first breathe in, then lengthen the out-breath and mentally direct it into and through that part. At the same time feel that the out-breath is taking away with it any tension or feelings of pain and discomfort. Repeat this two or three times. Return to normal breathing.
   (f) Now notice how you feel generally. Accept it without criticism or judgement. Just be with yourself for a few moments, quietly.
   (g) Now choose another part of your body that felt uncomfortable. Repeat the practice of breathing into

that part. Feel that as you breathe in you are taking in healing energy, while as you breathe out you are directing the healing energy into and through that part of you that feels uncomfortable. Repeat this for three to five breaths, then return to normal breathing.

(h) Pause to study how you feel. Notice any changes or lack of change, accepting what there is.

(i) When you are ready, breathe five times into your solar plexus. As you breathe in feel the breath moving through your nostrils, down your throat, to your lungs and down to your solar plexus region. As you breathe out, feel the breath radiating out from the solar plexus to all parts of your body, enlivening and energising them with the vital life force.

(j) Return to normal breathing, watching the breath flow in and out. Pause to experience the deep state of calm and stillness you have discovered within you. Feel that you will act now from the calm centre of peace and strength, rather than just from your head.

(k) Gradually bring yourself back to outward awareness by wiggling your toes, feet, fingers, hands. Rub your hands together. When you are ready, open your eyes. Accept what you have done and welcome what came to you. Be glad it spoke to you and you listened.

## Conducting a consultation and recording the case history

The initial consultation involves observation, verbal questioning and discussion with the patient and then recording information on a **patient record** or consultation sheet. The information is used by the practitioner to formulate the therapeutic strategy and choose appropriate essential oils and their method of application for the patient. This is put on the record sheet. Observations gained during the treatment are also recorded. The information forms a base line for evaluating any future changes and developments in the case. While it is important to obtain relevant information, be aware that in some cases even important information may not come out in the first session. This is not so unusual. Sometimes the patient just forgets or doesn't consider it worth mentioning. Sometimes the patient's trust is not yet enough that sensitive information can be divulged. Sometimes it just takes time for the layers of possibly years of experience to come to the surface.

### Personal history

Record the patient's personal details as in the sample record sheet provided on pages 76 and 77 or one that your tutor provides. While asking, be alert to any information relevant to the patient's state of mind or emotions that may come out at this point, such as how the patient feels about his or her situation or any difficult circumstances that are involved (unemployment, divorce, bereavement).

# Initial observations

## 1 First impressions

Observation really starts with the first contact with the patient. This can be a phone call, a letter, email or in person. Be sensitive to information conveyed by the voice expression, physical gestures or the appearance. Does the patient seem nervous? confident? extrovert or introvert? Does the patient seem 'weighed down'? Is the patient's manner talkative, quiet or disturbed? Is the breathing obviously laboured? Are there signs of tension such as clenched fists or nervous movements? Listen to the patient's voice for any obvious signs of imbalance.

## 2 Physical examination

Your tutor will instruct you in a good method of physical examination. Your tutor may use reflexology or muscle testing as an assessment aid, or other techniques, for example, from Chinese medicine. Whatever the model, looking carefully at the patient's physical condition can give important clues about their constitutional type or the *terrain*, and the possible root causes of any imbalances or the condition he or she is concerned about. Record observations on the patient's record sheet.

Skin and face should be examined and observations recorded. Observe for areas of:

- dryness, rash, acne, rosaceae
- redness or paleness: indicates either hyperaemia/inflammation or poor circulation
- yellow skin or pallor: suggests possible liver or kidney problems
- discoloration: suggests toxicity or bruising
- bluish tinge: indicates poor blood circulation
- varicose veins: indicates possible colon congestion, back problems, stagnant energy and blood and lymph circulation
- tense, spongy or congested tissue: indicates muscle tension, adhesions, poor circulation or fluid retention.

Observe if the patient is markedly over or underweight.

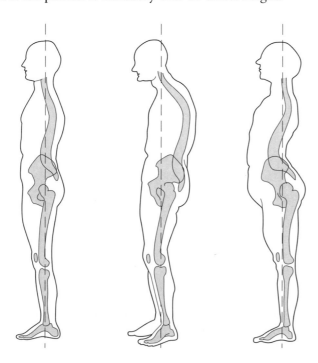

**Fig. 3.2a** *Balanced posture with correct pelvic tilt; kyphosis with pelvis tilted back; lordosis with pelvis tipped forward*

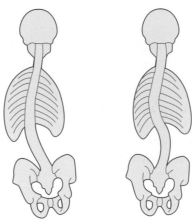

**Fig. 3.2b** *Forms of scoliosis: left, a single C-curve; right, a primary curve with a secondary compensation curve below*

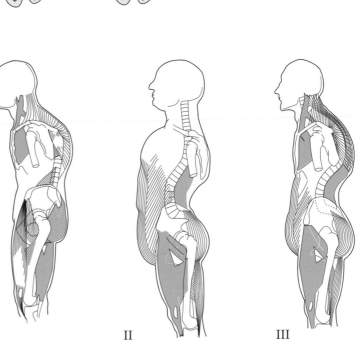

**Fig. 3.2c** *I Kyphosis results in lengthened muscles of posterior neck, back and anterior thighs and shortened antagonists of anterior neck, chest, buttocks and posterior thighs*
*II Lordosis results in lengthened muscles of abdomen and buttocks, posterior thighs and shortened muscles of posterior neck, back and anterior thighs*
*III A combination of rounded upper back and hollow lower back*

I                    II                    III

It is a good idea to perform a postural examination to become aware of any obvious imbalances along the spine such as lordosis, scoliosis (curvatures), deviations of the shoulder and pelvic girdle, or imbalance of head position.

---

### Possible figure imbalances

Head tilt
High shoulders (one or both)
Scapula abduction
Dowager's hump/osteoporosis
Adipose deposits on biceps or triceps muscles
Poor muscle tone on triceps muscles
Back: flat, rounded, kyphosis, lordosis, scoliosis

Abdomen: abdominal bulge
Buttocks
Pelvic tilt
Legs: muscular tone
Adipose deposits/cellulite

Knock knees, bow legs, hyper-extended knees
Feet: flat feet, ankles rolled in or out, feet turned in/out

## Verbal examination

Your tutor will instruct you in her chosen verbal examination procedure. The following is given only as an illustration of what is usually included in taking the case history.

### Complaint or inquiry

Ask about the reason for the consultation. This may only be one of general interest or simply for relaxation in an otherwise healthy person. But if there are specific concerns about symptoms, record and explore these with the patient. Here you may ask such questions as: what would the patient like most to have relief from, what exactly is bothering him or her? It may be that the patient has already received a medical diagnosis and wishes to explore an alternative approach, or support orthodox treatment with aromatherapy. Try to be clear with the patient what aromatherapy can and cannot offer.

> **GOOD PRACTICE**
>
> Explain briefly the need to ask questions for the case history. Be sensitive, tactful and discreet. Reassure the patient of the confidentiality of the information. Accept that the patient may not wish to confide some aspects with you at this time.

### Medical history

Ask about the following:

- Past medical conditions, including childhood diseases.
- Any medications used, past or present, e.g. antibiotics, anti-inflammatories, HRT, other.
- Family medical history: Is there a family history of heart, liver, pancreas, digestive, lung, nerve, kidney or other disease?
- Traumas/major or minor: falls/car accidents/significant emotional traumas such as loss of a loved one, loss of employment or moving house.
- Any operations, hospitalisations or serious illnesses.
- Any recent travel. Sometimes a symptom may have been acquired while travelling abroad.

### Systems assessment

Ask the patient specifically about each system of the body to discover how it is functioning. This often brings out information the patient doesn't consider significant, or has forgotten, but which has a bearing on the cause of the complaint. It is important for a holistic assessment. Asking about the quality of any symptoms can give information about the *terrain* and the constitutional type. Does a symptom show signs of heat, cold, dryness, excess moisture, tension, pain or spasm? Fine-tune your assessment, and differentiate from among the symptoms as to which area(s) may be the root cause of the imbalance. This is called making a differential diagnosis. It helps to show how the different systems are relating to each other. Is one system supplementing a weakness in another system?

The systems you ask about are as follows:

- Digestive: Is the appetite good, poor, excessive or erratic? Is there any heartburn, acidity, headache associated with eating, any flatulence? Record any constipation – less than one bowel movement a day – or diarrhoea. Ask the patient to say exactly what they eat and drink on a typical day, and at what times.

◊ Urinary: Ask about problems in the area such as cystitis, urinary tract infections, problems with urination, kidney disease, water retention. Ask if there has ever been blood in the urine (a sign of possible stones or Bright's disease) and if so refer the patient to GP for check up. Ask if any medications have been taken, e.g. antibiotics.

◊ Respiratory: Ask about any problems or history here such as sinus, shortness of breath, allergies, repeated or chronic infections, colds or flu. Record any medications taken.

◊ Lymphatic: Ask about any symptoms of swelling in lymph glands of neck, axilla or groin; any history of repeated tonsillitis, or infections, water retention or mononucleosis. Such history may indicate a weakness in the lymphatic system.

◊ Skin: Ask about the history of any skin problems or allergies, e.g. eczema, psoriasis, dry skin. Visually observe these if they are present. (See above guidelines.)

◊ Circulatory: Ask about presence of varicose veins (examine these visually), circulation problems such as excessive cold or heat (chilblains, unusual sweating); history of any heart disease. Ask if the patient knows if blood pressure is normal/high/low. Record any medications. As a constitutional consideration, does the patient typically feel hot or cold?

◊ Muscular–skeletal: Take the history of any muscular strains, sprains, of broken bones or spinal traumas, aches, pain; or stiffness in the joints.

◊ Nervous and endocrine: Enquire if the patient has frequent headaches, tension, spasms, pains or significant mood swings. Be sure to ask about the patient's energy levels: are they adequate, or low, and what is the sleep pattern like? Ask the patient to describe the sleep pattern. If it is poor or disturbed, this is often a telling indicator of imbalances.

◊ Reproductive: Asking about this area may require extra tact and sensitivity. For pre-menopausal women, enquire about the overall nature and the pattern of her menstrual cycle: abnormally light or heavy bleeding, PMS, fatigue? Was there any trauma associated with the menarche, any difficulties with pregnancies or childbirths? Has there been any difficulty with the menopause? Record any medications taken. For men, especially those over 40 (from about which time they become susceptible to prostate problems), ask if they have experienced any problems in the reproductive area or on urinating.

**GOOD PRACTICE**

Highlight in your record sheet (with stars, red marks, underlines) any signs that call for extra cautions when choosing or applying essential oils, such as allergies, skin sensitivities, high blood pressure.

## Lifestyle assessment

As you are taking the case history, areas relating to lifestyle may have already come up. Do note any relevant aspects or ask about the following:

- Activities: Whether very active, sedentary, 'workaholic', other.
- Rest and recreation: Whether regular and adequate, or needs attention. Hobbies and recreational activities are important to our general health, providing enjoyment and self-expression.
- Eating habits: Whether the patient has strong preferences for hot, spicy foods, sweets and puddings, savoury. Any special diets (e.g. vegan). Enquire if the patient takes adequate amounts of fresh fruits and vegetables; whether he or she eats regularly or tends to skip meals.

## Emotional, psychological and mental factors

It is important to understand if there are any mental–emotional factors affecting the patient or a condition. If such factors have not been expressed up to this point, it is worth asking about them. You can approach it directly, for example, 'Please tell me if there are any other factors, perhaps emotional or mental, that may be affecting you.' If you feel uncomfortable addressing the area, you can do so indirectly by inferring it from other information the patient gives, and from inquiring about sleep patterns and energy levels:

- Energy levels: Does the patient have enough energy for his or her life? Have energy levels changed significantly recently? Is the patient more active at a particular time of day or night? Such questions can suggest constitutional patterns or point to underlying stress patterns.
- Sleep pattern: Do ask about this as it can be an important indicator of health balance. If problems are reported, ask follow-up questions to identify any factors involved. Is there a constitutional pattern here?
- Stress: If it has not already come out in the consultation, ask if there are any particular stress factors in the person's life? How well is the patient coping or being supported? Is there a cause for concern?

> **REMEMBER**
> Disturbances or imbalance in lifestyle and emotional areas may affect the patient's condition and influence your choice of essential oils.

> **GOOD PRACTICE**
>
> Consider whether to select essential oils primarily for the psychological or the physical level of the patient's being, or as a secondary consideration, to support treatment of the primary physical area with psychological considerations being secondary.

> **ACTIVITY**
>
> 1. Take a case history of yourself. Record it in your health journal. Next, think about what you have recorded, evaluate the information for any patterns – positive or negative – that may exist, or any areas of weakness and strength. What steps can you take to improve or maintain your optimum health level? Record these.
> 2. On Figure 3.2c on page 64, label the muscle groups involved in postural imbalances.

1   What is the purpose of taking a case history?
2   Why might it be important to record medications taken? Operations? Skin conditions?
3   Why is it helpful to understand the diet and digestion of the patient?
4   What can sleep patterns indicate about the patient's overall health?

**GOOD PRACTICE**

Be able to tell the patient if what he or she is saying does not make sense to you. Ask follow-up questions to obtain precise information and ensure you have understood what the patient is expressing.

## The therapeutic strategy

After assessing the patient and taking the case history, you can form and plan your **therapeutic strategy**, or **treatment plan**. Your tutor will be advising you on a good method for this but in essence you are defining the objectives for treatment and the remedies to be used to meet these. You should consider the following questions:

- What is the primary or presenting condition? Is it acute or chronic? Primarily physical or psychological? Always include an essential oil to help with this aspect.
- Are there any constitutional factors that need balancing? If so, include an essential oil to help this if possible.
- Will treatment aim primarily at the physical level or the psychological level? If both are needed, which is more important today? Focus treatment in the area.
- Do eliminative channels need activation (diuretics, diaphoretics, laxatives)? Does the patient need relaxing (calming, sedative oils)? Do any tissues need to be strengthened or vital energy raised (astringents or tonics)?
- Does the patient need primarily stimulating, warming, cooling, relaxing, tonifying or regulating?
- Has the patient indicated a dislike or preference for a particular type of fragrance?
- Will I need to change the blend for the facial massage?
- Which carrier oil is best for the massage blend and why? Would the patient benefit from a particular enriching or balancing carrier oil? Why?
- Will I be giving a full body massage? Will I be concentrating or giving special attention to a particular body part?
- Will I be adjusting my touch, avoiding or taking precautions over any particular body part?
- Will I be using or recommending a method of application other than massage?

**REMEMBER**

A treatment plan involves consideration of the patient's condition, the selection of essential oils and carriers and reasons why, any cautions regarding the essential oils, the massage or other applications, any relevant psychological or lifestyle aspects. All these should be recorded.

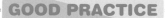

> To treat the patient on the physical level for a full body massage, blend a maximum of 7–10 drops. To treat primarily on the psychological level, for a full body massage, blend a maximum of 3–5 drops.

## Selecting essential oils

Your tutor will be giving you his or her method of selecting essential oils. The following are examples in use by aromatherapists to illustrate a sound method. Always record your initial selection and be prepared to change this at subsequent consultations according to how the patient responds.

Your work may look like this:

**Main condition:** osteo-arthritis   **Second condition:** poor sleep   **Third condition:** anxiety, coldness

| Top | Middle | Base | Top | Middle | Base | Top | Middle | Base |
|-----|--------|------|-----|--------|------|-----|--------|------|
| eucalyptus | juniper | benzoin | petigrain | lavender | frankincense | eucalyptus | ginger | frankincense |
|  |  |  |  | ylang |  |  |  |  |
|  |  |  |  | ylang |  |  |  |  |
|  |  |  |  |  |  |  |  |  |

Essential oils chosen: eucalyptus _____ drops, ginger _____ drops, frankincense _____ drops

NB: facial blend, substitute lavender for eucalyptus

Here is another scheme:

| Condition | Top notes | Middle notes | Base notes |
|-----------|-----------|--------------|------------|
| 1 osteo-arthritis in joints | eucalyptus* warming, anti-inflammatory | ginger*, warming, anti-inflammatory | benzoin |
| 2 poor sleep | petitgrain | lavender, ylang ylang calming, balancing | frankincense*, warming, calming |
| 3 energetically cold, anxious | eucalyptus* | ginger*, lavender, calming | frankincense* |
| Choice: eucalyptus, ginger, frankincense |  |  |  |
| NB: eucalyptus too strong for face, use lavender | Px has dry skin, use 5% wheatgerm oil in blend | massage full body, with attention to joint areas, finish with facial massage to relax the mind |  |

Oils with an * indicate ones chosen to be used in the blend.

Here is a third scheme:

| Conditions | 1 Stress/emotional | 2 Physical disorder | 3 Physical, skin or constitutional type |
|---|---|---|---|
| **Symptom 1** | feeling low | headache | phlegmatic, congested skin |
| **Symptom 2** | worries, anxiety | poor sleep | sedentary, low activity |
| **Possible oils** | **1** jasmine, lavender, petitgrain | **1** ylang ylang, rosemary, marjoram | **1** rosemary, cypress, geranium |
| | **2** lavender, ylang ylang, basil | **2** lavender, R. chamomile, ylang ylang | **2** juniper, cypress |
| **Final choice** | **1** ylang ylang, 1 drop | **2** lavender, 2 drops | **3** cypress, 2 drops |

(Note: whichever scheme you adopt, the same symptoms may be repeated, the same oils to help may also be repeated.)

## Recording the treatment plan and blend

Write down in the case notes:

- the essential oils chosen and the reasons
- the quantity of essential oils in drops
- the carrier oil(s) and the reasons
- any special notes on how you will adapt the massage.

For example:

Carrier oil: almond oil 10 ml, meadowsweet herbal oil, for arthritis, 5 ml.

Considerations: massage full body, with extra attention and care to joints. Finish with facial to relax the mind.

After doing an initial assessment and forming the aims and strategy for treatment, it is a good idea to take a moment to explain briefly the treatment plan (aims, oils and carriers chosen and why). The patient is presented with the blend to confirm it is pleasant to her.

## Record observations after massage

For example: 'Patient reported feeling v. relaxed after the massage. Tight muscles noted in the neck and shoulder areas.'

## After care advice and home treatment

As well as advising the patient on what to do and expect after a treatment, give the patient the benefit of any advice and experience you can that will help to balance the system as part of your **after care** advice. Record these in the patient record. For example: 'Px to try to get 10 minutes' exercise daily and eat less of acid forming foods.' If necessary, refer the patient to his or her GP or other health care professional if you consider the patient needs care beyond your skills. Be sure to record the advice in the case record notes.

Inform the patient of the following:

- Avoid bathing for 6–8 hours to allow full time for absorption of oils and carrier.
- Advise the patient to drink extra water over the next 24 hours to enhance the cleansing process, and help with elimination of toxins and wastes stimulated by the treatment. Offer the patient a glass of water immediately after the treatment.
- Avoid alcohol or a heavy or rich meal immediately after treatment.
- The patient may experience possible responses such as headache, mild tiredness, an increase in urine or bowel movements or muscle aches after treatment. Some, not all patients do. Reassure the patient that this is part of the elimination process activated by the treatment (healing crisis); that while uncomfortable, it is a positive sign: the body is working with the energy created by the treatment. Any discomfort will pass within 1–48 hours. If discomfort is experienced it is likely to be the result of positive healing activity in the body.
- Some patients report initial increase in energy followed by some fatigue and then a further increase in energy.
- The patient should listen to his or her intuition about what he or she needs to do: take more rest if tired, go for a walk if invigorated.
- The patient should take as much rest as possible to enhance the effects of the treatment.

Discuss with the patient any significant observations you have made, relating these to his or her condition.

Explain the cumulative effects of aromatherapy treatments – the fact that the greatest benefits may take three or more treatments to be noticed, as it may take time for any patterns of imbalanced energy flow to be altered. Also point out that some people naturally respond quickly to treatment, while others take a little longer. Recommend and prepare the home blend or treatment application, if any. Discuss and explain its use with patient. Answer any questions and also make any recommendations about further treatments, diet or lifestyle changes, and referrals if necessary.

## Home treatment

Home treatment is an important part of aromatherapy and often not given due weight in consultations. It helps in the following ways:

- Ensures the patient continues to get repeated daily doses of remedial essential oils for his or her condition, surrounding him or her with aromatic fragrance.
- Helps the patient take responsibility for the healing process.
- May prompt the patient to remember to act on your suggestions for lifestyle changes.

Home treatment you prescribe can include the following:

1   using a prepared blend of essential oils in carrier (cream, lotion, oil, gel, diffuser, other) for self-massage application, bath use or other, as needed

2 using an essential oil application to balance emotional moods, for example, have the patient put a drop of the blend on the inner wrist and smell this at regular intervals throughout the day, while engaging in positive thinking or practising a relaxation exercise.

### Instructing the patient

Give clear instructions to the patient on when and how to use the home remedy. Label these on the bottle. For example:

Contains 45 ml lotion and 5 ml comfrey oil

Apply to stiff joints 2–3 x daily

12 drops ginger

8 drops eucalyptus

5 drops frankincense

* External use only. Keep out of reach of children. Store away from light and heat.

## An example of advice/recommendations record

Advised on postural awareness, exercises and to avoid tensing shoulders when working.

Home remedy: Home blend (100 ml) of same essential oils to be rubbed into joints and shoulders 2 x daily. Smell from bottle and practise relaxed breathing before bedtime.

After care: Advised no tea or coffee after 6 p.m. and to avoid coffee altogether if possible. Use warming spices in foods: ginger, pepper, rosemary, sage. Take daily exercise to improve circulation, benefit osteo-arthritis.

## Therapeutic strategy and plan for further treatments

Unless aromatherapy is given for health maintenance, generally it is advisable for the patient to have a minimum of four treatments in weekly succession before any improvement can be expected, though this always depends on the complexity of the condition and the inherent health and constitution/*terrain* of the patient, as well as how well the patient follows any advice given and uses home treatments. The impact of essential oils on the organism can be quite instant or it may take time for a difference to be noticed. Also the effects are cumulative, so repeated treatment over time is advisable. Take time to discuss the topic with your patient, making sure he or she understands that a level of commitment is needed on his or her part, but that together you will assess the effectiveness at regular intervals and the patient is of course free to choose if and how often he or she has treatment. Make a note of how many treatments you ideally intend to give. For example:

Treatment recommendations: 1 massage treatment weekly for 4 weeks, then reassess with patient.

Continue treatment every 2 weeks, then every month if progress is made.

Patient agrees to use home blend on daily basis.

## Possible negative reactions

Don't feel discouraged if improvement is not swift or if things even seem to go backwards for a while; this may be a necessary part of the healing process. The patient may need time to become more open to the treatment. Even if there is no change the fact itself informs and can guide your next selection of essential oils. Keep a calm and open mind and trust in the body's ability to respond, given the right support and circumstances and necessary time.

## Follow-up treatments

At each follow-up appointment, ask the patient about his or her response. Review the symptoms, update your assessments if necessary and note any changes to the conditions presented, whether positive or negative. Record these and discuss them with the patient. Based on this and any new information the patient reports, formulate your therapeutic strategy or treatment plan for that session and record in the case history notes as before. Give the treatment and record observations and any home treatments as in the initial consultation.

> **REMEMBER**
>
> A good rule of thumb is: a month of treatment is needed for every year the patient has had the condition.

**Progress Check**

1 How can keeping clear records of the case help you in planning and evaluating the treatments?
2 Why is it helpful to conduct a careful check of each system?
3 How can forming a therapeutic strategy or treatment plan assist your patient?
4 Why is it important to record any recommendations and referrals you make to the patient?

## Contra-indications and precautions to aromatherapy treatment

Observe these precautions and avoid or adapt massage in the following circumstances:

- Abnormal temperature.
- Two days before or after menstrual cycle.
- After a heavy meal or significant period of not eating.
- Local areas of imbalance: inflammation, infection, broken skin, bruises, fractures, varicose veins, scars.
- Pregnancy: only give massage if trained in special techniques for early and late stages of pregnancy.
- Post-operative conditions:
  - Major surgery: obtain doctor's advice. Generally wait 6 weeks to 3 months before giving massage.
  - Minor surgery: do not massage over the area until completely healed. It is safe to massage lightly above, around the area after 1 week.
- Hyperthyroid: avoid over-stimulation by using a light, gentle massage technique.
- Highly strung patient: shorter treatment with calming, soothing movements.

- Medical conditions: have the patient seek medical advice if presenting with: asthma, diabetes, heart disease, cancer.
- Recent inoculations: no treatment within 36 hours of immunisation.
- Medications, recreational drugs, alcohol: caution the patient and be aware that due to increased circulation, effects of any drug may be magnified by massage or essential oil application. Depending on the prescription, the patient may wish to have the medication monitored by the GP. Often it is possible to reduce medication as the body's overall health improves. This is only done in consultation with the physician.
- Osteopathy/acupuncture: give no aromatherapy treatment on the same day.
- Homoeopathy: ask the patient to check with the homoeopath on contra-indication. Some essential oils may counteract homoeopathic prescriptions. Peppermint is one of these.
- Other: air travel or a heavy meal right after treatment may cause discomfort to the patient.

## Process in the therapeutic relationship

If we put together the essence of the discussions of the chapter, we can form a model for the process that occurs during an aromatherapy treatment session: we can visualise the consultation and treatment as a circle of healing, which the patient enters at the time of treatment.

### First stage: greeting
The patient enters and you make initial contact, greeting and introducing yourself. If the patient is new to aromatherapy, explain what aromatherapy involves or answer any questions, and make the patient feel at ease.

### Second stage: consultation
The practitioner listens to the patient's account of the complaint or reason for coming and takes the medical history and systems details. Here active listening, eliciting and recording skills are in play. The practitioner has a caring attitude and begins to process the information received.

### Third stage: treatment
Begin by making the patient comfortable. Allow a little free relaxation time at the beginning and end of the treatment. After treatment, while the patient is quiet, finish any notes, recording any observations and recommendations to be made.

## Fourth stage: after care and closing

When the patient has risen from the couch and/or is sitting comfortably, explain the after care advice and any home treatment recommendations. Answer questions and agree the next appointment. This rounds off and closes the session and the patient leaves.

Within the circle of time you have endeavoured to give your patient your best attention and care, confident in the healing power of aromatherapy. Within the circle the patient has benefited from a period of time and a place for deep relaxation, allowing the body to balance and be supported as it heals itself with its own vital force.

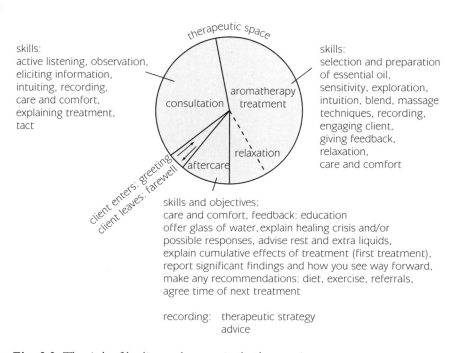

skills:
active listening, observation, eliciting information, intuiting, recording, care and comfort, explaining treatment, tact

therapeutic space

consultation

aromatherapy treatment

relaxation

aftercare

client enters: greeting
client leaves: farewell

skills:
selection and preparation of essential oil, sensitivity, exploration, intuition, blend, massage techniques, recording, engaging client, giving feedback, relaxation, care and comfort

skills and objectives:
care and comfort, feedback: education
offer glass of water, explain healing crisis and/or possible responses, advise rest and extra liquids, explain cumulative effects of treatment (first treatment), report significant findings and how you see way forward, make any recommendations: diet, exercise, referrals, agree time of next treatment

recording:   therapeutic strategy
             advice

**Fig. 3.3**  *The circle of healing and process in the therapeutic space*

---

## Key Terms

You need to know what these words mean. Go back through the chapter or check in the glossary to find out.

- after care
- case history
- contraindications and precautions
- integrity
- limits of training
- patient record
- therapeutic space
- therapeutic strategy/treatment plan
- transference

# A SAMPLE AROMATHERAPY CONSULTATION SHEET

Date_____ Practitioner Name_____

Patient name_____ Date of Birth_____

Address_____
_____

Telephone Home_____ Work_____

Marital Status_____ e-mail_____

Children_____

Occupation/retired_____ Physician_____ Tel_____

Enquiry/reason for
consultation_____
_____
_____
_____
_____

Medical History:

Have you suffered from medical conditions of:

Heart_____ Liver_____ Kidneys_____ Pancreas_____

Thyroid_____ Nervous system_____ Stomach_____

Bowels_____ Lungs_____ Other_____

Back or joints_____

Operations_____

Accidents_____ Areas affected_____

Medications currently taken or taken in the past, with dates_____

Allergies: skin_____ respiratory_____ food_____

[Details] Triggers/ how affects/how copes/medication_____

---

**Systems assessment:** [Tick if patient reports no problems, to indicate you have enquired about it]

**Digestive:**

Appetite: Good_____ Poor_____ Strong_____ Meals: regular_____ irregular_____

Digestion: Good_____ Heartburn/acid_____ Bloating_____

Other_____

A typical Daily Diet:

Breakfast_____

Mid-morning_____

Lunch_____

Mid-afternoon_____

Evening_____

Coffee/tea/alcohol per day_____

Bowels: No. movements per day_____ Constipation_____ Diarrhoea_____

Alternating_____ Pain_____ Bloating_____

---

**Urinary:** cystitis/prostate_____

**Respiratory:**_____

Asthma_____ Sinus_____

**Lymphatic:** swollen glands/ sore throats/ swollen ankles_____

**Circulation:** Good_____ Poor_____ Cold/warm_____ Varicose veins_____

Hypertension_____ Hypotension_____ Other_____

**Skin:** Normal_____ Dry/sensitive_____ Oily_____ Combination_____

Other_____

Eczema/psoroasis_____ Other_____

**Muscular–skeletal injuries:**_____ Stiffness_____ Pain_____ Arthritis_____ RA

**Reproductive:** Female: Menstrual cycle: Regular_____ Next date_____

Dysmenorrhoea/PMT_____ Amenorrhoea_____

Menopause difficulties_____ Hot flushes_____
Other_____
Male: Prostate_____ Impotence_____ Other_____

**Nervous:** Headaches_____ Epilepsy_____ Depression/anxiety_____
Sleep pattern_____
Energy level Good_____ Poor_____ Fatigue_____ Erratic_____
Stress/stressors_____

**Lifestyle:**
Exercise_____
Recreation/hobbies_____
Smoking_____

**Assessment:** [visual, tactile by practitioner]
Posture: Good_____ Lordosis_____ Scoliosis_____ Other_____
Circulation_____
Constitutional type_____
Skin:
Normal_____ Dry_____ Oily_____ Combination_____ Sensitive_____
Other [muscle testing, aromatherapy, TCM]_____

**Signature of patient**_____ Date_____
(authorising treatment)

**TREATMENT PLAN/THERAPEUTIC STRATEGY/AIMS**_____
Precautions:_____

Conditions assessed
1_____ 2_____
3_____ 4_____

Essential oils, for body massage, quantities and reasons
1._____
2._____
3._____
4._____

Carrier oil, reason_____

Essential oils for facial, if different_____
Carrier_____

Observations of treatment_____

Home treatment and method of application_____

After care recommendations/referrals _____

_____

Futher treatment recommended:
_____treatment for _____weeks then reassess

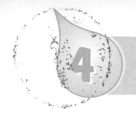

# PRACTICALITIES OF THE THERAPEUTIC SPACE

After working through this chapter you will be able to:
♦ understand the physical requirements of the treatment room
♦ understand the need for a professional appearance and manner
♦ implement the requirements of safety, hygiene and universal access
♦ understand the basics of first aid and the need for first aid training
♦ understand the requirements for essential oil safety in the beauty salon.

## The physical requirements of the treatment room

Giving careful consideration to the nature of the physical surroundings is important. Whether the treatments take place at a complementary medicine clinic, a beauty salon, a hospital, educational or other setting, the atmosphere that should be created is a positive, caring one characterised by calmness, clarity and a professional approach. In a professional setting certain arrangements are advised.

Ensure the setting is clean, well ventilated and heated, with some natural light. Ventilation is especially important for the health and safety of the practitioner. The ability to adjust the room temperature to some extent is helpful because many patients are cold or might become cooler as they relax, while others are more warm-natured. A treatment room should be well maintained and have a welcoming, relaxing and comforting atmosphere and decor: warm, softly coloured, with no strong, direct, overhead lighting.

If working in a hospital or salon where private space is not available, ensure the maximum of privacy possible, e.g. using screens or curtains.

Entry to a clinic, or therapy room in the home, should be kept freely accessible and safe for the patients. Wheelchair access should be available.

## Professional appearance

The style of dress you choose when working in your own clinic is an individual matter but a professional appearance is essential. Many practitioners wear a tunic, shirt or dress uniform to lend an air of distinction and professionalism. This may be especially appropriate when working in a hospital or similar setting. Others, by contrast, find a uniform creates a barrier between them and the patient, and prefer to dress less formally. The important factor is good grooming, which creates a positive impression, inspires the patient's confidence and reflects a professional approach.

Hair must be kept neatly out of the way of treatment. Hands should be washed before and after each treatment session or patient encounter. They should be warm when giving the massage. Nails need to be kept very short and clean. Rings, watches and dangling jewellery should be removed when giving treatment.

Some aromatherapists and salons like to have a quiet background of relaxing music. Others find this distracting, either for themselves or the patient as it hinders the patient being 'present' in the treatment process. Be aware that playing of music is subject to the Performing Rights restrictions (see Chapter 13).

**GOOD PRACTICE**

Ensure both your own and the patient's comfort and security.

## Equipment and furnishings

To ensure the patient's comfort and to enhance the therapeutic atmosphere, keep a supply of blankets, thick towels and cushions available. Support for head and neck should be offered, and even for under the knees, as this takes the strain off the lower back. Some patients also need support under the chest or shoulders. Use small cushions or rolled up towels for these areas. A box of tissues comes in handy for a variety of occasions.

### Treatment couches
There are many varieties of treatment couches available today. The couch should be stable, with a vinyl cover for ease of cleaning. Many practitioners like to use a couch with an extra headrest and/or with a backrest that can be raised. Some couches have adjustable legs, which allow the practitioner to have the right height of couch for his or her height and minimise strain. Such extras give maximum flexibility for treatments and minimise strain to the practitioner.

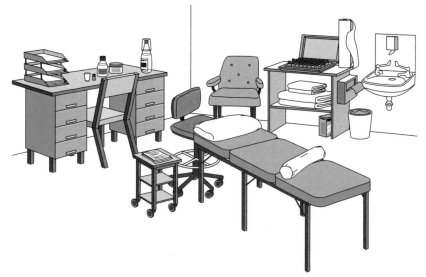

**Fig. 4.1** *A treatment room furnished with couch and accessories*

Some practitioners or salons use washable sheets to cover the couch. Couch roll paper can be used to protect sheets from oil. Either the paper or sheet itself should be changed between every patient.

**Additional equipment**

A small table or cupboard to house your essential oils, carriers, skin-cleansing items, sheets and towels is necessary. Some practitioners like to use a trolly one with wheels, which can be easily placed close to hand.

A cupboard, cabinet or portable file for your papers and patient records is needed. Any file or filing cabinet should be kept secure to protect confidentiality.

Choose comfortable chairs for the consultation. A separate chair with wheels for the practitioner's use is a good idea.

A stable footstool is advisable for assisting patients on and off the treatment couch.

A bottle of spring water and glasses should be available, so patients may have a drink after treatment if they wish. Practitioners should also drink several glasses of water during the day to cleanse the system and help maintain energy.

---

**GOOD PRACTICE**

To prevent sheets from oil stains, soak them in borax solution and/or wash them as soon as possible in warm water, gentle detergent.

---

## Hygiene

**REMEMBER**

The lives of many people are rushed and stressful. Try to provide an oasis of tranquillity for your patients, which relieves stress and nourishes inner well-being.

Ensure there are facilities for washing your hands. Professional clinics should have a wash basin available with antiseptic soap and paper towels. If this is not possible in other settings, have a stock of antiseptic wet-wipes or surgical spirit. The practitioner's hands should be cleaned before and after each treatment.

Toilet and washing facilities should be available for patients' use – ideally with a mirror. These need to be wheelchair accessible. It is a good idea for patients to void the bladder before treatment. Aromatherapy massage is gently stimulating to all the systems.

## After care

It should be possible to offer patients a drink of water or a cup of tea after treatment and, if possible, a place to sit for a moment before leaving. Water helps the cleansing process begun with the treatment and should be advised for all patients. This also helps reinforce the advice to take time to care for themselves. If treatments are given in an area other than a salon or clinic, a bottle of water and paper cups can be brought along.

**Progress Check**

1   What is the intention behind creating a therapeutic space?
2   What is as important, or even more important, than the physical setting?
3   What are some disadvantages and advantages of having background music playing during treatments?
4   What hygiene considerations must you implement for your patients and yourself?
5   What arrangements must you make for securing patient records?

## Safety and first aid

When working from your home, in a clinic, or travelling to a patient's residence, a first aid box should be available, equipped and kept up to date. To comply with the Health and Safety (First Aid) Regulations 1981 and the revised Approved Code of Practice 2 July 1990, aromatherapists will require the following as a minimum in their first aid box:

- guidance card explaining how to use the contents
- 20 individually wrapped sterile adhesive dressings
- 2 sterile eye pads, no. 16
- 6 individually wrapped triangular bandages, preferably sterile
- a pair of disposable gloves
- 6 safety pins
- 6 medium, sterile, unmedicated wound dressings, no. 8 or 13
- 2 large, sterile, unmedicated wound dressings, no. 9, 14 or amb. no. 1
- 3 extra large, unmedicated wound dressings, amb. no. 3.

In addition, soap, water and disposable drying materials should be available for first aid purposes. Where soap and water cannot be available, individually wrapped, moist cleansing wipes, which are not impregnated with alcohol, may be used. The use of antiseptics is not necessary for treating wounds. It is also a good idea to keep a stock of sugar lumps or sweet biscuits on hand in case a patient has an emergency hypoglycaemic episode.

Sterile water or normal sterile saline solution should be available in sealed, disposable containers for eye irrigation in cases where mains tap water is not available. A total of 900 ml should be provided and each container should hold at least 300 ml and should never be reused once the seal is broken. Do not use eye cups, baths or refillable containers for eye irrigation.

### The travelling first aid kit

This should contain the following:

- guidance card explaining how to use the contents
- 6 individually wrapped, sterile adhesive dressings
- 2 triangular bandages
- 2 safety pins
- 1 large, sterile, unmedicated wound dressing, no. 9, 14 or amb. no.1
- individually wrapped, moist cleansing wipes
- a pair of disposable gloves.

---

**ACTIVITY**

Research and make notes on the appropriate first aid response to the following events, which may occur in your clinic:

nose bleed          faint          asthma attack

---

### Risk assessments

First aid trainers recommend that a **risk assessment** should be carried out on the premises to minimise the risk of accidents. The idea is to think ahead about what could go wrong, implement corrective measures and also to think how you can make emergencies easier to deal with. Some questions you might consider include:

- Are all electrical outlets safe?
- Is access into and out of the premises safe?
- Is it easy to get an ambulance to the site?
- Are the premises well sign-posted?
- What is the grid reference on local maps?
- Is the telephone always in working order?

### Emergency action

In the event of an emergency, the following procedure is recommended if you are on your own.

### 1 Assess the scene

Obtain help if needed by telephoning 999. With help coming or if it is delayed proceed as follows and use the **ABC** procedure. ABC stands for Airway, Breathing, and Circulation.

Make the area safe for the victim and anyone in the immediate vicinity (clear anything hazardous).

Check for injuries, remove all potential sources of injury.

Reassess at intervals.

### 2 Assess the casualty

Check if the patient is conscious by shaking him or her or shouting to raise a response. Then:

---

**REMEMBER**

ABC stands for Airway, Breathing, Circulation.

---

A:  check the **ai**rway. Remove any obvious obstructions. Open with chin lift and head tilt.
B:  check **b**reathing by looking, listening and feeling for 5 seconds.
C:  check **c**irculation by feeling the pulse in the neck for 5 seconds.

### 3 Act on the assessment

If victim is breathing, has a pulse but is unconscious, place in the **recovery position**, and continue to monitor until help arrives. The recovery position helps airways to remain open, prevents the tongue blocking the throat, yet allows vomit or liquid to drain from the mouth.

If victim is not breathing but has a pulse, then open and clear the airway and give resuscitation as trained.

If victim is not breathing and there is no pulse, open and clear the airway and start chest compression or cardio-pulmonary resuscitation as trained.

---

**GOOD PRACTICE**

Keep your first aid skills intact by taking refresher training every year.

---

## Special circumstances

In the case of a patient having an epileptic seizure:

- Do nothing, except remove any danger to the person from items in the area.
- When the patient has come out of the seizure, ask if this is his or her first fit and, if yes, call an ambulance by dialling 999. If not, ask how you may further assist the patient.

In the case of an asthma attack:

- Ask if this is more than a normal attack and, if yes, call an ambulance by dialling 999.
- If no, ask if the patient wants to go to hospital and assist.

In the case of an episode of hypoglycaemia:

- You may notice or the patient may complain of one or more of the following: weakness or faintness, hunger, palpitations, confusion or loss of consciousness, sweating, pallor, cold, clammy skin, a bounding pulse, shallow breathing, violent or strange behaviour.
- Help the patient to lie or sit down and give them a sugary drink (fruit juice) or food (sugar lump or sweet biscuit). As the condition improves you can give more sweet food or drink. Allow the patient to rest until fully recovered and advise a visit to the doctor.

**REMEMBER**
Keep calm and follow procedures as trained.

---

**ACTIVITY**

With a group of fellow students discuss how you might react to emergency situations. Express your concerns and listen and learn from each other's experiences.

Find out about local first aid training courses: how often they are run and by whom; what is involved?

---

1 Why is it a good idea to carry out a risk assessment before you set up your practice? How often would you review this assessment?
2 What safety precautions do you need to consider for the place of your practice?
3 What should be the contents of a first aid box?
4 What does ABC stand for in first aid?
5 What are the objectives of the recovery position?

## Essential oil safety in the beauty salon

- Because essential oils are flammable, extra caution must be exercised when using them in a sauna or near heating equipment. Do not store essential oils near heat or direct sunlight.
- Keep prepared, sterile eye washes or an eye bath and distilled water available to wash out the patient's eyes should they be accidentally splashed with an aromatherapy product or essential oil.
- For persons who are sensitive or allergic to highly perfumed products and essential oils or have highly sensitive skin, essential oils are contra-indicated for use after hair removal.
- If a patient is planning to undergo facial peeling or laser treatment, which prohibit use of preoperative products, essential oils should not be used.
- Persons preparing aromatherapy blends, even if individual and for immediate use, should be insured for product liability.

### Key Terms

You need to know what these words mean. Go back through the chapter or check in the glossary to find out.

- ABC
- Recovery position
- Risk assessment

# ORIGINS: BOTANY AND THE PRODUCTION OF ESSENTIAL OILS

**5**

'I know a bank whereon the wild thyme grows.'

*A Midsummer Night's Dream*, Shakespeare

---

After working through this chapter you will be able to:

- identify the different parts of a plant
- understand the basic anatomy and physiology of plant life
- appreciate the way plants are classified
- understand the production of essential oils by plants
- relate this knowledge to the understanding of the properties of essential oils.

---

## Plant–human relationships

Aromatherapy is more than wonderful scents that come from liquids in dark-coloured bottles. Its healing power is based on the deep relationship between humans and plants and the intelligence that nature has placed within each. Knowledge of how a plant is formed, how it functions, why and how it creates volatile oils brings us closer to the essence of the plant, and to its embodiment of the *vis medicatrix naturae*, the healing power of nature. It is a way of communing with and paying respect to a life form with which we have a most intimate relationship. Knowing about the source of our *materia medica*, the material of our medicine, is an important grounding for aromatherapy practice.

Plant life is necessary for our survival and a complement to human life. Plants make our lives possible as they are our primary source for food, shelter, clothing, fuel and medicine. Through the process of **photosynthesis** they make available sugar and many other nutrients. They make oxygen available and help remove excess carbon dioxide from the atmosphere, helping to reduce global warming. If this were not enough, they give even more: the beauty of their form, colour and fragrance delight and inspire our deepest thoughts and feelings, our highest spiritual aspirations. Plants themselves need good conditions in order to thrive: essential minerals, carbon dioxide, water, sunlight and protection from extreme weather and predators.

Animal and plant cells are actually quite similar. Plant cells are distinguished from animal cells by the following extra features:

- Plant cells have a relatively rigid cell wall outside the cell surface membrane. This keeps the cell membrane from bursting when water enters by **osmosis**. Animal cells have a membrane but not the rigid cell wall.
- Mature plant cells often possess a large central vacuole, containing a solution of salts, minerals, oxygen, carbon dioxide, pigments, enzymes and other compounds and waste products.
- Plant cells conducting photosynthesis contain **chloroplasts**. Chloroplasts are organelles containing chlorophyll.

---

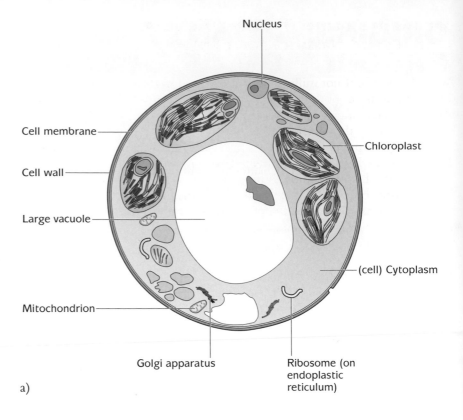

Nucleus

Cell membrane

Chloroplast

Cell wall

Large vacuole

(cell) Cytoplasm

Mitochondrion

Golgi apparatus

Ribosome (on endoplastic reticulum)

a)

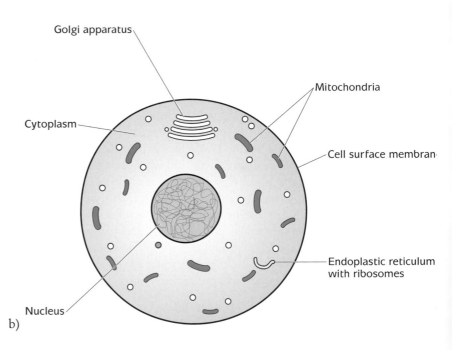

Golgi apparatus

Mitochondria

Cytoplasm

Cell surface membrane

Nucleus

Endoplastic reticulum with ribosomes

b)

**Fig. 5.1** *a) A plant cell. A plant cell may contain stored starch grains or volatile oil droplets. b) An animal cell*

# What's in a name? The identification, naming and classification of plants

With thousands, if not millions of plant species in the world, it is important to have some systematic way of identifying and ordering them. Attempts at naming and classifying plants date back to the study of nature begun by the ancient Greeks. Aristotle (384–322 BC) and particularly his pupil Theophrastus (370–285 BC), author of *Enquiry into Plants,* were perhaps the first to record systematic observations of plants and to group them according to their similarities of form and habitats. Theophrastus observed, for example, that plants differ according to whether they are annual, biennial or perennial. **Taxonomy** is the name given to this science of classification, which enables us to identify and name plants, and see how they are related.

In the 18th century, taxonomy was taken many stages further by the work of Carolus Linnaeus (1707–78). He perceived that plants could be grouped according to similarities in the formation of their reproductive organs, the flowers, and specifically according to the number of their stamens and styles. Although this was an 'artificial' system, in that it did not allow for the grouping of related species, it did allow anyone to identify and classify a previously unknown plant by observing the structure of the flower. Linnaeus classified and described as many species as he could, both local European ones and ones that plant finders sent him from abroad.

He also, importantly, began the method of naming plants, the Latin binomial system, which was later adopted by all scientists: each plant has a two-word Latin name or 'binomial'. The first Latin word is a noun and names the plant's **genus** (see below); it is written with a capital letter. The second is a descriptive word or epithet. It describes something distinctive about the plant, for example, its colour or form; or it gives in Latin form the name of a person associated with it in some way; or it may capture something about its history. *Artemesia alba* indicates the white flowering species of the genus *Artemesia. Rosmarina officinalis* indicates the species used by medical monks in their *officium* or surgery. The two Latin words are generally italicised or underlined when printed.

Increased knowledge of plant forms, varieties and behaviours has meant some plants are given a third name or trinomial. In aromatic plants the third name often denotes the **chemotype**. A chemotype is a subclass of the species that varies in its chemical composition, featuring a particular chemical component; it remains identical in all other ways with the species. The appellation *Thymus vulgaris* ct. thymol is an example, using 'ct.' to abbreviate 'chemotype', and 'thymol' to identify the prominent molecule.

In the 19th century Charles Darwin put forward the idea that all life evolves by successive steps from earlier, more primitive forms. This has prompted botanists to study, identify and classify plants according to how they are related genetically because relatives will share similar characteristics of form or reproductive process. This is known as 'natural' classification.

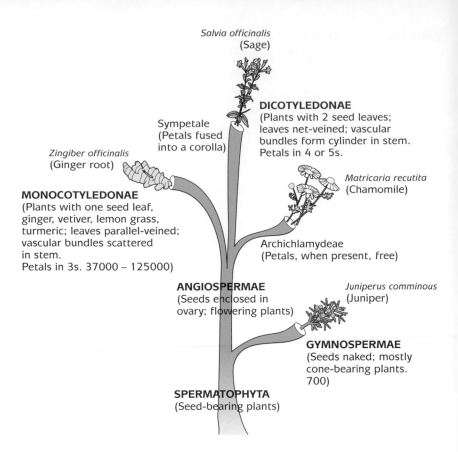

Salvia officinalis
(Sage)

**DICOTYLEDONAE**
(Plants with 2 seed leaves;
leaves net-veined; vascular
bundles form cylinder in stem.
Petals in 4 or 5s.

Sympetale
(Petals fused
into a corolla)

Zingiber officinalis
(Ginger root)

Matricaria recutita
(Chamomile)

**MONOCOTYLEDONAE**
(Plants with one seed leaf,
ginger, vetiver, lemon grass,
turmeric; leaves parallel-veined;
vascular bundles scattered
in stem.
Petals in 3s. 37000 – 125000)

Archichlamydeae
(Petals, when present, free)

**ANGIOSPERMAE**
(Seeds enclosed in
ovary; flowering plants)

Juniperus comminous
(Juniper)

**GYMNOSPERMAE**
(Seeds naked; mostly
cone-bearing plants.
700)

**SPERMATOPHYTA**
(Seed-bearing plants)

**Fig. 5.2** *Flow chart of plant classification*

Plant classification organises plants from the most simple organisms, lower organisms like algae, to the flowering plants, the most complex. Plants are grouped together according to their similarities; the guide is that members of a group have more structural similarities than differences.

The first and widest category of classification is the division or *phylum*, followed by the class, then the order (see Figure 5.2 above). In aromatherapy we only use plants of the spermatophyte division, the ones that produce seeds.

Of importance to the aromatherapist is the distinction between angiosperm (plants whose seeds are covered and which produce flower) and gymnosperm (plants with naked seeds and whose reproductive body is a cone of overlapping scales). Conifers are the only group belonging to the gymnosperm which produce essential oils.

Apart from the conifers, essential oils are only found in the higher, flowering plants or angiosperm. Among the angiosperm, plants are further identified according to whether the seedling or cotyledon (pronounced 'cot-i-lee-don') produces one or two seed leaves: a **monocotyledon** produces one seed leaf ; a **dicotyledon** produces two seed leaves. Monocotelydons develop narrow leaves with parallel veins. In their stems are vascular tissues of tubular cells (xylem cells carry water from roots to upper parts, phloem cells carry nutrients from where they are made to where they are needed, such as in leaves). In addition, their flowers are multiples of three. Examples include ginger, onions, palms and grasses, lilies and orchids. Dicotelydons will develop broad leaves with web-like vein structure and vascular bundles form cylinders in the stem. Flowers are in fours or fives, and the primary root is woody and sometimes swells as a food store. Among numerous examples are chamomile, roses and mints.

Within an order there are different families. A **family** is a group of plants having a strong particular resemblance; for example, Umbelliferae, the carrot family, is distinguished by the umbrella-like form of their inflorescence.

## Plant species i.d.

Within a family there are different genera, or groups. A single group is known as a genus. The different members of a genus are known as **species**, abbreviated as 'sp.' (singular) 'spp.' (plural). Each species within a genus shares a similarity in the variation of a particular genus feature. For example, a variation in the colour and/or shape of a structure such as flower, leaves, roots or in their reproduction, pollination or fruiting. Plants within the same family and/or genus, as well as being similar in form, will often – though not always – have similar chemical constituents and healing properties.

Within the Lamiaceae/Labiatae family are such genera as thymes (*Thymus*), sages (*Salvia*), basils (*Ocimum*) and so on. These share the family characteristic of four-sided stems, with leaves arranged oppositely, and a basic flower form of five united sepals, five united petals forming a tube, four stamen and two carpels (see Fig. 5.6 on page 97). A genus can have many member species or only a few or just one. The *Salvia* genus has many members: *S. scleria, S. officinalis, S. lavandulaefolia* and many others (not all are fragrant). *Gingko biloba* is the only species known in the genus *Gingko*.

> **ACTIVITY**
>
> Obtain a sample or photograph, or visit a garden in which basil, thyme and sage are growing and are in flower. Examine their stems, leaves and flowers and notice features they have in common and features that are different. Use a magnifying glass.

### Subspecies and chemotypes

Within the species grouping there may be subgroups and these will be given a third word in their name. Sometimes the abbreviation 'ssp.' is included. A chemotype is a type of subspecies and indicates that although a plant belongs to a particular genus and species, and has the same morphology (form) as the others in the species, its chemical composition will be different, often with a higher proportion of a component (same form, different composition). This chemical variation happens naturally among wild species, especially of the Lamiaceae/Labiatae family in the Mediterranean, and is thought to be created by different altitude, light or other environmental factors. *Thymus vulgaris* has over a hundred chemotypes, though only about seven are used in aromatherapy. *Rosmarinus officinalis* ct. camphor features more camphor ketones, whereas *R. officinalis* ct. verbenone has a higher proportion of the ketone verbenone, and *R. officinalis* ct.1,8-cineole (once called eucalyptol) features that oxide.

> **REMEMBER**
>
> Taxonomists, scientists who specialise in plant classification, are continually revising and refining their work in the light of new knowledge and they do change names and classifications accordingly. Hence don't expect names to remain the same. The Labatiae family is now called the Lamiaceae family; the Compositate family is now called the Asteraceae family. Quite often a name is changed if the plant is reclassified into a new group. This is also a reason you see a different name for the same plant (or family) in different books. One book may be older or the author may not have put in the most up-to-date name, scientifically speaking.

A variety name indicates there is a major subdivision within the species whose members display a variation of certain features, such as form or colour, in common. Varieties can happen naturally but often are of horticultural origin or importance. The abbreviation 'var.' appears and then the name of the variant: *Rosemarinus officinalis* var. *angustifolia*.

Cultivar is a term used to show a new variety that has been developed by a particular grower. Often they bear his or her name, and the name is sometimes placed within quotation marks, e.g. *Lavandula angustifolia* 'Maillete'.

A hybrid can happen either naturally in the wild or be developed by growers. It is a cross between two species and bears some characteristics of each. The Latin name includes an 'x'. *Lavandula* x *intermedia* is a cross between *L. angustifolia* and *L. latifolia* (synonym *L. spica*). Cultivars can be developed from hybrids. So the name *L.* x *intermedia* 'Super' indicates a cultivar of a hybrid from a cross between two lavenders.

Plant classification is much like making a genealogy chart of your own ancestry, showing your relationship with family members past and present: first in your immediate family, then with your extended family of aunts, uncles and cousins; further back your grandparents and their families and so on. It shows how each species is related to the wider groupings of plants, which are believed to be the plant's ancestors.

> ### REMEMBER
> An aromatherapist can identify a plant according to its family, genus, species and variety and chemotype, if one exists.

Knowing the correct name and identification for the essential oils we use is very important for the aromatherapist. The therapeutic properties desired will be based on the chemistry of the essence from a particular species, so we must know we are using an extraction from the correct species whose oil has those properties. In conducting or making use of research it is also important that the essential oil used is from a traceable botanical source and the Latin name is clearly specified for the results to be meaningful and useful.

> ### GOOD PRACTICE
> Plants have two names, both derived from Latin or Latinised Greek. If a third word is part of the name, use the appropriate abbreviation, such as 'ct.', 'spp.', 'x', 'var.', before the word. Try to learn the Latin names of essential oils for correct identification and use them whenever you write the name.

> ### REMEMBER
> Each plant species belongs to a larger group, genus and then family, that shares many essential features of form and function.

## Chart of aromatic plant families

The natural habitats in which a plant family likes to grow can give pointers to its character because its member plants have had to adapt themselves to such habitats, and this influences its form and internal chemistry. Of the approximately 280 families, those with aromatic members include:

| Family | Characteristics |
|--------|-----------------|
| Betulaceae, the birch family | Trees and shrubs, which are wind-pollinated; with male and female flowers separate in the same plant. The male is a catkin and the flowers have six stamens. The female flowers, grouped at the shoot tip, have a single carpel attached to a tri-lobed bract. The fruit is a small ridged nut. Examples: birch |
| Burceraceae | Grow in desert or tropical habitats of intense sunlight; form gum resins. Plants adapted to the arid conditions tend to produce gum-resins with strong antiseptic, antiputrescent, and decay- or age-inhibiting properties. Essential oils of the family are used for ulcers, gangrene, gastric and intestinal fermentation, skin preservation, rejuvenation. Mentally they purify the mind and induce clarity and inner calm. Examples: desert: frankincense, myrrh; tropics: elemi, *Canarium luzonicum* |
| Annonaceae | Some species are found in tropical America, most in Asia and Australia. Most are small trees, e.g. Ylang Ylang. Examples: *Cananga odorata,* ylang ylang; syn.*Unona odorantissumum* |
| Asteraceae/Compositae | Distinguished by a flowering head containing many small florets, either rays (e.g. dandelion), discs (groundsel) or both (the outer ring contains rays, the inner ring has discs, e.g. *Chamomile* spp.). Displays great diversity of form, widest range of habitat (seashore, mountain, desert, swamp). Have the largest number of members, 800 genera and 13,000 species, which often occur together in large 'settlements' preferring open spaces exposed to light (meadows and steppes). Examples: Chamomile species, *Helechrysum italicum* |
| Cupressaceae | Gymnosperm trees and shrubs, of great longevity with typically no vessels in the secondary xylem, but with resin canals. Habitat is frigid and temperate zones of both hemispheres, or tropical zones at high altitudes. Structure is vertical, linear. Oils and resins abundant in trunks, branches, cones, needles; sometimes exuding naturally. Intensely warming oils and resins to balance a cold habitat suggest an affinity for the 'cold' nervous system. Examples: *Cedrus atlantica, Cupressus sempervirens, Juniper communis, Thuja occidentalis* |
| Geraniaceae | Herbs or low shrubs often in spreading flower heads or single flowers. The genus perlangonium has 250 species, e.g. rose geranium. Examples: *Pelargonium graveolens* and *roseum* |
| Gramineae/Poaceae, the grass family | Widest of habitats, from polar to equatorial, swamp to desert. Highly adaptable and diverse with powerful root systems. Leaf structure is linear. Examples: *Cymbopogon nardus, C. citratus, C. martini, Litsea cubeba, Vetiver zizamoides* |
| Lamiaceae/Labiateae | Herbs or small shrubs with notably square stems, leaves in opposite pairs; often hairy with glands producing volatile oil. Flowers irregular and lipped. Many species are healing. Prefer and love heat; high, open, often rocky spaces where they absorb ultraviolet light, e.g. rock slopes of the Mediterranean. Examples: *Ocimum basilicum, Scleria salvia, Hyssopus off., Lavandula off., Lavandula spica, Lavandin, Origanum marjorana, M. hortnsi, Melissa off., Mentha spp. Oreganum vulgare, O. compactum, Patchouli, Rosmarinus off., Salvia spp., Thymus spp.* |
| Lauraceae | Tropical/subtropical trees, shrubs; evergreen. Example: *Cinnamomun zeylanicum* |
| Myrtaceae | Tropical zones of every continent. Evergreen leaves, strong and simple. The family produces sweet spices and sweet fruits, e.g. pomegranate, guava, cloves. Examples: *Eugenia aromatica, Eucalyptus spp., Melaleuca leucadendron, M. alternifolia, M. viridiflora, Eugenia caryophyllata, Myrtus communis* |
| Myristicaceae | Species are found in tropical Asia. Flowers are dioecious (male and female on separate plants) with an inconspicuous 3-lobed perianth; fruit a fleshy drupe, splitting on both sides to release a single seed. Examples: *Myristica fragrans*, nutmeg |

| | |
|---|---|
| Pinaceae | Tall conical trees with resinous wood, branches in whorls – a blend of the linear and circular. Abundant in the northern hemisphere, though also found in the southern hemisphere. Needle-like leaves in clusters or solitary. The flower is a cone, male and female, with scales in a spiral arrangement; males have anthers on the lower side; females with two ovules on upper side swell after fertilisation, changing from green to woody brown before the scales separate to release winged seeds. Examples: *Pinus sylvestris*, pine, *Picea mariana* |
| Piperaceae | Comprised of four genera found in the tropical ranges. Most are climbers with swollen nodes and fleshy spikes of flowers. Leaves contain oil cells. Fruits are often aromatic. Examples: *Piper nigrum*, black pepper |
| Rosaceae | Members large in number and variety: herbs, shrubs and trees – many of food or ornamental value. Flowers are typically open and scented, Examples: *Rosa, damascena, R.* x *centifolia* |
| Rutaceae | Thrive in tropical heat. Mostly small, thorny trees with hard wood, often resinous, firm green leaves. Flowers in symmetrical stars; fruits juicy or small hot, spicy berries. Examples: *Citrus bergamia, C. paradisi, C. limetta, C. vulgaris, C. auruantium, C. recutita* |
| Santalaceae | A small family of herbs, trees or shrubs with individual leaves. Flowers are very small, often greenish, formed as a calyx of 4–5 often fleshy parts fused to the ovary; fruit is 1-seeded. Examples: *Santalum album*, sandalwood |
| Umbelliferaceae (Apiaceae) | Typical umbel inflorescence; stems stout with hollow internodes; leaves much or extremely divided; strong root or vigorous rhizome, which stays underground for one or more years; vegetation grows rapidly; seeds hollow. Many members used for food or aromatic seasoning (seeds, roots, leaves), e.g. caraway, fennel, carrot. Mucilages and gums are characteristic. Aromas less refined than floral scents. *Pimpinella anisum, Carum carvi, Daucus carota, Coriandum sativum, Cuminum cyminum* |
| Verbenaceae | A family of herbs, shrubs, trees or woody climbers; leaves are usually opposite, without stipules. Fruit is often a berry or drupe with one or more stones. Examples: *Lippia citriodora*, Lemon verbena |
| Zingiberaceae | A family of perennial aromatic herbs with fleshy rhizomes and tuberous roots, e.g. tumeric, ginger, cardomom. Examples: *Zingiber officinalis, Elettaria cardamomum* |

**GOOD PRACTICE**

Make a label for each of your essential oils that gives the family to which it belongs. From time to time arrange your bottles of essential oils according to their families and review the common features they share.

**ACTIVITY**

1  Create a 'genealogy' chart for five essential oil plants. Include notes on the important features at each level of classification, e.g. 'flowers tubules', 'flowers with lips' and 'leaves adapted for hot climate'.
2  Find out which aromatic plant(s) belong to the family Orchidaceae.
3  Make notes on the similar characteristics of four species within the Lamiaceae/Labiatae family. What features do they all share?
4  Using a herbal or plant name dictionary, explain the meaning of ('translate') the following names: *Eugenia aromatica, Boswellia carterii, Melaleuca viridiflora.*
5  Research the characteristics of the Zingiberaceae, Verbenaceae, Santalceae and other families, and make notes on the similarities shared by their genera and species.

# Plant anatomy: knowing plants by their form and structure

## The parts of a plant
### Underground parts
*Root*

This underground part anchors the plant in the earth; absorbs water and minerals from the soil, stores nutrients and initiates their transport to the upper plant. Tissues include an outer, protective bark, and inside xylem for transporting water to leaves, and phloem for transporting glucose to other parts of the plants. Root systems vary among plants. Some have a main taproot going down deeply, some have creeping, spreading roots. Roots have many side hairs for absorbing water and nutrients. The root is the plant's nutritive centre. Aromatic compounds of roots are typically base notes.

Aromatic example: parsley root.

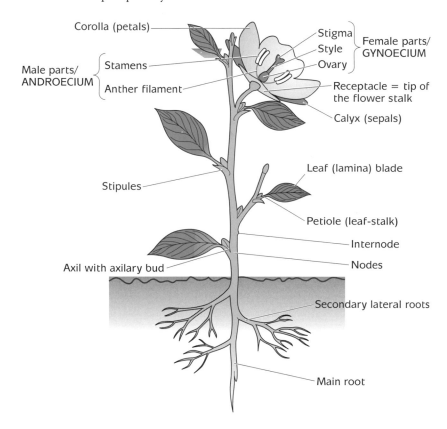

**Fig. 5.3** *The parts of a flowering plant*

*Rhizome*

The rhizome is not a root but a modified stem (see below) growing just beneath the soil surface. It has a series of nodes where leaves form (often with roots coming out). Buds are produced at the leaf axils.

Aromatic example: ginger, turmeric.

*Tuber*

This is a stem modified for food storage with minute scale-like leaves and buds or 'eyes' from which new shoots grow.

The potato is a tuber.

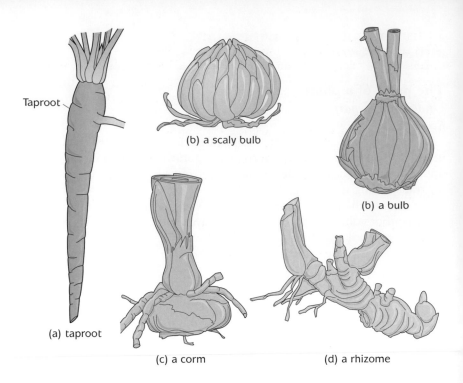

Taproot

(b) a scaly bulb

(b) a bulb

(a) taproot

(c) a corm

(d) a rhizome

**Fig. 5.4** *The underground parts of a plant: (a) taproot; (b) two types of bulb; (c) corn; (d) rhizome. Bulbs, tubers, corms and rhizomes are underground stems modified for food storage*

*Corm*
This is a stem swollen to a very thick, short, firm, fleshy part, usually more broad than high. It produces roots from the base, and leaves and flowering stems from the top.

Aromatic example: *Iris florentina*, orris root; used in pot pourri.

*Bulb*
This is a flattened stem, and the leaves growing from it are swollen and sheathing.

Aromatic example: lily family (onion, hyacinths, bluebells).

### Above ground parts
*Stem*
This is the axis of a plant, its trunk or stalk; it provides structure to support the leaf, flower and fruit and contains the inner vessels for transportation of water, minerals and glucose. It links the roots with the leaves; its xylem and phloem are continuous with those of root and leaf. It has food storage tissues also. In some plants stems are above ground runners (strawberry) from which roots emerge, or support a climbing plant by twining. In some plants, the stem serves as a food store and lies underground.

Aromatic examples: some Lamiacae/Labiatae plants have aromatic stems as well as leaves and flowers: mints. In cinnamon, the outer bark is fragrant. In sandalwood the inner bark is fragrant.

*Leaf*
This is the organ of respiration, transpiration and photosynthesis. It relates to the human lung in that it is also used for gaseous exchange. Leaves can also absorb water to a certain extent. The structure, the many shapes, sizes, textures of leaves are determined by their particular adaptations: for photosynthesis, but also for water metabolism, food storage or defence. For example, the needles of conifers aid survival in cold and dry conditions. They have a deep groove along their length to minimise water loss. Needles remain in winter so photosynthesis can continue even in winter months of little light.

Aromatic examples: leaves of rosemary and lavender are also narrow to minimise water loss in a hot, dry climate.

Leaves may be classified by the overall shape of the lamina or blade and by the shape of the lamina's tip (apex), its margin or its base. Descriptions include by shape: linear, oval, elliptical, rounded; by margins: serrated or entire; by base: cunate or truncate; by apex: acute, acuminate or mucronate.

Aromatic examples: these are numerous and include oregano, sage, eucalyptus, pine.

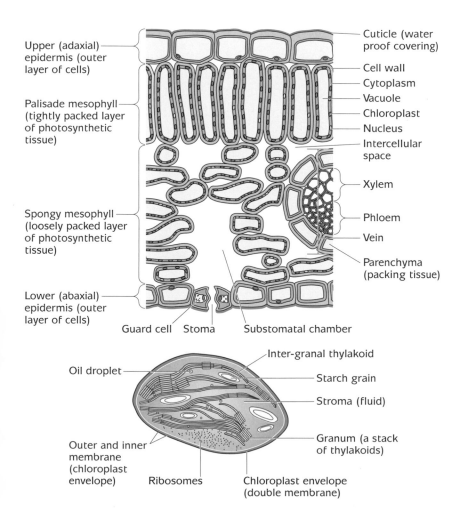

**Fig. 5.5a** *The parts of a leaf and a chloroplast*

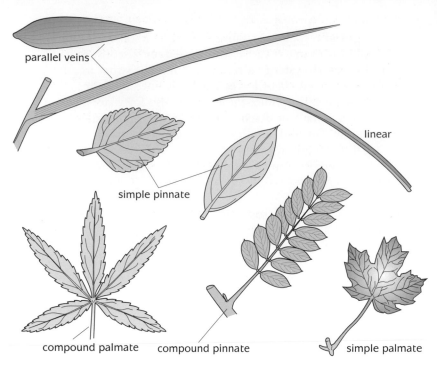

**Fig. 5.5b** *Some leaf types and shapes. Simple – the leaf blade (lamina) is a single unit. Compound pinnate – the pinnae (leaflets) occur on both sides of a main axis (rachis)*

Phyllotaxy is the study and classification of the arrangement of leaves on the plant stem. The overall arrangement is often a spiral so as to minimise any shading and maximise exposure of each leaf to sunlight. Arrangements include spiral, alternate, opposite (two leaves arise from the same node), whorled (three or more leaves arise from the same node).

*Flower*
This is the reproductive organ containing male and/or female parts. The form, colour and texture of the petals in some way assist fertilisation, e.g. by attracting pollinating insects. Aromas produced in some flowers are thought to attract pollinators or ward off pests, which would threaten species survival. They may also be meant to attract or deter human interaction!

## The parts of a flower
The main parts of a flower (see Figure 5.6) include:

- Sepals (calyx): a calyx is a ring of usually green inconspicuous sepals just below the petals (sometimes coloured and enlarged). Sepals are like modified leaves which form a protective envelope for the developing flower and become less conspicuous when it blooms.
- Petals (corolla): the conspicuous organs above the sepals and surrounding the reproductive parts. 'Corolla' refers to the petals as a whole, which may be separate or joined together, sometimes to form a tube. Petals surround the reproductive organs and usually act to attract pollinators by their colour, scent or nectar. The petals

may have nectaries, or may be wholly modified from netaries. Wind-pollinated flowers have less conspicuous petals and rely on producing large amounts of pollen grains, which are easily dispersed by the wind.

- ◦ Stamen: the male organ usually surrounding the carpels lying outside the centre of the female part or pistil, in a rim; stamens are comprised of a filament tipped by anthers containing pollen and are usually coloured.
- ◦ Carpel: female reproductive part made of an ovary, with an upper end or stigma to catch and germinate pollen grains prior to fertilisation and, sometimes, a narrow 'neck' or style separating the stigma from the ovary.
- ◦ Bract: a modified leaf associated with the inflourescence. In some plants the bracts are colourful and can be mistaken for flowers. Their placement is so close to the flower that they seem part of it, especially when the floral, reproductive organs are less showy than the bract. Examples include begonia, poinsettia and bougainvillaea.
- ◦ Perianth: this is the term for a corolla and calyx (sepals and petals) that cannot be distinguished from each other, typically in Monocytyledons.

Some flowers are arranged singly on a stalk or pedicle. Others occur in a group on the stalk, which is then called an inflorescence. Examples of inflorescence include spike and umbel shapes. Regular flowers have several planes of symmetry. Irregular flowers have only one plane of symmetry. If you turn a regular flower around and view it from different angles, it will appear the same; any halves will be mirror images of each other. An irregular flower can only be split once through the middle to get two halves.

Aromatic examples of flowers: Single flowers: geranium. Inflorescence: elderflower. Regular: rose, Verbenaceae species. Irregular: Violaceae species, violets.

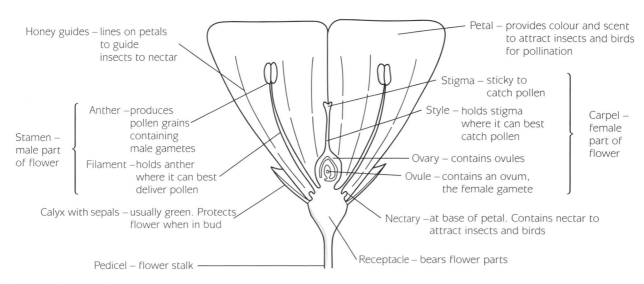

**Fig. 5.6** *The parts of a flower*

## Fruit

This is the seed-bearing organ, the product of the fertilised, ripened ovary. Fruit form is adapted to help the distribution of the seeds. A nut is actually a dry, indehiscent fruit, a single seed within a woody wall.

Aromatic examples: *Citrus* spp.

Types of fruit are:

- ⬥ Fleshy – attractive to animals, which eat the fruit and disperse the seed away from the parent plant
  - • Drupe: seed inside a stony layer surrounded by fleshy fruit – peach
  - • Berry: one or more seeds from one ovary – blackberry
- ⬥ Dehiscent dry – the seed sac splits open for release of seeds for wind dispersal, e.g. a pea pod
- ⬥ Indehiscent – seed sac does not split by itself, e.g. nut, grain. Dry seeds may also be eaten by birds and dispersed, or be dispersed by the wind, or hook on to animal fur for dispersal.

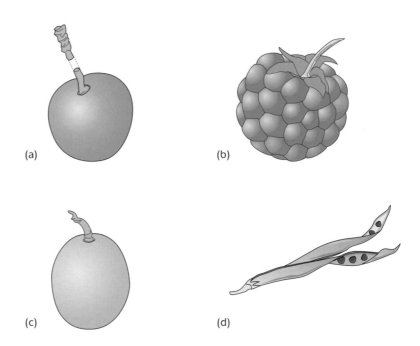

**Fig. 5.7** *Types of fruit: (a) drupe with seed inside a stone within the flesh; (b) berry with many seeds from one ovary; (c) berry with one seed from the ovary; (d) dehiscent fruit*

## Seed

This is the fertilised, mature ovule and the origin of the new plant. Seed parts comprise: an outer protective husk or testa; an inner layer called the endoderm; an inner germ that contains the embryo, a proto root and the cotyledon, the one or two proto leaves that become the seedling on germination.

Aromatic example: fennel, cardamom, coriander, cumin.

1   Find and name three further examples of plants, which produce aromatic compounds in their roots or modified stems, stems or bark, leaves, flowers, fruits, seeds.
2   Draw and label the parts of an aromatic plant species from three genera of different families: root/modified stem, stem, leaves, flower parts, fruit, seed. Draw from life if at all possible.
3   Collect and press and label an example of the following: simple leaf, compound pinnate leaf, compound palmate leaf.

**Progress Check**

1   What are the differences between a monocotyledon and a dicotyledon?
2   Which families are found in the widest ranges of habitats?
3   What is the meaning of the terms angiosperm and gymnosperm?
4   What is the difference between a genus and a species?
5   What is a chemotype? Give two examples.
6   What is the calyx?
7   What parts of a flower are contained in the androecium or male organ? In the gynoecium or female organ?

## Plant metabolism and physiology

As we noted, plants share many requirements with animal and human life. However there are important differences at the most fundamental level, that of the cell. Both animal and plant cells have a cell membrane, which contains the cytoplasm with its different organelles (nucleus, rough and smooth endoplastic reticulum, golgi body, mitochondria). In plants the cell membrane has a rigid wall outside it, which gives the cell a definite shape and, importantly, prevents moisture from bursting the cell when water enters by osmosis and puts pressure on the membrane. Also, plant cells have an additional central vacuole and special cells for photosynthesis containing a chloroplast.

The chorophyll in the choloroplast in the cells of the leaf absorb the sun's energy and use it to join together carbon dioxide and water to form sugar/glucose. Glucose is the energy source for the plant's metabolism. Leaves have pores (stomata) to allow oxygen and carbon dioxide to pass out and in. Veins bring water to the leaves and transport the glucose to the rest of the plant.

The important plant processes are:

●   photosynthesis (see overleaf)
●   metabolism – **anabolism** and **catabolism**
●   growth
●   transportation – of water and dissolved minerals from root through the plant

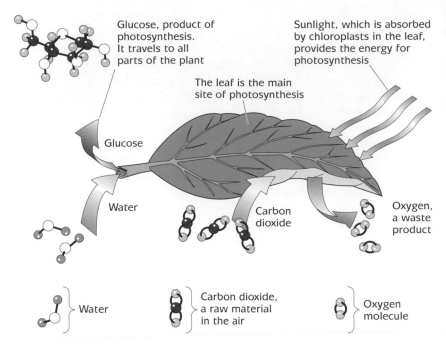

Glucose, product of photosynthesis. It travels to all parts of the plant

Sunlight, which is absorbed by chloroplasts in the leaf, provides the energy for photosynthesis

The leaf is the main site of photosynthesis

Glucose

Water

Carbon dioxide

Oxygen, a waste product

Water

Carbon dioxide, a raw material in the air

Oxygen molecule

**Fig. 5.8** *Sunlight is absorbed by the leaf and provides energy for photosynthesis*

- translocation – movement of the products of photosynthesis to the other parts of the plant
- transpiration – loss of water by evaporation in the epidermis of the leaves
- respiration
- gaseous exchange
- reproduction.

## A glossary of plant processes

- Photosynthesis takes place in the leaves by means of the chlorophyll, which captures sunlight, and the chloroplasts within leaf cells. It is not fully understood yet but is known to comprise two phases:

  1 Light reaction: sunlight is used to split water into oxygen, protons (hydrogen ions/ H+) and electrons (negative charge). Oxygen is released.

  2 Dark reaction: the protons and electrons are then used to convert carbon dioxide into carbohydrates, the fuel the plant needs for its metabolism.

  $$6CO_2 + 6H_2O + light \rightarrow C_6H_{12}O_6 + 6O_2$$

  carbon dioxide + water + light produce ($\rightarrow$) glucose + oxygen

- Metabolism is the constant work of a cell and alternates between anabolism and catabolism. In anabolism the cell builds up complex organic substances and tissues from simpler substances, i.e. carbon dioxide and water using photosynthesis. In catabolism the cell breaks down complex substances into simpler ones, releasing energy.

- Meristematic tissue allows for growth to occur. It contains cells that are actively dividing to produce new tissue. They are found at the tip of roots and stems and in the cambium of perennial plants to increase their girth.

- Transportation is the term used for the movement of water into and through the plant. It is made possible by the principle of osmosis acting between the interior and exterior of cells in the root, stem and leaves. The root, stem and leaves have vascular xylem structures to transport water and minerals from the root to the stem, leaves and flowers. These vessels have a hollow centre or lumen with thick, strong walls, made of dead cells (lignans), which give structure and support. They are grouped in vascular bundles (also containing phloem tubes) within the stem (see Fig 5.5).
- Osmosis occurs when the pressure of the fluid/solute inside the cell is lower than that outside. The water outside will be able to diffuse through the semi-permeable cell membrane. This continues until the pressure inside the cell equals that on the outside. When the pressure outside the cell becomes lower, the water inside the cell will move to the outside. *See* transpiration (below). It is by means of osmosis that water is drawn into the plant from the soil by the root (facilitated by the presence of minerals). Then again it is by osmosis (helped by some root pressure) that water is drawn into the vascular tissues in the centre of the root and up through the stem xylem to the leaf. The cohesion of water molecules is also thought to help draw water up from the roots by osmosis.
- Nutrition: minerals and nitrates in the soil are absorbed by the root hairs and, once in the roots' vascular tissue, are transported to the leaves along with water.
- Translocation is movement of the soluble products of photosynthesis, i.e. glucose, along with proteins, fatty acids and hormones. This occurs in the phloem. Phloem vessels have sieve tubes or cylindrical columns of cells in which the end walls are perforated. The food products from the leaves pass from cell to cell along the sieve tubes. Phloem vessels (as well as xylem) are located in vascular bundles within the stem, root and leaves.
- Transpiration is the release of water from the leaves. It is thought to help cool the leaves (important in hot conditions), and it plays a role in transport by causing a pull on the water coming in and up from the roots. Water molecules in the leaf leave the spongy mesophyll and spread out to the stomata, the pores by which water is released through the leaf surface. This loss triggers water from adjacent cells to spread in, drawing water from the xylem.
- Gaseous exchange in plants takes place through the stomata or pores in leaves. Carbon dioxide is absorbed through the cuticle via stomata and enters the spongy mesophyll cells. In photosynthesis oxygen is produced and is released through the stomata.
- Respiration is the chemical breakdown of carbohydrates with oxygen inside the cells and tissues of animals and plants to provide energy and release carbon dioxide and water.
- The **carbon cycle**: using photosynthesis plants convert the carbon dioxide in the atmosphere to carbohydrates to supply the energy they need. When the plants respire, decay or are burned, the carbon dioxide is released again into the atmosphere. Living plants extract carbon from their environment and animals depend on carbohydrate and other nutrients produced by plants. The concentration of carbon in living matter (18 per cent) is almost 100 times greater than its concentration in the earth (0.19 per cent). This carbon must be recycled for life to continue.

• **Nitrogen cycle**: plants need nitrogen for metabolism and obtain it from soil. They use nitrogen to produce amino acids and protein after soil micro-organisms have first converted the nitrogen into soluble nitrogen compounds (nitrites or nitrates), which the plant can absorb. Animals depend on protein from plants as their source of nitrogen.

**ACTIVITY**

1   Draw a figure illustrating a plant cell containing a chloroplast. Label the cell's wall, membrane, vacuole and structures involved in photosynthesis.
2   Draw a figure illustrating an animal cell. Label the cell's membrane, nucleus and mitochondria.

## Plant production of volatile oils

Why do some plants produce these aromatic compounds? The purpose of volatile oils in the plant's life is not fully understood as yet. They may perform a different function in different species. They can be viewed as a form of information that the plant uses to communicate within itself and beyond itself to its environment. The known or assumed roles of volatile oils include:

• defence against animals or insects
• resistance to bacterial, viral or fungal invasion
• wound healing
• attraction of insects or animals for pollination
• survival in difficult conditions
• unknown.

### Plant – animal /human communication

In some plants the aromatic compounds function as a method of deterring predator insects, or animals. For example, evaporating molecules may irritate the mouth or eyes of a grazing animal, or repel insects. Termites do not attack sandalwood. In other plants the compounds attract pollinating insects, helping to ensure successful reproduction. Bees seem to love the lemon balm and other mints. It is even possible, though largely uninvestigated, that some plants want to attract humans to interact with them as well. After all, our attraction to lavender and roses has inspired us to propagate them widely.

### Intra-plant communication

While not true phyto-hormones volatile oils may help regulate the plant's own hormones, which in turn trigger growth and reproduction. They could be part of a plant's internal signalling system, important initiators of metabolic functions within the plant.

Stress has been shown to increase the production of particular aromatic compounds in some plants, suggesting that volatile compounds are part of the adaptive response of self-preservation. In hot, dry summers, aromatic plants of the Mediterranean, such as sage, thyme, lavender, rosemary and oregano, release essential oils, which form a surrounding haze that helps reduce water loss and coats the leaves with a thin, protective film. The aromatic vapour from sage and thyme leaves also

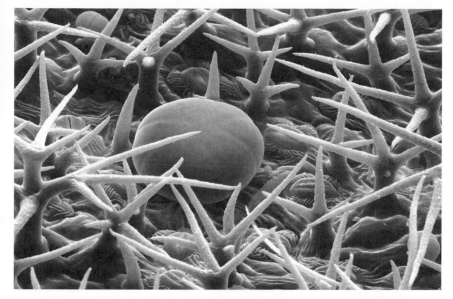

*(a) Lavender: lower leaf surface with secretory gland and non-secretory trichomes (hairs)*

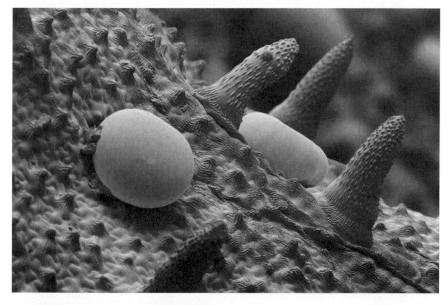

*(b) peppermint: calyx surface with secretory glands and non-secretory trichomes*

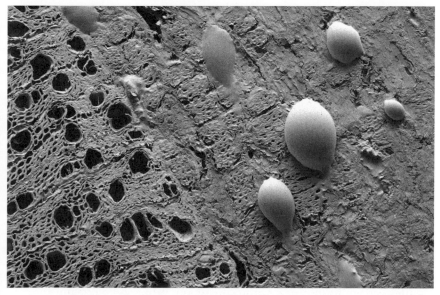

*(c) Frankincense: stem with resin globules oozing from ducts*

**Fig. 5.9a, b and c** *Secretory structures in plants*

retards the growth of nearby seedlings, ensuring that these plants are widely separated and so must compete less for scarce water. Oregano has been observed to increase production of methyl chavicol and linalool while lowering production of sesquiterpenes when conditions are too dry. The gum resin produced by conifers and other trees is secreted when their bark is damaged, suggesting a wound-healing function. Formation of aromatic compounds has been related to photosynthesis since, in some plants, monoterpenes use sugars as a source of carbon (Battaglia, 1995).

### Inter-plant communication

Some recent research has shown that some plants produce essential oils for release as a means of communicating with each other. For example, the American sagebrush, when under attack by predator beetles releases methyl jasmonate, which turns on the genes that make an insecticide-deterring chemical (proteinase inhibitor). As the odour is released it also triggers surrounding plants to do the same. The effect is to trick other beetles, which will detect the chemical, into avoiding the other plants. The first plant preyed upon has communicated danger to its fellow species using aromatic particles in the air.

## Origin and metabolism of essential oils.

So far as is known, aromatic compounds are not essential for primary metabolism, i.e. vital functions, such as photosynthesis. But they act like trace elements: tiny amounts are thought necessary for the successful completion of metabolic functions. Chemically speaking, volatile oils are products of secondary metabolism (non-essential reactions). They are thought to be important to defence.

The compounds originate in secretory cells or structures located on the surface of the plant or within it (Figure 5.9). The type of structure is specific to a family or a species. This fact is used in identification and authentication of plants. Types of structures producing volatile oils include the following:

- Single-cell structures – only the content distinguishes them from neighbouring cells, e.g. ginger, nutmeg.
- Secretory cavities – usually spherical spaces, lined with secretory cells that produce the compounds (citrus and eucalyptus spp.), though they can be elongated, e.g. clove, frankincense.
- Ducts – formed from elongated cavities that join up; often branching to a network, from root to leaf, flower and fruit (Umbelliferae/Apiaceae, Compositae/Asteraceae, Pinaceae), e.g. fennel, chamomile, pine.
- Glandular trichomes or hairs – modified epidermal hairs on leaves, stems and floral calyx, which are covered by a cuticle (Lamiaceae Labiatae), e.g. lavender, peppermint, oregano.
- Epidermal cells – aromatic compounds originate here and then diffuse through the cytoplasm, cell wall and cuticle to evaporate, e.g. *Rosa* spp., jasmine, acacia. (Yield of essential oil is very low in these species.)

In the buds of some species, epidermal cells, beneath their cuticle, secrete essences mixed with other substances, such as flavones, e.g. *Betula* spp., *Prunus* spp.

Conifers create resin canals within the wood, probably to contain the molecules, which may be toxic to other plant tissues.

**REMEMBER**

The production of volatile oils by the plant is a dynamic and varies according to the plant's needs and to environmental conditions. This is why harvesting at the right time is an important judgement.

## Growing conditions affecting the plant's production of essential oils

As living beings plants are constantly responding to environmental conditions in their habitat:

- climate/weather – temperature, sunlight, rainfall, wind factors
- altitude and orientation
- soil type and fertility.

In response to such conditions, aromatic plants can vary the production and composition of their aromatic compounds. Water stress provokes change in chemistry. Too much rain or unseasonable cold or heat can also affect the quantity of compounds produced. Exposure to sunlight at high altitude is an important factor. It is thought that plants growing in the high arid conditions of the Mediterranean are exposed to more ultraviolet light and that this has a beneficial effect on the composition of their oils. The same species of *Lavandula angustifolia* grown at different altitudes shows a different composition of essential oils. Other aromatic plants prefer a more tropical type of heat and sun. It is known that the best rose otto comes from roses grown in Bulgaria, and that the highest quality cinnamon is from Sri Lanka.

Environment also has an effect on reproductive activity and essential oil production. Genera in the Lamiaceae/ Labiatae family are greatly prone to hybridisation (cross-pollination between two species with sterile offspring) and to producing subspecies and chemotypes. These events are probably responses to local environmental factors.

> **REMEMBER**
>
> Variation in growing conditions affects the chemistry, quality and yield of the essential oil produced by the plant. In aromatherapy this is seen as indicating a dynamism that is reflected in their healing properties.

### Progress Check

1 Name four reasons why plants may produce aromatic compounds.
2 Name three ways in which plants create or store aromatic compounds.
3 Describe the variables in a plant's habitat, which can affect the composition of its aromatic compounds. Give an example of a plant that varies its composition in response to environmental stressors.
4 Which family is known to produce many hybrids, subspecies and chemotypes?

### Key Terms

You need to know what these words mean. Go back through the chapter or check in the glossary to find out.

- anabolism
- carbon cycle
- catabolism
- chemotype
- chloroplast
- dicotyledon
- family
- genus
- monocotyledon
- nitrogen cycle
- osmosis
- photosynthesis
- respiration
- secretory cells or structures
- species
- taxonomy
- translocation
- transpiration
- variety

# 6 THE PROVENANCE OF ESSENTIAL OILS

After working through this chapter you will be able to:

♦ appreciate the factors that affect the quality of a therapeutic essential oil
♦ understand the different extraction methods for essential oils
♦ understand the basics of quality tests for essential oils
♦ distinguish a reliable from an unreliable source of essential oils.

**Provenance** means where something comes from. In aromatherapy terms, an essential oil's provenance tells what has taken place to bring the plants' aromatic compounds to the bottle of essential oil you hold in your hands. What factors influence the plant's cultivation and harvesting, the extraction methods, and the storage conditions before an essential oil is brought to the wholesale or retail market?

Historically, for the most part essential oils have been produced for the food flavouring, perfumery, cosmetics and toiletries industries. Their intended use has been not therapeutic but industrial – where standardisation of fragrance or taste is required, and the blending of essential oils from different plants with the aim of obtaining a correct flavour or scent is accepted. In aromatherapy the purpose is therapeutic and for this reason aromatherapists need to be careful to source essential oils from suppliers who are extracting them with their therapeutic use in mind.

## Cultivation and harvest

As discussed in Chapter 5, growing conditions influence the quantity and composition of plant aromatic compounds. Unless 'wildcrafted', the source plants will have been cultivated and so influenced by the grower to a considerable extent, for example: the selection of species, choice of location, time of planting and decision to farm organically or not.

The majority of plants are harvested according to traditional knowledge gained over centuries as to the optimum time and the part of the plant used for the **distillation**. Only recently have scientific investigations been applied to compare the different yields and qualities of different harvesting times and only a few oils have been studied. Some of those that have been studied have revealed the following (Battaglia, 1995):

♦ *Salvia officinalis* contains more α-thujone after flowering, so it is better harvested before flowering.
♦ *Ocimum basilicum* flower heads rather than whole plant produce an essential oil richer in linalool and lower in methyl chavicol; distillation from the flower head is preferred for aromatherapy.
♦ *Mentha piperita* produces a greater yield if harvested when flowers are just at budding stage.

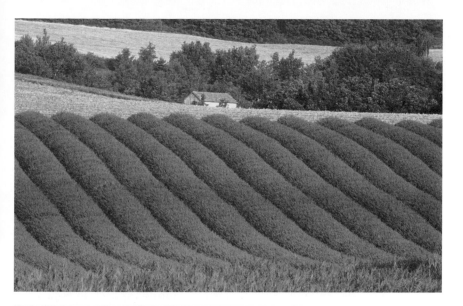

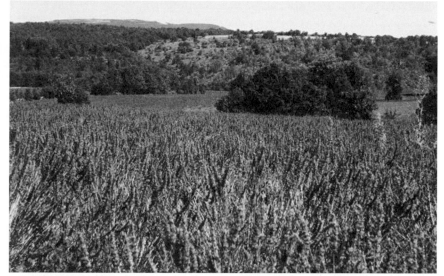

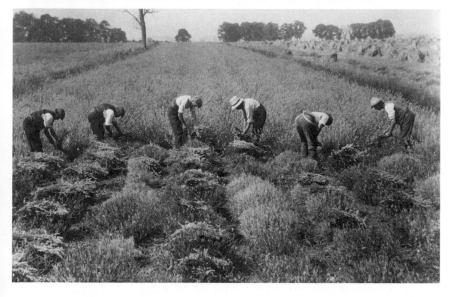

**Fig. 6.1a, b and c** *Cultivation of lavender: (a) clonal lavender bred for uniformity and ease of cultivation and harvest; (b) mixtures of wild populations; (c) lavender harvest near Hitchin, Hertfordshire in the 1930s*

# Extraction methods

Traditionally extraction has been conducted by small scale artisan distillers committed to their craft and to producing highest quality essential oils. In Europe, for native or naturalised species, extraction can take place close to the area of cultivation. This is particularly important for leaves and flowers. For seeds, roots and barks, material can stand some storage and much herbal material originates in other countries and then is brought to Europe or another country for extraction. Extraction also takes place in the country of origin.

As the vast majority of essential oils are extracted to meet the requirements of the food-flavour or perfume-cosmetic industries and it is not important to distil for the whole oil the addition of synthetic compounds is commonplace and accepted. Such partial distillations and addition of synthetic compounds is not acceptable in the case of essential oils for aromatherapy. For aromatherapy, the aim of extraction is to obtain the whole essential oil. Such extractions take more time and care so as to obtain an oil as 'close to nature' as possible. It is important that suppliers to aromatherapists source only from those producers willing to provide therapeutic quality essential oils. Fortunately, with the growth of demand by highly qualified aromatherapists, it has been possible to support such producers and genuine, authentic *therapeutic* quality oils are available.

## Distillation

Distillation is a centuries old technique for obtaining the aromatic essences of plants. It is an artisan's craft. Some improvements and modifications have been made to the process, such as the use of stainless steel equipment and electrical steam generators, but the process itself remains basically the same and is shown in Figure 6.2. In parts of France and some other countries distillation is still carried out by itinerant distillers with portable stills close to the site of harvest. The material of the still can be important. Stainless steel is generally the best for the purpose, although copper is still used by some artisan distillers.

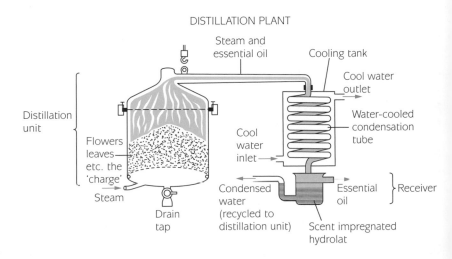

**Fig. 6.2** *A generalised scheme of the distillation process*

## Distillation methods

### Water distillation

The **charge** (plant matter) is completely covered in water in the still and then brought to the boil. The heat compels the essences in the plant to evaporate. They rise to the top of the container tank and enter a tube there, which coils and descends cooling the vapours and prompting their condensation to liquid form. The essential oil impregnated water is collected in a vessel. Since essential oil compounds are lighter than water, they rise to the top and this yield is separated from the water, which is now known as hydrolat, or flower water. (There are exceptions, for example, clove oil compounds, being heavier than water, collect at the bottom of the vessel.)

Since the charge is covered with water, the exposure temperature is lower than in steam distillation. This has the advantage of protecting the essential oils from overheating and the method is used for such oils as neroli and rose. However, the distillation time is longer, so the method is not recommended for plants such as lavender whose esters are damaged by long exposure to hot water (Battaglia, 1995).

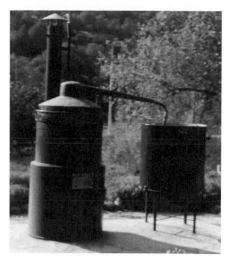

**Fig. 6.3a** *A traditional still*

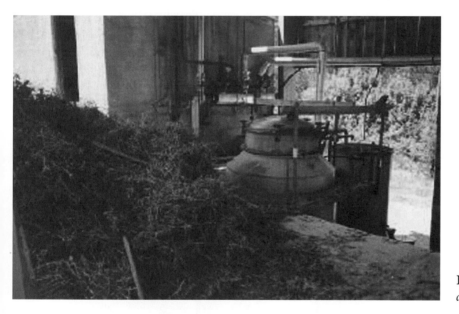

**Fig. 6.3b** *A modern but small distillation unit with rosemary*

### Steam distillation

Steam is generated outside and is directed into the charge. Ideally the temperature of the steam is just enough to provoke the essential oils to evaporate and the atmospheric pressure is as low as possible. If the temperature or pressure is too high, there will be a loss of quality as molecules can be damaged. This method is used for the majority of essential oil plants, particularly for material that is subject to deteriorisation soon after harvest, such as many flowers, leaves and stems. Steam distillation takes from between 1 and 48 hours, depending on the charge, and always leaves some residue in the condensation water and some substances are changed – hydrolysed or oxidised in the process. This is not always a bad thing. For example, azulene is not a natural component of chamomile but is produced during distillation.

In water and steam distillation, steam is generated at some distance from the plant matter, and fed to the distillation tank.

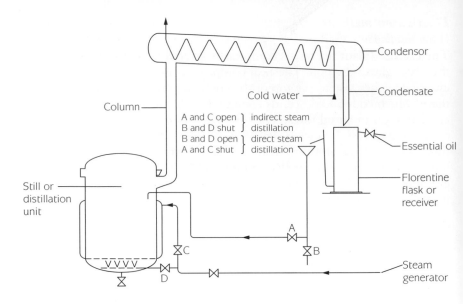

**Fig. 6.4** *Steam distillation*

*Percolation or hydro-diffusion*

In this method steam is introduced into the top of the tank containing the charge. It percolates down through the charge, picking up the volatile compounds, which are collected and cooled at the bottom of the same tank. The advantages are that a lower temperature is needed so minimising exposure of volatiles to heat and it is a speedier process, i.e. 4 hours compared to 12–48 hours. In addition the yield is greater. Percolation is most often used for tougher plant material such as woods or seeds, e.g. fennel, dill, cumin.

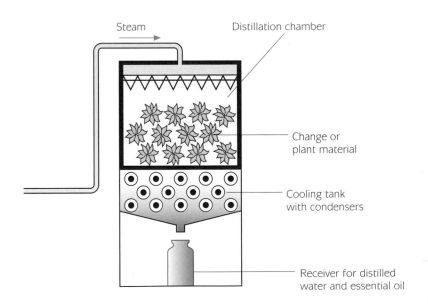

**Fig. 6.5** *Percolation or hydro-diffusion*

*Fractional distillation*

This process is used for certain essential oils, such as ylang ylang. Instead of recovering the essence continually from the cooling tank, it is recovered in batches as the distillation process proceeds. The first batch is called 'extra' and is the finest essential oil. Then come grades 1, 2, 3.

*Cohobation*
This is a process used mainly for the extraction of rose species. In normal distillation the phenyl-ethyl-alcohol fraction is not recovered from the cooled water of steam distillation. So the distilled rose water is distilled again to recover the phenyl-ethyl-alcohol and this is then returned to the original distillate to produce the full-spectrum essential oil. This process is used only to produce rose otto.

## Quality in distillation
Ideally distillation is conducted at the lowest possible temperatures to protect the volatile molecules from being destroyed or oxidised by heat. But this does take longer, especially if one desires the full complement of the essential oil. For example, about 75 per cent of the total yield of a lavender batch comes in the first 25 minutes of distillation and will have – to the untrained nose – a good fragrance of lavender. This is how commercial grade lavender essential oil is produced ('lavender 40/42'). However, this does not include all the molecules. Coumarins, for example, take another 50–80 minutes and while they aren't so obvious in the scent, of course do make a difference to the therapeutic effect. Genuine, therapeutic quality lavender must come from the yield of full distillation.

## Hydrolats
A valuable traditional by-product of the distillation process is the hydrolat or hydrosol. The recovered water, which has itself been distilled and purified, is now impregnated with minute amounts of weak acids and water-soluble components from the aromatic molecules. Hydrolats have been used for centuries as the finest facial cleansers – lavender, rose and orange blossom water. Today hydrolats are also produced for their own sake through a dedicated, gentle water distillation of plant material. These fine, aroma-impregnated waters have excellent healing properties. Actually the fact that the healing properties are already in an aqueous medium means they are better absorbed by our cells. They are particularly recommended for children, elderly people and those with sensitive constitutions or conditions.

Some products marketed as 'floral waters' are not genuine and useful for therapy because either they are just reconstituted by adding essential oil to water or, if produced by a distillation, more essential oils are added to the distillate with a soluble, e.g. alcohol or a detergent. Such oils are used for food flavouring or scenting clothes.

> **REMEMBER**
> A valuable product of distillation is the genuine hydrolat. It can be used therapeutically.

## Expression
**Expression** is used to extract the aromatic compounds, which are found in the peel of citrus fruits. Traditionally this was done manually by two methods, sponge and *éculle à piquer*. These traditional methods have almost completely gone out of use and citrus essential oils are now produced as a by-product of the citrus juice industry only.

## Sponge method
First the fruit is halved and the pulp removed. The peel is softened in warm water, then dried off slightly in air. Next it is *everted* (turned inside out) so that the essential oil-containing flavedo part of the peel can be placed against the sponge. The peel is then compressed to release the oil, which the sponge absorbs. The sponge is periodically squeezed and the essential oil collected and decanted.

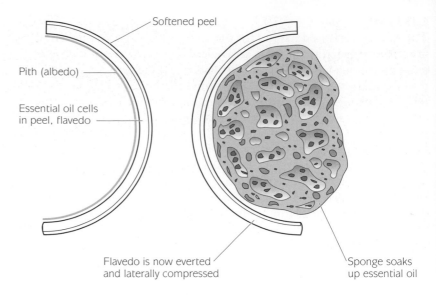

Softened peel

Pith (albedo)

Essential oil cells
in peel, flavedo

Flavedo is now everted
and laterally compressed

Sponge soaks
up essential oil

**Fig. 6.6** *Detail of fruit peel prepared for simple expression. Peel is everted then pressed against a sponge*

### Éculle à piquer

This is another semi-manual method in which the whole fruit is rotated in a vessel with spikes that pierce the oil cells. The broken up pulp and juice with the released oil is collected and allowed to settle, separating the essential oil, which is then decanted.

Abrasion is a mechanised form of the *éculle* process using a rotating drum with spikes, which pierce the peel.

## Solvent extraction methods
### Enfleurage

This is the traditional, manual and labour-intensive method used in past centuries. It is used for plants that are too delicate and contain too small a quantity of essential oils to withstand the heat of distillation. In **enfleurage** the solvent is a rendered animal fat or vegetable oil, which is spread on framed sheets of glass, the chassis. Fresh blossoms of flowers are gathered in early morning and spread on to the chassis and over the next 12–24 hours the essential oils dissolve in the lipid medium. At the right time the flowers are removed and, as the harvest proceeds, more flowers are added and left to wither in the fat until it becomes saturated with the essential oil. This stage produces the enfleurage **pomade**. The pomade will also contain small amounts of plant waxes and fixed oils.

Next the pomade is 'washed' with an alcohol solvent such as ethanol, in temperatures warm enough to melt the fat, and is stirred. The essential oil now leaves the fat and dissolves in the alcohol. This solution is then chilled, which precipitates out the residue plant matter, leaving only an essential oil-rich alcohol. This is then filtered and distilled at very low temperatures to evaporate the alcohol and leave only the **absolute** – the essential oil concentrate.

This method used to be used for flowers such as jasmine, rose and tuberose, whose essential oil content is small but of great delicacy and intense fragrance. However, because it is so labour intensive it is used rarely today.

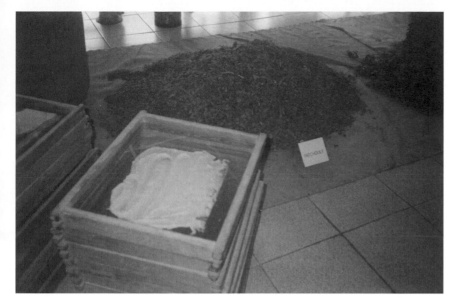

**Fig. 6.7** *A stack of chassis smeared with fat ready to receive blossoms for enfleurage*

In his fascinating novel *Perfume* from 1986, Peter Susskind has authentically described how in the 18th century an absolute is made from delicate jonquil blossoms. A cauldron of rendered fat is used instead of a chassis:

> The blossoms were . . . emptied out in the workshop. Meanwhile, in a large cauldron Druot melted pork lard and beef tallow to make a creamy soup into which he pitched shovelfuls of fresh blossoms while Grenouille constantly had to stir it all with a spatula as long as a broom. . . . Now and then the soup got too thick and they had to pour it quickly through a sieve, freeing it of macerated cadavers to make room for fresh blossoms. Then they dumped and mixed and sieved some more . . . until as evening approached all the piles of blossoms had passed through the cauldron of oil. . . . The following day the maceration continued. . . . This went on for several days. . . . After a while Druot would decide that the oil was finally saturated and could absorb no more scent. He would . . . sieve the viscous soup one last time and pour it into stoneware crocks where almost immediately it solidified to a wonderfully fragrant pomade. . . . Perfumed pomades, when stored in a cool place, keep for a long time . . . the pomade would be brought up again from the cellar, carefully warmed in tightly covered pots, diluted with rectified spirits, and thoroughly blended and washed. . . . Returned to the cellar, this mixture quickly cooled; the alcohol separated from the congealed oil of the pomade and could be drained off into a bottle. . . . Thus the fragrance of the blossoms had been transferred to yet another medium. But the operation was still not at an end. After carefully filtering the perfumed alcohol through gauze . . . Druot fill a small alembic and distilled it slowly over a minimum flame. . . . What remained in the matrass was a tiny quantity of a pale-hued liquid . . . its polished scent concentrated a hundred times over to a little puddle of *essence absolue*. . . . Its smell was almost painfully intense, pungent and acrid. And yet one single drop, when dissolved in a quart of alcohol, sufficed to revitalise it and resurrect a whole field of flowers.

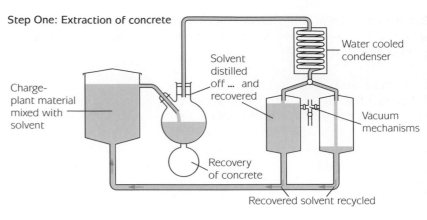

**Step One: Extraction of concrete**

Charge-plant material mixed with solvent

Solvent distilled off ... and recovered

Water cooled condenser

Vacuum mechanisms

Recovery of concrete

Recovered solvent recycled

**Step Two:** Alcohol mixed with concrete, stirred and warmed to dissolve non-volatile plant components (e.g. waxes)

Gentle heat

**Step Three:** Alcohol distilled off in vacuum unit leaving absolute

Alcohol

Recovery of absolute

**Fig. 6.8** *A simplified scheme of solvent extraction*

### Modern solvent extraction

This is a modern form of the enfleurage method. Instead of a chassis of fat, the flowers are placed in a tank with a hydrocarbon solvent, such as hexane, into which the delicate flowers deliver their aromatic compounds along with waxes and fixed oils. This extract is then distilled over very low heat to release the solvent and leave an extract known as a **concrete**. Some plant residues, such as waxes, remain, from 50–80 per cent depending on the plant, along with a small portion of solvent. Concretes are more stable and concentrated than distilled essential oils; they may be kept for longer in this form and only when needed are they processed in the final stage to separate the essential oil from the solvent and alcohol.

As with the enfleurage pomade, the concrete is next mixed and warmed in ethanol alcohol to separate the alcohol and essential oils from the solvent and plant residues. Then the alcohol is evaporated off in a vacuum at low temperature leaving the fragrant, rich absolute – a concentrated viscous liquid, solid or semi-solid depending on the source plant.

**Solvent extraction** is used to produce rose and jasmine absolutes, for example. A small amount of hydrocarbon solvent residues will always be left, and also absolutes contain all the fragrant molecules of the charge, including essential oils. So it is different from a distilled essential oil. For this reason, absolutes are not recommended for skin application, except on those patients in general good health, as these residues might irritate. However, they can be very beneficial used in the form of inhalations for psychological conditions.

Solvent extraction of resinous plants is also used to obtain resinoids. In this case the plant material used comes from plants producing resin, balsam, oleo-resins and oleo-gum-resins, such as benzoin, turpentine, frankincense and myrrh. The product is typically more viscous and often solid at cool temperatures. Myrrh and frankincense are sometimes also extracted by distillation.

## CO₂ extraction

In the past few decades a new method of extraction by carbon dioxide has been developed. $CO_2$ can be either a liquid or a gas depending on the pressure and temperature it is subjected to. At a certain temperature and pressure – called hypercritical state – it can act like a gas and a liquid at the same time: can be dispersing and also have solvent properties. Hypercritical $CO_2$ extraction combines the advantages of low temperature (no heat damage) and speed with that of a solvent that is inert, so there is no residue – the solvent is removed simply by releasing the pressure. Nor is there a residue or by-product left from the reaction. While it does recover a product as close as one can get to the plant's original aromatic substance, the process is at present too expensive to be used on a large scale, putting the price of essences by this method beyond the reach of the average aromatherapist.

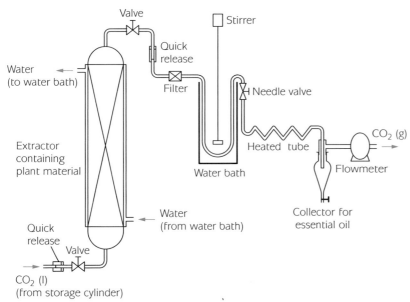

Continuous dense phase extraction apparatus

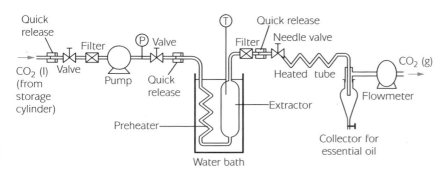

Continuous supercritical extraction apparatus.
(P = pressure gauge, T = temperature measurement).

**Fig. 6.9** $CO_2$ extraction

## Storage

The method of storage can also affect the quality of an essential oil. On extraction, essential oils are decanted and stored in different types containers from plastic barrels to vitrified aluminium, the later being preferred for essential oils destined for aromatherapy. Exposure to light and heat and variations in temperature should be avoided during storage. Under correct storage conditions an essential oil will be dynamic for from one to several years depending on the essential oil. Some oils even improve on ageing, for example, rose or vetiver. Citrus oils keep for a shorter period of time, from one to two years to be at their best, longer if they are extracted traditionally, though these are now difficult to find.

 **Progress Check**

1 Describe the traditional methods of expression. What type of plant material is used?
2 What flowers are considered too delicate for steam distillation? Why?
3 Describe what happens in the following: the still (alembic), the condensation tube, the receiver or florentine.
4 What is cohobation? When is it used?
5 What solvent is often used in solvent extraction?
6 Define the following terms: concrete, absolute, pomade, charge.

## Quality controls

The quality of an essential oil used in aromatherapy will depend on the quality of the original plant material, the quality of the extraction process and on subsequent handling and storage. In addition to quality in the extraction process, the essential oil should only come from one batch or harvest of a particular crop of an identifiable botanical species. The batch number and date of extraction should be labelled. A reputable wholesaler will make sure that suppliers can give documentation of the handling of each consignment.

It is also important that therapeutic oils are not adulterated. There are at least four means of adulterating a batch of essential oils, with the aim of gaining more payment per kilogram:

◆ By 'cutting', i.e. substituting, diluting or extending a product with a cheaper oil whose odour is similar and so its presence is not easily detected. Spanish sage has been used to cut lavender, for example. Yet its chemical make-up has different molecules to lavender, so the healing effects will not be exactly those of lavender.
◆ By diluting with a cheaper oil from the same species but from plants grown other than in the preferred growing conditions. *Pelargonium graveolens* Bourbon, produced in Réunion, may be extended by addition of essential oils of the species grown in other parts of the world. Their chemical make up will be different.
◆ By cutting with a synthetic odour molecule. For example, synthesised camphor can be used to adulterate spike lavender,

giving it a greater quantity of camphor, and different quality than it would naturally have.

- By adding reconstituted amounts of essential oils or mixing essential oils from other distillations to a yield of essential oil. This is done to obtain a standardised composition, or to disguise the lower quality of a product.
- By rectifying, i.e. certain chemical components are removed for industrial purposes.

These practices are accepted in the industries that use essential oils. They have their own standards and guidelines for the composition of their odourants, be they natural or synthetic. They are not acceptable in aromatherapy.

In a therapeutic setting the healing power of the essence comes through its unique blend of constituents, many of which may be known and could be copied, but others that are not yet identified or present in minute amounts. Through the principles of holism and synergy these none the less play their role in the therapeutic properties of that essential oil, often quenching, balancing or enhancing the effects of the known or well-researched constituents.

What is often labelled 'natural' or 'pure' for the purpose of commercial products may in reality only be 'nature identical' – composed from natural products, but not as close to nature as possible because naturally occurring odorants from other plants or varieties have been added to an extracted essential oil. It has been manipulated. This is not good enough for therapeutic purposes where the healing effects depend on the nature-given chemistry, synergy and vitality of the original plant itself.

Therefore it is important that wholesalers of essential oils for aromatherapy have their oils checked for adulteration and the results of these tests should be made available to the buyer.

To detect such practices and help judge the quality of an essential oil, quality control tests are carried out. The main ones are:

- **gas chromatography** or gas-liquid chromatography (GC or GLC)
- mass spectrometry MS
- optical rotation
- refraction index.

## Gas chromatography

A vaporised substance – the essential oil – is mixed with hydrogen and passed into an absorbent column. Heat is applied rising from 70° to 270°C by increments of 2°C every minute. The chemical constituents will evaporate off at different rates and as each does, a sensor (flame ionisation detector) registers this on a chart – the **chromatogram** – in a series of peaks and toughs corresponding to the quantity and evaporation rate of each component or fraction. Although not all the many components of essential oils are known, some have been identified as characteristic of each oil and these produce a certain pattern on the chromatogram, like a fingerprint. The pattern of these peaks and troughs from the test oil is compared to that of the agreed standard and if the oil is genuine it will match. For all its worth, the chromatogram needs a lot of expertise to be properly interpreted and it is not able to be a complete assessment. It has its limitations.

Sample ID    : Lavender Bul 8191

*********** Star Chromatography Workstation ****** Version 4.5 ******

Chart Speed = 0.37 cm/min    Attenuation = 900          Zero Offset
Start Time  = 0.000   min    End Time   = 53.000  min   Min / Tick

a pinene — 3.362

Myrcene — 6.277
Limonene — 7.349   7.663

cis Ocimene — 8.878
Octan-3-one — 9.721   9.478

Camphor — 21.391

Linalool — 24.342 / 24.838
b caryophyll — 25.732
lavandulyl a — 26.635   26.347

tr beta farn — 29.035
Lavandulol — 29.900
borneol — 30.360   30.756

Run Mode        : Analysis
Peak Measurement: Peak Area
Calculation Type: Percent

| Peak No. | Peak Name | Result (%) | Ret. Time (min) | Time Offset (min) | Area (counts) | Sep. Code | Width 1/2 (sec) | St Co |
|---|---|---|---|---|---|---|---|---|
| 1 | a pinene | 0.18 | 3.362 | 0.002 | 67259 | VV | 2.3 | |
| 2 | Myrcene | 0.65 | 6.277 | 0.007 | 249049 | PB | 3.4 | |
| 3 | Limonene | 0.36 | 7.349 | 0.049 | 139814 | BV | 4.0 | |
| 4 | 1,8- Cineole | 0.29 | 7.663 | -0.037 | 112290 | VV | 4.2 | |
| 5 | cis Ocimene | 5.13 | 8.878 | 0.008 | 1969121 | BV | 6.7 | |
| 6 | trans ocimen | 2.47 | 9.478 | -0.022 | 948285 | VV | 5.0 | |
| 7 | Octan-3-one | 0.90 | 9.721 | 0.021 | 343986 | VV | 3.7 | |
| 8 | Camphor | 0.20 | 21.391 | -0.009 | 77074 | BV | 6.4 | |
| 9 | Linalool | 31.70 | 24.342 | 0.042 | 12174349 | BV | 17.6 | |
| 10 | Linalyl acet | 36.60 | 24.838 | 0.038 | 14053909 | VV | 20.8 | |
| 11 | b caryophyll | 3.65 | 25.732 | 0.032 | 1402211 | VV | 7.6 | |
| 12 | Terpineol-4 | 2.86 | 26.347 | 0.047 | 1097656 | VV | 6.2 | |
| 13 | lavandulyl a | 3.18 | 26.635 | 0.035 | 1220533 | VV | 7.3 | |
| 14 | tr beta farn | 2.00 | 29.035 | 0.035 | 767742 | VV | 8.4 | |
| 15 | Lavandulol | 0.67 | 29.900 | 0.000 | 257471 | VV | 4.7 | |
| 16 | alpha terpin | 0.40 | 30.360 | -0.000 | 152656 | VV | 5.9 | |
| 17 | borneol | 1.55 | 30.756 | -0.044 | 595068 | VP | 5.0 | |
| | Totals: | 92.79 | | 0.204 | 35628473 | | | |

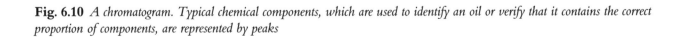

**Fig. 6.10** *A chromatogram. Typical chemical components, which are used to identify an oil or verify that it contains the correct proportion of components, are represented by peaks*

## Mass spectrometry or GC-MS

In this test, the results of a gas chromatogram are further analysed by mass spectrometry. As the molecules emerge from the GC column they are fractured (by bombardment with electrons). Since each molecule forms a characteristic pattern, the spectometer identifies each component by its pattern. Thus, for example, true rosemary essential oil contains a certain proportion of borneol in a particular molecular form (isomer). If a sample has been adulterated by addition of a natural borneol constituent from a cheaper source, this can still be detected because the structural pattern of the substituted borneol will be different.

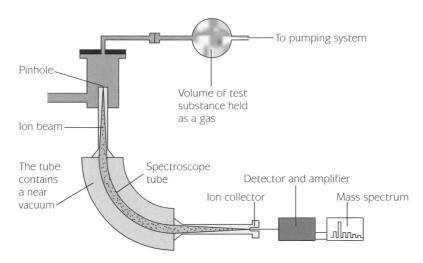

**Fig. 6.11** *A mass spectrometer. A vapour is converted into ions and shot into the curved tube where a magnetic field deflects those ions with a specific mass and charge into the detector. The various ion are detected and the reading printed out*

## Optical rotation

The majority of essential oils have the ability to bend polarised light; they are optically active. By measuring the angle through which the light is rotated by the test material and comparing this to the standard for that essential oil, its integrity can be determined.

## Refraction index

When light is passed through an essential oil in its liquid state it becomes refracted in a measurable way. If the refracted light in a test sample matches that of the standard, it helps to authenticate that essential oil.

## Other tests

Other tests that can be used to authenticate essential oils include checks for their specific gravity (weight), infrared fingerprinting, solubility in alcohol and colour.

**REMEMBER**

European regulations require the producer to publish the composition of an essential oil. This documentation should be checked by wholesale suppliers and made available to buyers if requested.

# Developing an intuitive sense of quality

Technical tests are useful to ensure that suppliers of essential oils are marketing products of integrity and therapeutic value. Producers conduct tests on a sample from each batch and the record is made available on request to buyers. However, let us remember there are limitations to science and technology and such tests do not tell us everything about an essential oil. For many essences, science has not yet even detected and let alone measured the proportion of all the known constituents. These lesser quantities and undetected compounds also contribute to the genuine oil's therapeutic effect. Their presence can be detected by an experienced **'nose'**.

## Developing your 'nose'

It is still important, therefore, for the aromatherapist to develop his or her own intuitive sense of the integrity of an oil based on experience and observation. This is developed over time. As the therapist uses the *materia medica*, he or she gets to know and can compare different examples of the same essential oil. The ability can be developed and is a sense that a therapist can learn to trust. It is developing his or her own 'nose'.

> **REMEMBER**
>
> The fragrance industry employs the professional 'nose' to help create perfumes. A nose can detect over 3,000 individual scents using organoleptic assessment. Such experts can detect certain molecules at levels that are too low for the measuring equipment to read.

> **ACTIVITY**
>
> 1 Write a letter to three essential oil suppliers and request a copy of a GC or GC-MS test for a particular oil. Compare the responses you receive. If possible purchase or request a sample of the same essential oil from each supplier and perform a scent test on each as in activity 3 below. Assess the quality of each oil. Record and write up a discussion of your results.
> 2 Conduct an organoleptic exercise – see page 46 – on three essential oils that are rich in a particular molecule, for example, cineol. See if you can detect that molecule in each. Then evaluate the overall scent of each one using descriptive terms. Now compare the three. Record your observations.
> 3 Obtain (purchase if necessary) three samples of an essential oil from three different suppliers, for example, one from a professional aromatherapy supplier, one each from two different high street suppliers. Test and evaluate each for their quality according to colour and scent using your own observation skills. Write up your results. Compare them with those of your fellow students.

## Progress Check

1 Why is it important to conduct tests of quality?
2 Describe two ways an essential oil might be adulterated.
3 What is a 'nose'?
4 Describe a gas chromatogram test process.
5 What information should a supplier be able to give to buyers to document the quality of an essential oil?

## Key Terms

You need to know what these words mean. Go back through the
chapter or check in the glossary to find out.

- absolute
- charge
- chromatogram
- concrete
- distillation
- enfleurage
- expression
- gas chromatography
- 'nose'
- pomade
- provenance
- solvent extraction

# 7 ESSENTIAL OIL CHEMISTRY FOR AROMATHERAPY

After working through this chapter you will be able to:

◆ understand the terms of chemistry most relevant to essential oils

◆ understand the basic chemistry of essential oil molecules and how this influences their bio-activity

◆ be familiar with the main types of molecules found in essential oils

◆ appreciate the role the chemistry plays in aromatherapy's use of essential oils and the limitations of this role

◆ apply this knowledge to the selection and application of essential oils in a clinical setting

◆ relate essential oil chemistry to constitutional models of health and disease.

## Chemistry and aromatherapy

Essential oils have been characterised as a 'cocktail of chemicals'. Some of us find anything to do with chemistry disconcerting, but we can learn to handle the basics necessary for understanding essential oils in aromatherapy. Let's remember that the science is there to serve the therapy, to help us help our clients. Chemistry provides another language that can help explain what we therapists experience in practice. It can suggest which essential oils could be appropriate in a particular context and why. The language of chemistry is one health professionals understand, so if we are familiar with some basic, relevant science, this facilitates communication with other professionals. In turn, this promotes confidence and credibility in our profession. Some basic vocabulary also helps us to evaluate any research published in our field. Finally, we would not be holistic in our approach if we did not also try to embrace the scientific. The founders of modern aromatherapy, from Gattefosse and Valnet to Maury, have all appreciated this.

Science in its true sense strives to understand nature. The more we understand nature the better we can follow nature's lead in our work with patients.

## Chemical messengers

The chemistry relevant to essential oils has mainly to do with the types of molecules that form them, and how these behave. In terms of their effects on the body, molecules are like messengers. Once applied, they communicate information that stimulates or influences, directly or indirectly, our own molecules, the basis of human tissue cells and systems. First we will look at how essential oil molecules are structured and how they behave in terms of bio-electricity. Many of their known properties, the effects aromatherapists find in practice, can be explained in this way.

## Atoms, the building blocks of molecules

Atoms are the basic units that make up all substances in the physical world. Although there are only 100 or so different types of atom they can join up (bond) to each other to form innumerable different substances. Within the atom's centre or nucleus there are one or more protons (positively charged particles) and zero or more neutrons (particles of no charge). Around the nucleus electrons or negatively charged particles are arranged in layers or shells (see Figure 7.1). Some atoms, such as hydrogen, have only an electron and one shell. Others have more electrons, building up more shells around the nucleus. For example, carbon has six electrons arranged in two shells, with four electrons in its outer shell. Atoms rarely exist on their own; they have a natural tendency to link together in order to achieve outer shells that are filled with the maximum number of electrons.

## Molecules, the structure formed by atoms

Molecules are formed by atoms sharing electrons. In essential oil molecules this is called co-valent bonding. If one pair of electrons is shared, it's called a single bond; if two pairs are shared, it's a double bond; if three, a triple bond. There are different degrees of sharing. If carbon bonds with certain atoms, such as hydrogen, the bond is balanced in terms of the shared electrons within the bond. But if carbon bonds with oxygen, an imbalance exists. The electrons in the bond are found, on average, nearer to the oxygen atom. This makes a partial negative charge on the oxygen atom and a partial positive charge on the carbon atom, creating a force or pull. This type of bond is called a **polar** bond.

Of all the 115 currently known elements or atoms (ever more are discovered), there are only a few found in essential oil molecules to a significant extent: oxygen, hydrogen, carbon, nitrogen, sulphur and potassium. The first three are the most common in essential oil molecules. Of these three, carbon is the most important. It is a very special atom.

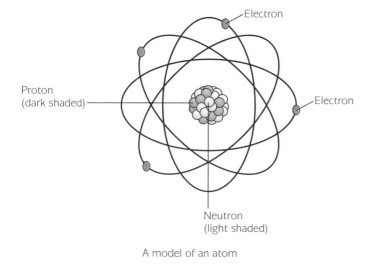

Proton (dark shaded)

Electron

Electron

Neutron (light shaded)

A model of an atom

**Fig. 7.1** *An atom showing the nucleus with protons and neutrons and shells with electrons. Neutrons have no electrical charge, protons have a positive charge and electrons have a negative electrical charge. There are always the same number of electrons and protons so their opposite charges are neutralised making an atom's total charge zero. The mass of an atom is concentrated in its nucleus and is determined by the sum of its number of protons and neutrons*

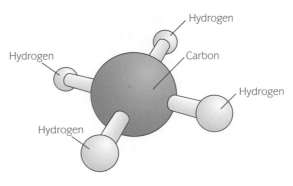

CH₄ methane

**Fig. 7.2** *A methane molecule. Atoms of non-metallic elements bond to each other by sharing their electrons. The outer shells of their atoms overlap. This is called a co-valent bond*

### Carbon the 'TLC' element

Carbon has some unique properties. It is the basis of the almost infinite variety and number of substances inside our bodies and around us in the natural world. This is because of the following characteristics:

◆ Carbon has six electrons, two in one shell and four in the next but the second shell has space for four more. So carbon can form four bonds (share electrons) at once, more than either oxygen or hydrogen.

◆ Carbon can form not only single, but also double and triple bonds. Double and triple bonds of carbon are stronger than single bonds but subject to attack by other atoms, particularly oxygen.

◆ Carbon atoms can bond to each other to form the skeleton of organic molecules that can be structured either as a **chain** or a **ring**. The chain can be rather simple and short or more complex and long. On to this skeleton other atoms and molecules can bond, forming branches off the skeleton. This makes possible a wide variety of **compounds**.

Carbon has been called the 'love atom' because it so naturally and actively attracts and bonds to other atoms. It bonds and connects other

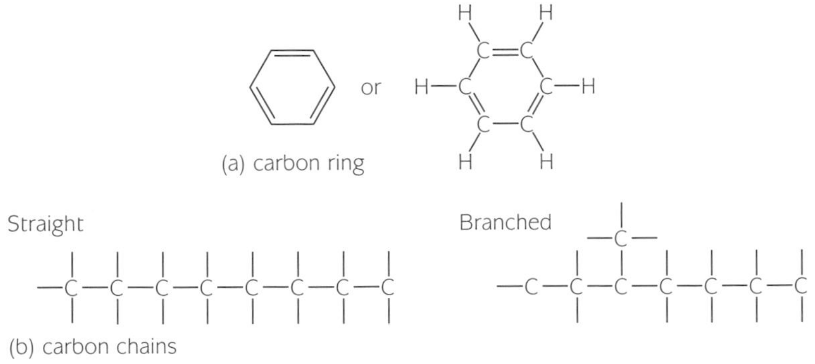

(a) carbon ring

Straight

Branched

(b) carbon chains

**Fig. 7.3a and b** *By the bonding of other atoms or groups of atoms to the carbon skeleton a wide variety of substances are formed: haemoglobin, sugars or saccharides, hormones, peptides and the molecules found in the essential oils of plants, such as* **terpenes, phenols, alcohols, aldehydes**

**REMEMBER**

Molecules based on carbon are the basis of both animal and plant chemistry, so our bodies and essential oils have carbon in common. This bio-compatibility helps explain the therapeutic effectiveness of essential oils.

atoms, making possible all the substances of the living world (the study of which is called organic chemistry). It is a chemical way of saying love makes the world go round!

## Compounds and mixtures

Molecules comprised of more than one type of atom are known as compounds. Molecular compounds can be as solid as a rock, as fluid as water or as light as a gaseous substance – like a fragrance. For example, a molecule of water is made of two hydrogen atoms joined to one oxygen atom but this molecule can be a solid (ice), a liquid (water) or a gas (steam), depending on the conditions in which it exists, such as temperature and pressure.

Molecules can exist together without forming bonds to each other. Muddy water or sea water are examples of a **mixture**: molecules of different substances (compounds) can mix together without bonding chemically. Essential oils themselves are also mixtures of different molecular compounds – the chemical families discussed below. They 'hang together' because of the conditions under which they exist. If these conditions change, for example, if the temperature rises, the molecules separate easily from each other and evaporate. A base cream is also an example of a mixture – two compounds, oil and water, come together. The two are not bonded chemically, but are suspended together by the action of mixing and the adding of emulsifiers such as lecithin.

### *Molecular properties*

The electrons within molecules are in constant motion and this results in tiny imbalances of electrical charge, even in **non-polar** molecules. It is through the charge of their electrons that they are interacting with other molecules around them. Each molecule generates an electro-magnetic field around itself, which means its chemistry also involves aspects of physics. The electrical potential enables it to interact and 'communicate' with its environment (e.g. other molecules) by the transfer of information. Science does not yet fully understand all the implications of this bio-electrical energy.

- Molecules have size; they can be large and complex or quite simple and small. Their size also gives them a certain weight, depending on the number and weight of the atoms of which they are made. (The mass of an atom is the sum of its protons and neutrons.) Essential oil molecules are incredibly small. They are so small that a single drop of an essential oil can contain up to 40 thousand million million million molecules (Price and Price, 1999). This helps explain why even a single drop of an essential oil can have therapeutic effects.
- Molecules also have shape. Don't be misled by two-dimensional diagrams: molecules really exist in 3D! The shorthand diagrams of molecules may give the impression that a molecule's shape, the position of the atoms in the structure, is flat and fixed. In fact aromatic molecules have the ability to change shapes. Parts of them can bend, fold, twist and rotate because of their bonds – especially the single bonds, which behave like springs rather than rigid sticks.

Beneath the surface of all life there is enormous activity as atoms inside molecules are constantly shifting in response to their environment.

> **REMEMBER**
> Having some flexibility in their bonds allows essential oil molecules to bend and 'wiggle'. For example, when applied to the skin they can move between the cells and penetrate to lower levels and enter lymph circulation.

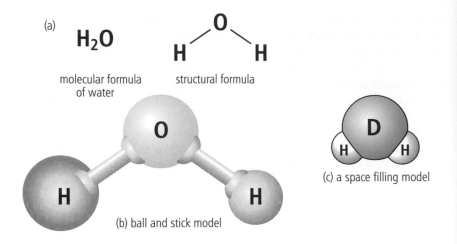

molecular formula of water

structural formula

(c) a space filling model

(b) ball and stick model

**Fig. 7.4a, b and c** *Molecules are represented graphically in different ways: (a) a structural representation shows letters denoting each type of atom and lines showing the types of bonds (single, double, triple); (b) a ball and stick model aims to show the pattern of the bonds and their angles; (c) a space-filling model shows how the atoms overlap as they share electrons*

Energy is constantly being exchanged and information communicated. This gives essential oil molecules a great variety in their applications.

### Molecular isomers

Some of nature's molecules display **isomerism**. Two compounds can have exactly the same chemical formula in terms of their kinds and numbers of atoms, but their atoms can be arranged differently within their molecules. For example, both neral and geranial contain the same number of carbon, hydrogen and oxygen atoms but their atoms are

(a)

an ether
(dimethyl ether)

an alcohol
(ethanol)

(c)

Geranial
(trans)

Neral
(cis)

(b)

cis

trans

(d)

mirror image

a, c and d represent functional groups

**Fig. 7.5a, b, c, and d** *Types and examples of isomers: (a) structural isomers – the formula $C_2H_6O$ can indicate two compounds, each with a different arrangement of the same atoms; (b) cis/trans isomers – there has to be a double bond $C=C$ in the molecule. There are the same types of atoms and the same number and types of bonds but the arrangement in space is different. The atoms or groups of atoms cannot rotate about the double bond and the positions of the groups are fixed differently in space. Each position produces different properties. The positions are cis (same) if the identical groups are on the same side of the double bond, trans (across) if they are on opposite sides. (c) Isomers of neral and geranial showing cis-trans isomerism; (d) optical isomers – the molecules are mirror images of each other. Optical isomerism may explain the harmful effects of thalidomide. A harmful isomer rather than a benevolent isomer was present in the drug (Battaglia, 1995, page 71)*

arranged in very different ways. It is distinct arrangements of the same atoms that create **isomers.** The different shapes will give isomers different properties. In essential oils, several isomers of a molecule can exist. While one isomer may have potentially toxic effects, others can have therapeutic effects. This may be the explanation of why sage essential oil, which contains a potentially hazardous molecule called thujone, has not been found in aromatherapy practice to be particularly hazardous: it has the isomers of thujone, which are not harmful (Price and Price, 1999). Isomers of thujone in sage include: α-thujone (pronounced alpha-thujone); β-thujone (pronounced beta-thujone).

What is important in aromatherapy is that the biological interaction of different isomers with our body cells can be different. For example, cells can react differently to the two forms of an optical isomer. Sometimes one isomer is biologically active; the other shows no activity. Sometimes one isomer is therapeutic and its mirror image is potentially hazardous.

## GOOD PRACTICE

When purchasing an essential oil, be aware of any isomers that are important in influencing its biological activity.

## ACTIVITY

1   Purchase some small polystyrene balls from a craft shop and some toothpicks. Label or better still colour them to represent different molecules found in essential oils: carbon, oxygen, hydrogen. Using these construct a molecule of nerol and one of geraniol.
2   Research three essential oils that have isomers and compare their known effects.

## REMEMBER

Because aromatherapy is holistic and uses the whole aromatic complex extracted from the plant, side effects are rare. One reason is because while an isolated molecule may on its own irritate the system, when the whole essential oil is used, the other molecules buffer or control this effect. This phenomenon is called **quenching**. The potentially harmful effect of one isolated constituent is quenched by the beneficial effects of others present with it.

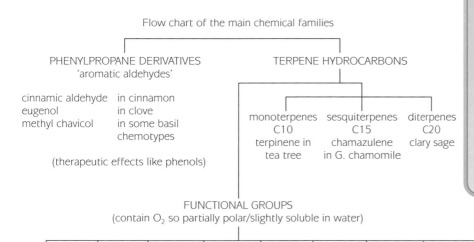

Flow chart of the main chemical families

PHENYLPROPANE DERIVATIVES
'aromatic aldehydes'

| cinnamic aldehyde | in cinnamon |
| eugenol | in clove |
| methyl chavicol | in some basil chemotypes |

(therapeutic effects like phenols)

TERPENE HYDROCARBONS

| monoterpenes C10 | sesquiterpenes C15 | diterpenes C20 |
| terpinene in tea tree | chamazulene in G. chamomile | clary sage |

FUNCTIONAL GROUPS
(contain O₂ so partially polar/slightly soluble in water)

| alcohols | phenols | (alipatic) | ketones | esters | oxides | ethers | lactones | sesquiterpene |
| linalool | thymol | aldehydes | menthone | linalyl | cineol | eugenol | coumarins | alcohols |
| in lavender | in thyme | citral | in | acetate in | in | methyl | bergaptene | sanatol in |
| | | in melissa | peppermint | petitgrain | eucalyptus | ether in | in bergamot | sandalwood |
| | | | | | | tropical basil | | |

**Fig. 7.6** *Flow chart of chemical families*

# Chemical families: constituents of essential oils and their therapeutic properties

With the basic understanding that essential oils are composed of molecules whose properties allow them to be biologically active, we are ready to explore the main molecules currently known to constitute our essential oils. We can consider these constituents as chemical families, each having certain properties. Their properties influence their therapeutic effects. If an essential oil is particularly rich in one or two chemical families we can say that these are determining the oil's effects to a large extent – bearing in mind the important point that even small amounts of a particular chemical, such as **esters**, also contribute to the effect. (Esters buffer or balance the effects of other, more assertive constituents). Trace elements and elements not yet discovered are also affecting the properties of the essential oil.

The aim of choosing the essential oil(s) most suited to the individual's mind–body–spirit wholeness, becomes informed with our knowledge of biochemistry. This approach works particularly well when combined with the biogram developed by Pierre Franchome and with knowledge of the patient's **constitutional type** (see Chapter 1 and page 137).

## Structure and function

Essential oil molecules are composed mostly of three atoms, carbon, hydrogen and oxygen, bonded in a variety of ways. Due to the way they are synthesised (formed) in plants, the component molecules fall into two main groups:

- terpene **hydrocarbons** – **monoterpenes** and **sesquiterpenes** – and terpenes that have been modified by oxygen – called oxygenated, or terpenes with a functional group
- phenylpropane derivatives.

However, since phenylpropane derivatives behave like terpenes, for practical therapeutic purposes, aromatherapists need only learn the different molecule families according to *activity*. For this we organise them into two groups:

- terpene hydrocarbons and phenylpropane derivatives
- functional groups – terpenes modified by oxygen.

The figures used to illustrate these compounds and their properties are taken from the aromatic biogram on page 146.

## Terpene hydrocarbons, monoterpenes, sesquiterpenes and diterpenes

Terpene hydrocarbons – often just called hydrocarbons or terpenes – contain only carbon and hydrogen formed as a molecular unit called isoprene. The basic unit isoprene is itself made of 5 carbon atoms. So the number of carbon atoms a terpene will have is always a multiple of 5:

- a monoterpene contains 2 isoprene units or 10 carbon atoms
- a sesquiterpene (*sesqui* indicates $1\frac{1}{2}$ times the original, e.g. 2 units plus 1) contains 3 units or 15 carbons
- a diterpene (*di* indicates 2 times the original) 2 times 2 isoprene units: 4 units or 20 carbon atoms.

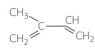

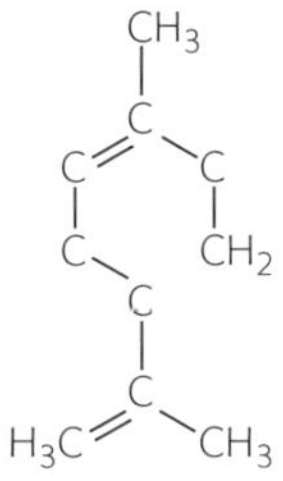

**Fig. 7.7a** *An isoprene unit $C_5H_8$*

**Fig. 7.7b** *A molecule built up of two isoprene units $C_{10}H_{10}$ ocimene*

The greater the number of carbon atoms, the greater the weight of the molecule, the less volatile it becomes and the more difficult to distil. So only a very few essential oils contain diterpenes, and their presence in the oil is a small percentage of the whole. Clary sage (*Salvia sclaria*) is an example. Essential oil molecules are never larger than diterpene. Larger molecules present in plants include starches, waxes, proteins and cannot be distilled.

## Hydrocarbons/terpenes/terpenoids: monterpenes and sesquiterpenes

### Hydrocarbons and monoterpenes

#### Basic formation
The core of the terpene hydrocarbon is the structure of a carbon-to-carbon bonded chain. It is thought that approximately 90 per cent of the effects of essential oils is due to the presence of terpenes. So, understanding the effects of this group carries us a long way. The presence of terpenes, once considered hazardous, is now known to be beneficial since they quench the potentially toxic or irritating effects of some other molecules. Their potential toxicity is offset either by their low concentrations in an essential oil or the presence of other, quenching molecules.

### Monoterpenes (C10=2 isoprene units)
Name: It ends in '-ene'. It sometimes has a Greek letter prefix of *alpha*, *beta*, *gamma*, *delta* or *rho*: $\alpha$, $\beta$, $\gamma$, $\Delta$, $\rho$ to indicate an isomer.

Formation: The terpene carbon-carbon chain is formed of only two isoprene units. In a typical hydrocarbon these bonds are relatively strong because they are non-polar and hence stable. The atoms in these bonds do not react easily with other molecules.

The monoterpene hydrocarbons are present to some extent in all oils. They are particularly concentrated in the citrus oils. (Even so, interestingly, the aroma of citrus oils is not due to the monoterpenes but to other molecules present only in trace amounts.) Lemon, orange, grapefruit, bergamot and mandarin contain up to 90 per cent of the terpene limonene. Pinene, camphene and myrcene are other monoterpenes. When present in a high percentage monoterpenes tend to make an essential oil clear, and very fluid (low viscosity) and of high volatility. Eucalyptus is high in monoterpenes.

Properties: Monoterpenes and hydrocarbons are antiseptic and antimicrobial (some antibacterial, some antiviral), and antiparacidal. They are anti-inflammatory, with cortisone-like effects. They are stimulating to eliminative processes. They are drying, draining and decongestant; they help reduce excess moisture in the body, whether it is in the upper body/respiratory tract where they help eliminate excess mucus and congestion (eucalyptus, pine, myrtle), or in the lower body, helping to eliminate fluid via the urinary tract (juniper berry). Limonene, $\alpha$-sabenene and $\gamma$-terpinene have antiviral properties.

(Caution: Some monoterpenes have caused skin irritation in some people.)

Examples:
- $\alpha$-pinene in pine, abies, cypress
- limomeme in bitter orange
- phyllandrene in angelica
- terpinene in tea tree.

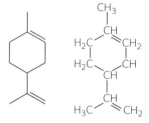

**Fig. 7.8** *Limonene molecule* $C_{10}H_{16}$ *represented in two ways. In the notation scheme chemists use, often the hydrocarbon core is simplified. The symbols for hydrogen and carbon are left blank since carbon is understood to be at the end points and corners of the pattern and hydrogen to be attached to the remaining carbon bonds. Only additional atoms such as oxygen and nitrogen need be labelled. Here are two kinds of notation for limonene. Since we know carbon can bond four times, we can replace the symbols correctly for a full representation*

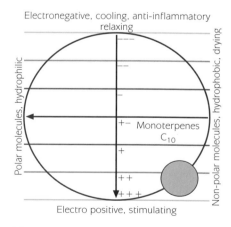

**Fig. 7.9** *Monoterpenes placed on the biogram*

For people with ME (myalgic encephalomyelitis) use gentler immune stimulants first (e.g. alcohols), as terpenes may be too strong for a weakened system.

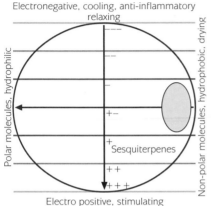

**Fig. 7.10** *Sesquiterpenes*

*Electronegative, cooling, anti-inflammatory relaxing*

*Polar molecules, hydrophilic*

*Non-polar molecules, hydrophobic, drying*

*Sesquiterpenes*

*Electro positive, stimulating*

### Sesquiterpenes (C15=3 isoprene units)

Name: It ends in '-ene'. A Greek letter prefix indicates an isomer.

Formation: The carbon-carbon chain has three isoprene units.

Sesquiterpene molecules are present in smaller concentrations in essential oils than are monoterpenes. They are heavier and less able to be distilled. They occur most often in woody structures, seeds or roots of plants – sandalwood, cypress, clove bud, ginger, vetiver – and in plants of the Asteraceae family – angelica, German chamomile, helichrysum/immortelle. While they may have functional groups (see below) attached to them, these do not seem to directly influence their properties. The hydrocarbon core is larger (C 15) and thus also influential so any activity displayed may be due to the whole complex, rather than one particular component. So, as a group, the properties of sesquiterpenes are not easily to classify.

Properties: Generally they are antihistaminic and anti-allergenic; and like other terpenes they are antiseptic and antibacterial to a degree. The feature of this group is that each one is individual when it comes to its structure and thus to therapeutic effects. Some may be also antispasmodic, some anti-inflammatory, such as German chamomile. Some are sedative and hypotensive. We have to learn each one's properties individually, rather than as a group

Few have been well researched but those that have, such as German chamomile, show marked anti-inflammatory properties.

Significantly, chamazulene is produced from *Matricaria recutita* (German chamomile) only during the distillation process, as matricene in the flowers decomposes. It is not present in the plant's original aromatic complex.

Sesquiterpene alcohols will be discussed under alcohols.

Examples:

- chamazulene – German chamomile (produced only during distillation), yarrow
- caryophyllene – clove, rose
- zingerberine – ginger
- farnescene – rose.

### Functional groups: terpene hydrocarbons modified by a group containing oxygen

Terpene hydrocarbons can be modified if one or more hydrogen atoms are replaced with a group containing oxygen, often hydrogen-oxygen

(-OH) called a **hydroxyl** group. In this functional group, oxygen and carbon form a polar bond (in contrast to the non-polar bonds of the isoprene core). This means the molecule has an imbalance of electrical charge, which makes part of it partly negative and part of it partially positive, and so can exert a greater influence on neighbouring molecules. In other words, these polar bonds are chemically – and thus therapeutically – more active. When a molecule is quite small, C10–C15, the influence of the functional group (oxygen-carbon bond part of the molecule) on its activity is greater. The fact that the molecule contains some oxygen makes it slightly soluble in water and considerably soluble in alcohol.

The six functional groups in the monoterpenes of essential oils are:

| | |
|---|---|
| alcohols | phenols |
| aldehydes | ketones |
| esters | oxides |

### Alcohols

Name: It ends in '-ol'.

Formation: One or more hydroxyl groups are bonded to the carbon chain.

Properties: Their chief charactcristics are that they are strongly anti-infections, antimicrobial and immuno-stimulant and very safe. They are of low toxicity and non-irritating to the skin. This makes them very valuable for treating infections, for daily hygiene, as ingredients in skin care products. They are also tonic. Essential oils high in alcohols have a very pleasant scent. According to Pierre Franchome, alcohols have molecular ions that are strongly electropositive.

Examples:

- linalool in petitgrain, lavender, rose, geranium
- geraniol in palmarosa
- borneol in abies
- menthol in peppermint, cornmint
- terpeneol-4-ol in tea tree, juniper and marjoram
- sclareol in clary sage
- citronellol in rose, geranium.

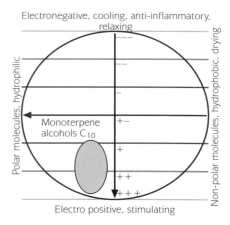

**Fig. 7.11** *Alcohols*

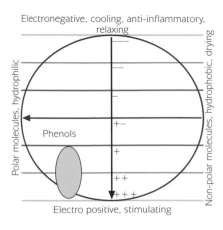

**Fig. 7.12** *Phenols*

### Phenols

Name: It ends in '-ol'.

Formation: The hydroxyl group attaches to a benzene (aromatic) ring rather than a carbon chain structure.

Properties: The –OH/hydroxyl group in the molecule is very reactive and therefore phenols are potentially irritating. Phenols are strongly anti-infectious, bactericidal, vermicidal and immuno-stimulant. The ions are strongly electropositive.

Examples:

- carvacrol in thyme, savoury, oregano
- thymol in thyme.

**GOOD PRACTICE**

Phenols in large amounts are potentially damaging to the liver (hepatotoxic), because the liver must convert them to sulfonates to be excreted, work that can weaken the liver. They can be skin and mucous membrane irritants. So, while particularly good for infections (e.g. respiratory), they should only be used for short periods of time and in low concentrations/high dilutions.

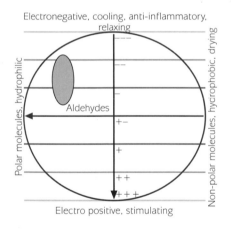

**Fig. 7.13** *Aldehydes*

### Aldehydes (also called aliphatic aldehydes)

Names: They either end in '–al' or '–aldehyde' is part of the name.

Formation: A carbon-oxygen group attaches to hydrogen (-CHO) and this attaches to a carbon atom in the basic structure.

Properties: They have a strong aroma. Channel No. 5 perfume has a characteristic aldehyde scent. In addition to being anti-infectious, they are antiviral, refrigerant or antipyretic, litholytic (break up stones), anti-inflammatory. They are also calming, sedative, relaxing, hypotensive. Significantly their sedative and antispasmodic properties are more effective at lower doses. They can be skin irritant or cause a rash reaction. This can be avoided by using lower doses. However, once someone is sensitised to an aldehyde, it is likely that any essential oil containing it will cause a reaction.

Examples:

- citral in melissa, may chang
- citronellal in citronella
- geranial in lemongrass, lemon, lime, melissa.

### Ketones

Name: It normally ends in '–one' but note that a few other molecules sometimes also end the same, so there are exceptions. For example, asarone is a phenolic ether, not a ketone.

Formation: A carbon-oxygen group, or **carboxyl** group, attaches to a carbon chain.

Properties: They are stimulating, strongly mucolytic and lipolytic; excellent for wound healing and skin problems as they stimulate cell and tissue regeneration (vulnerary or cicatrisant); sedative. Some are also anticoagulant, analgesic, anti-inflammatory, digestive and expectorant.

Caution: They are potentially neuro-toxic and abortificant if ingested. Restrict use to low dose and short term.

Examples:

- menthone in peppermint
- verbenone in rosemary, chemotype verbenone
- camphone in rosemary, chemotype camphor
- carvone in spearmint, dill, caraway
- thujone in sage, thuja
- jasmone in jasmine, helichrysum
- thujone in thuja.

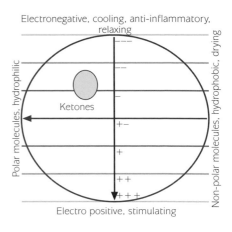

**Fig. 7.14** *Ketones*

## *Esters*

Note: Essential oils with a high proportion of alcohols also contain the esters formed from these.

Name: It usually forms a double name with the first part of the name ending in '–yl' and the second word ending in '–ate'. Or 'ester' is part of the name.

Formation: When an alcohol reacts with an acid, an ester is created; it is like a marriage. The acid and alcohol are joined to each other via a –COO– linkage.

Properties: **Amphoteric,** i.e. esters, are generally balancing and harmonising, no matter whether there is hypo- or hyperactivity. They can be highly relaxing, sedative or gently stimulating depending on the person's state. Some are antispasmodic or antifungal. The greater the number of carbon atoms, up to seven, the greater the antispasmodic or calming quality. The fewer carbons, the more subtle are the effects. The presence of esters makes the oil's fragrance pronounced and pleasant, often fruity. Even small amounts are important for the fragrance, giving it refinement. It is the large concentration of esters in lavender that help give its calming, regulating effect and make it safe to use on the skin.

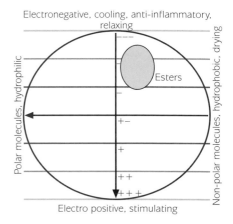

**Fig. 7.15** *Esters*

Examples:

- geranyl formiate (geraniol + formic acid) in geranium (1C)
- linalyl acetate (linalool + acetic acid) in lavender (48–52%), bergamot (30%), clary sage (60–80%), petitgrain (55%)

- benzyl acetate (benzol + acetic acid) in ylang ylang (7C)
- neryl acetate (nerol + acetic acid) in helechrysum (75%)
- bornyl acetate (borneol + acetic acid) in rosemary chemotype vebenone (15%) (2C)
- myrtenyl acetate (myrtenol + acetic acid) in red myrtle
- butyl angelate in Roman chamomile (80%) (5C)
- methyl salicylate (methyl + salicylic acid) in yellow birch.

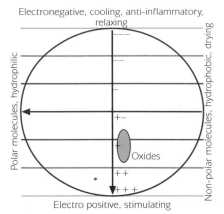

**Fig. 7.16** *Oxides*

## Oxides: cineol

Name: It ends in '–ol' or '–ole'. Oxides are named like an alcohol since they usually derive from an alcohol.

Formation: Oxygen links to two carbons and is at the same time part of a carbon ring. There is only one oxide of great significance in essential oils, 1,8 cineol, also called eucalyptol (linalool oxide is found, for example, in basil and hyssop).

Properties: This single component plays a large role in the effectiveness of eucalyptus. Cineol is expectorant and decongestant; strongly anti-infectious, antibacterial and vermicidal.

## Sesquiterpenols (sesquiterpene alcohols)

Name: It ends in '–ol'.

Formation: Some alcohols are based on a sesquiterpene.

Properties: They are like the sequiterpenes (see above; having no functional group), so their effects vary among the different molecules, but include the following: muscles and nerve antispasmodic, lymphatic decongestants, anti-allergenic, liver stimulating, anti-inflammatory and stimulant to glandular secretions. α-Bisabol, in German chamomile (*Matricaria recutita*) has been shown to be even more anti-inflammatory than the chamazulene.

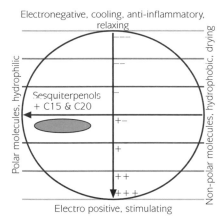

**Fig. 7.17** *Sesquiterpenols*

Examples:

- α-bisabol
- farnesol in rose
- sanatol in sandalwood (15C)
- zingerberol in ginger
- vetiverol in vetiver
- viridiflorol in naioli, sage (This has oestrogen-like effects.)
- cedrol in atlas cedar – tonifies veins
- caratol in carrot seed – stimulates regeneration of liver cells.

## Ethers

Name: 'Ether' or sometimes '–ethyl' appears in the name if a two-carbon chain is on one side of the oxygen.

Formation: They are formed from the hydroxyl group of either a phenol or an alcohol when hydrogen is replaced with a short carbon chain (as in methyl chavicol).

> **REMEMBER**
>
> For the best anti-inflammatory effect with German chamomile, choose one that contains α-bisabolol. Sometimes this is not present.

Properties: They are antispasmodic and relaxing, but are less subtle than esters in this effect, i.e their action seems more restricted to the physical level (less effect on mental–emotional). They help nervous spasms such as digestive or muscle cramps. According to Pierre Franchome their ions carry primarily a positive charge.

Examples:

- methyl chavicol – tropical basil (*Ocimum basilicum* var. *basilicum*), tarragon
- eugenol methyl ether – bay (*Laurus nobilis*), tropical basil

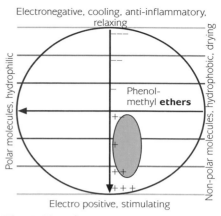

**Fig. 7.18** *Ethers*

## Coumarins and lactones
Name: The names vary. They can end in '–in', '–ene' or '–one'.

Formation: An ester group is attached to a carbon ring, and there is also a functional group on oxygen. They can be simple, such as coumarin, or more complex, such as bergaptene (a fouranocoumarin). They occur only in expressed oils and in jasmine absolute, as their molecular weight is too great for extraction by distillation.

Properties: They are found to be refrigerant and excellent expectorants and mucolytics, even more effective than ketones. Some are antiviral and antifungal. However, fouranocoumarins, such as bergaptene, cause photo-toxicity.

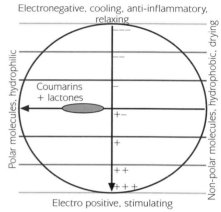

**Fig. 7.19** *Coumarins and lactones*

**GOOD PRACTICE**

Bergaptene increases the penetration of UV light, so should not be used on patients who will be exposing themselves to sunlight shortly after treatment or who have a history of skin cancer. It is found in significant quantities in bergamot, but also to some extent in all citrus essential oil.

## Acids
Name: It ends in '–oic'.

Formation: Usually COOH group.

Properties: Acids are rare in essential oils because they are of low volatility and do not survive distillation. One that does and forms during distillation is the potentially toxic, inorganic hydrocyanic acid found in bitter almond. Bitter almond is distilled for the flavouring and perfume industries, and should not be used in aromatherapy.

## Phenylpropane derivatives: phenyl aldehydes/aromatic aldehydes
Name: It ends in '–ol' or contains '–aldehyde'.

Formation: A few molecules found in essential oils are formed differently by the parent plant. They are based on the **aromatic or benzene ring** rather than the carbon chain. Additional groups of atoms

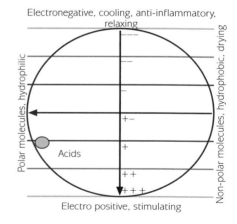

**Fig. 7.20** *Acids*

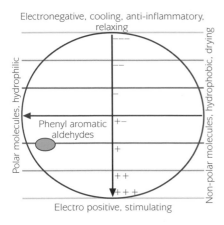

Electronegative, cooling, anti-inflammatory, relaxing

Polar molecules, hydrophilic

Phenyl aromatic aldehydes

Non-polar molecules, hydrophobic, drying

Electro positive, stimulating

**Fig. 7.21** *Phenyl/aromatic aldehydes*

are attached to it. Sometimes the oxygen is not integrated to the ring system but links between two unconnected carbon chains (anethol).

Properties: Like the phenols, they are pharmacologically highly active. They can be thought of as in the same class as the above phenols from the pharmacological point of view: strongly anti-infectious but also potentially irritant and hazardous to the central nervous system Historically, abuse of anise liqueurs caused neurological damage. Use essential oils rich in them for infections but only short term. Some authors class these as 'aromatic aldehydes' and with the phenols.

Examples:

- ♦ cinnamic aldehyde in cinnamon
- ♦ eugenol in clove
- ♦ apiol in parsley
- ♦ safrol in camphor
- ♦ anethol in aniseed.

### Sulphur compounds
Name: It contains 'sulph–' or '–thio–'.

Formation: These are not formed from hydrocarbons and as the name suggests contain sulphur compounds. An example is diallyl disulphide in garlic. They belong to neither the terpene-functional group nor the phenylpropane classes. They are found only in a few essential oils.

Examples:

- ♦ diallyl disulphide in garlic.

### Nitrogen
This is only found in small amounts in essential oils.

### Trace constituents
There may be many other constituents of essential oils than those discussed here, but to date they have either not been identified or not researched as to their properties. In a holistic sense, even these trace elements are playing their part in the effect the oil has on our bodies. They also contribute to the synergy of the whole essential oil.

> **REMEMBER**
>
> Cinnamic aldehyde, eugenol and methyl chavicol act like a phenol. They are strongly anti-infectious but their use carries restrictions: low doses and short term use only.

## Progress Check

1 What does amphoteric mean?
2 What does quenching mean?
3 Why is an essential oil an example of mixture rather than compound?
4 What are the special properties of carbon?
5 What does a Greek letter prefix before a molecule's name indicate?
6 How does a functional group/oxygen affect a terpene hydrocarbon molecule?
7 Which essential oil molecules should be used only in small doses and for short terms?
8 Which essential oil molecules can be potentially neurotoxic unless used carefully?
9 Which essential oil molecules can be skin or mucous membrane irritants?

# Franchome's aromatic biogram – an elegant and practical innovation

Building on the work of Paul Belaiche (*Traite de Phytotherapie et d'Aromatique*, 1979), Pierre Franchome made an important contribution to our understanding of how essential oils work when he investigated some of the properties of chemical families of essential oils. We introduce here only the basics of the work he published, with Dr Daniel Pénöel, in *L'Aromatherapie Exactement* (1990). Franchome found that the properties of an essential oil are due to the electrical charge of the electrons and to the polarity of the main molecules that constitute it. He plotted these on a graph or biogram. The biogram simplifies and makes more accessible to the aromatherapist the chemistry of the molecular families.

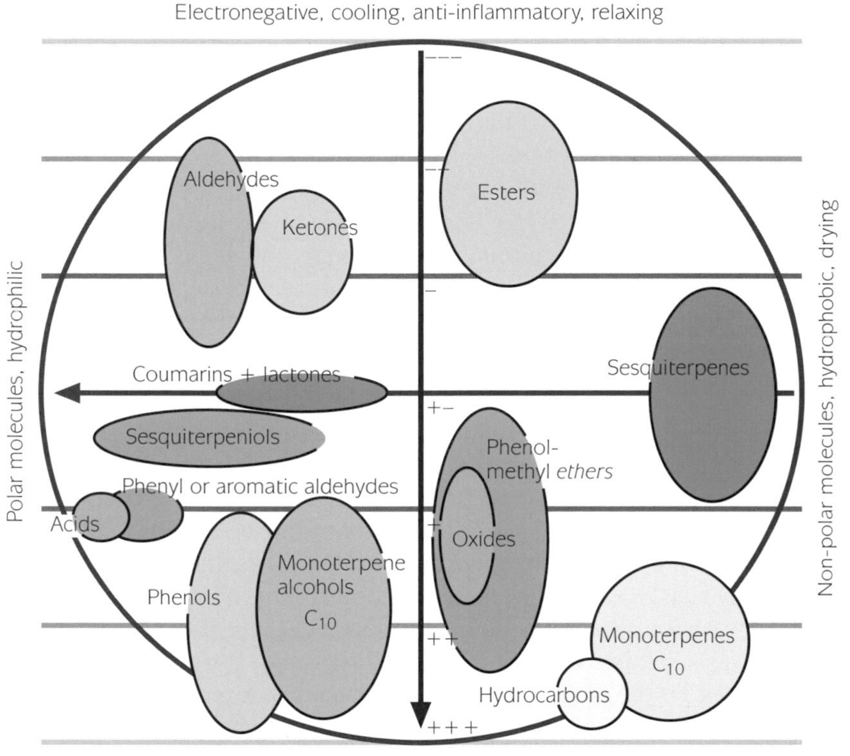

**Fig. 7.22** *The aromatic biogram*

## GOOD PRACTICE

Use the biogram to select the therapeutic action needed, correlating the action with the properties of the **chemical family**. Assess the condition of the patient, then refer to the biogram to choose the essential oil(s) rich in the molecules having the needed therapeutic effect for that condition.

## The electrical referential

An essential oil molecule has the potential to donate or receive electrons. If a molecule loses one or more electrons, it becomes a positively charged ion. If it gains one or more electrons it becomes a negatively charged ion. Franchome found that molecular ions with a positive charge are strongly anti-infectious and stimulating of their environment, e.g. body cells when introduced to them. They inhibit bacterial growth or kill bacteria outright; they are warming. Postively charged molecular ions are found in terpenes, alcohols and phenols. Molecular ions that have a negative charge are found in esters and sesquiterpenes, and produce relaxing and anti-inflammatory effects; they are more cooling.

These properties can be plotted vertically on an axis, called the electrical referential, according to the degree of their electrical charge. This method gives a physically measurable indication of the effects of the chief molecules present in an essential oil. The more electro-positive or electro-negative a chemical family is the further away from the centre it is placed on the chart. (See Figure 7.22 on page 137, vertical axis.)

### Polarity

Another property of molecules is whether they are polar or **apolar** (sometimes also called non-polar). Carbon and oxygen (a carbonyl group, $C=O$) form a polar bond and if this bond is part of a molecule it affects how the molecule behaves, making it more reactive. When in the presence of water, while all essential oils are mostly insoluble, if a portion of an essential oil's molecules has a polar bond it will be slightly soluble to a certain extent. This can also be measured and plotted on a horizontal axis. Apolar or non-polar molecules are hydrophobic (water-hating), or very insoluble in water and they tend to be more drying and draining in their effects on the body. Examples are terpenes and oxides. Polar molecules are hydrophilic (water-loving), and slightly soluble in water. Examples are aldehydes, ketones, alcohols. These are attracted to moist environments where they can exert their mucolytic effects: dissolving, breaking down mucus. (See Figure 7.22, horizontal axis.) Hydrolats contain hydrophilic molecules.

Using the Franchome model gives the aromatherapist a very practical, visual and more accessible way of linking an essential oil's chemical constituents to its properties and its uses. It orders the basic chemistry in a helpful way. For example, for a condition of infection with a lot of phlegm/catarrh and heat, the biogram shows that essential oils particularly rich in molecules that are more drying (non-polar) and anti-infectious, such as terpenes, along with those that are strongly mucolytic and cooling – ketones or aldehydes – are indicated. For a condition characterised by the organism being under stress, or tense and manifesting an allergic inflammation, the biogram shows that essential oils rich in cooling molecules – aldehydes, sequiterpenes, and relaxing molecules – esters and antispasmodic oxides – are indicated.

The Franchome model is a scientific one because it assesses the quantity (and thus strength) of an essential oil molecule's property by measuring the electrical charge of its ions and its polarity.

Rosemary Cady has added another dimension to the usefulness of the biogram by introducing colour coding. Molecular groups that are stimulating are coded yellow to red, while those that are relaxing are coded blue. Balancing molecules (able to relax or stimulate according to what is needed) are coded green. This system gives a visual imprint of an essential oil's combination of properties.

### ACTIVITY

1. Draw the aromatic biogram by hand and place the chemical families on it.
2. Write on the diagram names of some essential oils rich in each chemical family.

3 Colour in the biogram according to the Cady colour system: red for phenols; deep pink for alcohols; orange for monoterpenes; yellow for oxides; dark green for lactones-coumarins; bright-light green for sesquiterpenes; sky blue for ketones; darker blue for esters; very deep, dark blue for aldehydes; brown for aromatic aldehyde.

4 Think of an infectious ailment that you have had and the symptoms you experienced (temperature, inflammation, catarrh, swelling, pain, restlessness or nervousness, other).
  (a) Which chemical family or families would be therapeutically most beneficial for the ailment?
  (b) Which essential oil(s) are rich in these families?
  (c) What cautions if any would you bear in mind when using these essential oils?

## Progress Check

1 Which chemical families are strongly electro-positive and non-polar (drying or draining)?
2 Which chemical families are strongly electro-positive and polar?
3 Which chemical families are more electro-negative, ketones or aldehydes?
4 Which chemical families are placed close to the centre of the biogram and are more relaxing?
5 Which chemical families have anti-allergenic properties?

## Constitutional aromatherapy and the aromatic biogram

Another use of the biogram is to integrate it with a qualitative approach and use it with constitutional types as explained in Chapter 1.

Each constitutional type or **temperament** – phlegmatic/lymphatic, sanguine, choleric, melancholic/neurogenic – can also be placed on the biogram according to their typical qualitites. A phlegmatic/ lymphatic type is characterised by more moisture and coolness; a sanguine type by moisture and warmth; a choleric (bilious) type by heat and dryness; and a melancholic/neurogentic type by cold and dryness.

In very acute ailments, choosing oils according to the constitutional type is probably not that important, as the main focus is to first eliminate or inhibit the pathogen and relieve acute symptoms. Afterwards constitutional aspects can be considered to help full recovery.

In chronic ailments choosing essential oils in order to balance the person according to excesses or deficiencies in their constitutional predispositions can be very helpful, along with essential oils for the condition. Consider the patient from a physical point of view (heat, moisture, cold, dryness) and also from a psychological point of view: 'hot emotions' include irritation, frustration, anger, rage; 'cold' emotions – sadness, grief, anxiety, fear. Moisture may show as lack of motivation or attachment; dryness as indifference or isolation.

> **REMEMBER**
> Selecting essential oils to harmonise to the patient's inherent constitutional pattern lying beneath the symptoms of disease helps restore balance the system as a whole, the *terrain*.

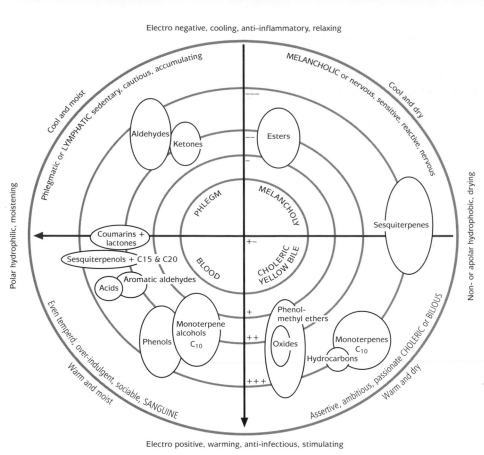

**Fig. 7.23** *Essential oils can be used to balance the constitution of the patient, as well as the individual condition. Chemical families and relevant essential oils in each quadrant can be used to balance excesses of each humour by choosing oils from its diagonally opposite or neighbouring quadrant. (Note: everyone has all four humours and can suffer any combination of imbalances. The figure shows the main tendencies.)*

> **GOOD PRACTICE**
>
> For emotional and mental conditions, use a method traditional to Unani Tibb medicine – the medicine of Avicenna and Muslim peoples today – to balance or adjust the subtle essence of humours at the cellular and atomic level. Place one or two drops of the appropriate essential oil on a small piece of cotton wool. Have the patient place this in the ridge – not in the ear canal – of the right ear. The application is left for from 1–3 hours, and repeated for 2 to several days. Often sandalwood is used for men and jasmine for women.

There is an energetic chart of essential oils which organises information about the therapeutic properties of essential oils and their energetic qualities in Appendix 4 (see page 349).

To use constitutional aromatherapy:

- First assess the patient to determine her basic type and assess any imbalances using the Humoural Assessment table on p. 23.
- Next examine the chart and chapter 11 to see which essential oils are rich in a certain molecule or which molecules would be best for balancing that constitution.
- Then refer to Appendix 4 Essential Oil Energetic and Therapeutic Chart to further refine your selection according to qualities and therapeutic actions needed to balance the patient's constitution.

# TEMPERAMENTS OF THE HERBS.

I. **A**LL medicines simply considered in themselves are either hot, cold, moist, dry, or temperate.

The qualities of medicines are considered in respect of man, not of themselves; for those simples are called hot, which heat our bodies; those cold, which cool them; and those temperate which work no change at all in them, in respect of either heat, cold, dryness, or moisture. And these may be temperate, as being neither hot nor cold; yet, may be moist or dry; or being neither moist nor dry, yet may be hot or cold: or, lastly, being neither hot, cold, moist, nor dry.

II. In temperature there is no degree of difference; the differences of the other qualities are divided into four degrees, beginning at temperature; so that a medicine may be said to be hot, cold, moist, or dry, in the first, second, third, or fourth degree.

The use of temperate medicines is in those cases where there is no apparent excess of the first qualities, to preserve the body temperate, to conserve strength, and to repair decayed nature. And observe, that those medicines which we call cold, are not so called because that they are really cold in themselves, but because the degree of their heat falls below the heat of our bodies, and so only in respect of our temperature are said to be cold, while they are in themselves really hot; for without heat there could be no vegetation, springing, nor life.

III. Such as are hot in the first degree, are of equal heat with our bodies, and they only add a natural heat thereto, if it be cooled by nature or by accident, thereby cherishing the natural heat when weak, and restoring it when it is wanting.

Their use is, 1. to make the offending humours thin, that they may be expelled by sweat or perspiration. 2. By outward application to abate inflammations and fevers by opening the pores of the skin. 3. To help concoction, and keep the blood in its just temperature.

IV. Such as are hot in the second degree, as much exceed the first, as our natural heat exceeds a temperature.

Their use is, to open the pores, and take away obstructions, by cutting tough humours through, and by their own essential force and strength, when nature cannot do it.

V. Such as are hot in the third degree are more powerful in heating, they being able to inflame and cause fevers.

Their use is to provoke sweat or perspiration extremely, and cut tough humours; and therefore all of them resist poison.

VI. Such as are hot in the fourth degree do burn the body if outwardly applied.

Their use is to cause inflammations, raise blisters, and corrode the skin.

VII. Such as are cold in the first degree, fall as much on the one side of temperature as hot doth on the other.

Their use is, 1. to qualify the heat of the stomach, and cause digestion. 2. To abate the heat in fevers; and, 3. To refresh the spirits, being suffocated.

VIII. Such as are cold in the third degree are such as have a repercussive force.

And their use is, 1. To drive back the matter, and stop defluctions; 2. To make the humours thick; and 3. To limit the violence of choler, repress perspiration, and keep the spirits from fainting.

IX. Such as are cold in the fourth degree are such as stupify the senses.

They are used, 1. In violent pains; and 2. In extreme watchings, and the like cases, where life is despaired of.

X. Drying medicines consume the humours, stop fluxes, stiffen the parts, and strengthen nature.

But if the humidity be exhausted already, then those consume the natural strength.

XII. Such as are dry in the first degree strengthen; in the second degree bind; in the third, stop fluxes, but spoil the nourishment, and bring consumptions; in the fourth, dry up the radical moisture, which being exhausted, the body must needs perish.

XIII. Moist medicines are opposed to drying, they are lenitive, and make slippery.

These cannot exceed the third degree: for all things are either hot or cold. Now heat dries up, and cold congeals, both which destroy moisture.

XIV. Such as are moist in the first degree, ease coughs, and help the roughness of the windpipe; in the second, loosen the belly; in the third, make the whole habit of body watery and phlegmatic; filling it with dropsies, lethargies, and such like diseases.

XV. Thus medicines alter according to their temperature, whose active qualities are heat and cold, and whose passive are dryness and moisture.

XVI. The active qualities eradicate diseases, the passive are subservient to nature.

So hot medicines may cure the dropsy, by opening obstructions; and the same may also cure the yellow jaundice, by its attractive quality in sympathizing with the humour abounding: and contrariwise cold medicines may compress or abate a fever, by condensing the hot vapours, and the same may stop any defluxion or looseness.

**Fig. 7.24** *An Explanation of the Temperaments of the herbs by Nicolas Culpeper (after Galen)*

This approach enables us to connect modern scientific knowledge with the healing traditions of European culture – of Hippocrates, Galen, Culpeper and others. It integrates information about the therapeutic properties of some of the molecules in essential oils, the energetic qualities and the known actions of the whole essential oil with the constitutional profile of the patient.

## Key Terms

You need to know what these words mean. Go back through the chapter or check in the glossary to find out.

- alcohol
- aldehyde
- amphoteric
- aromatic/benzene ring
- carbon chain
- carbon skeleton
- carboxyl
- chemical family
- compound
- covalent bond
- electrical charge
- ester
- ether
- temperament
- hydrocarbon
- hydroxyl
- isomer
- ketone
- mixture
- monoterpene
- oxide
- phenol
- polar/non-polar or apolar
- quenching
- sesquiterpene
- terpene

# CARRIER MATERIALS

**8**

After reading this chapter you will be able to:

◆ understand the different types of materials used to apply essential oils

◆ understand the provenance of vegetable oils used as carriers

◆ appreciate the therapeutic properties of vegetable oils based on oil nutrients

◆ choose the appropriate carrier for the intended purpose to meet the needs of the patient.

Essential oils are always applied in dilution in professional practice. The type of material used to dilute and apply them is known as a **carrier**. It is a substance in which the essential oil is soluble, and is often a vegetable oil, or oil based product like a cream or ointment. Other materials include clays and gels. Water and steam can also be considered carriers and used therapeutically. In spite of its name, a carrier is more than an inert, passive vehicle. Carriers have their own therapeutic properties and these are used to extend the benefits of the application. The carrier itself is chosen with due consideration.

## Vegetable oils

Cultures world wide have always valued and used vegetable oils. They are valued for cleansing practices, for ritual and ceremonies, for healing. Anointing with oil is mentioned often in the Bible. Hippocrates, in the 5th-century BC prescribed massage with olive oil. The Romans used olive oil as a cleanser in their public bath houses: it was applied before bathers entered the steam rooms and when they emerged it was scraped off by an attendant with a strigil (a curved scraper), after which fresh oil would be reapplied. Ayurveda uses oils applied in copious amounts for treatment of nervous and arthritic disorders, as part of pancha karma to eliminate ama (toxins), and for health maintenance. Martial artists of Kerala receive daily massage before practice to strengthen their skin and muscles.

Vegetable oils are called **fixed oils** to distinguish them from the volatile oils found in plants, as they do not evaporate. In aromatherapy they are also known as base oils, as they form the base for the essential oils in a blend. Aromatherapy uses them to minimise friction in a massage (general and local), but also for much more.

### Uses of vegetable oils in aromatherapy
Vegetable oils themselves have their own therapeutic properties and make their own contribution to a treatment:

◆ They contain vitamins, minerals and lipids or fats – biologically active substances that nourish and protect the skin, and counteract imbalances of the skin such as inflammation. Oils are added to creams and **lotions** for topical treatment.

◆ They act literally to carry the volatile essential oils, which naturally tend to evaporate away from the body, down into the skin and facilitate their penetration.

◆ They nourish the whole body. Their **phospholipids**, such as lecithin, penetrate quickly through the skin layers, interact with skin cells and pass into the circulation, where they can be further metabolised and nourish the body. Phospholipids are scavengers for free radicals. Price and Price (1999) and Leslie Kenton (1985) reference instances in which percutaneous (skin application) of vegetable oil was able to supplement for nutritional deficiencies of **essential fatty acids** in some people.

◆ They can assist in bath applications (see Chapter 9).

(In contrast, mineral oil, though a good lubricant, provides no nutrients, is not absorbed through deeper layers of skin, but remains on the surface. It is can be use in dressings as a barrier application.)

### Vegetable oils and the skin

Vegetable oils provide nourishment for our skin cells. The skin's natural bacteria feed on the vegetable oil and begin to break it down, making its components, e.g. vitamin D, available to the blood and lymph, thus actively nourishing the skin. The enzymes present in vegetable oils catalyse the synthesis of vitamin A. As carriers, vegetable oil bases of aromatherapy blends are bio-compatible with the skin. They can stimulate the natural production of collagens by stimulating the activity of the skin's immune cells, the **Langerhans cells**.

## Provenance and extraction

Vegetable oils come from nuts and seeds of a variety of plants, such as sunflowers, walnuts, wheat, roses and coconut palms. It is amazing to realise that what appears as quite dry, with nothing of a liquid nature in it, is actually the source of this marvellous liquid substance. The plant creates the oil as a food or fuel store for the seed to use on germination. It is the vitality in the oil that makes possible the new life of a seedling. The quality of any carrier oil will of course depend on the quality of the starting material before extraction. It must not be old, mouldy or contaminated.

Extraction of this vital substance from the seed is of two basic kinds: **cold pressing** from prepared seed material; and solvent or **heat extraction**, which is a further processing of the first pressing. These two methods produce what are known as unrefined and refined oils. Each method is done for a particular end purpose.

### Cold pressing

The nut or seed is prepared by mechanical crushing and gentle warming to draw the oil from cells. Then the oil is expelled by pressing, then collected and filtered. Although called 'cold' pressing, oil cannot be extracted without some heat, for where there is friction (as in crushing) there is heat, but this is kept below 60°C to minimise heat damage. No additional heat is used. The first extraction is usually called 'extra virgin', the next 'virgin'.

A cold-pressed oil is most often the best oil for aromatherapy – as well as for cooking and eating – though it will be more expensive. Some cold-pressed oils will be darker in colour and retain a stronger odour. Cold-pressed oils will turn rancid more quickly than refined products, so if used they should be purchased in small quantities and used in good time. Like all oils, they need to be kept in airtight and cool conditions away from light to minimise oxidation, which turns them rancid.

A **solvent extraction**, using hexane, is also considered a cold extraction in the sense that high temperature is avoided. However, this extraction is usually a preliminary to a further refinement for an industrial oil, and is not intended for sale as a cold-pressed oil. The seeds are not crushed first but macerated in a solvent. No extra heat is introduced. The solvent is subsequently distilled off at low temperature.

> **GOOD PRACTICE**
>
> Adding a little wheatgerm oil to a blend increases its shelf life because this oil is high in anti-oxidant Vitamin E.

### Heat extraction

Heat is deliberately introduced into the extraction, either before or during pressing, in order to maximise yield. It also may be applied after extraction to refine the product. Heat destroys the integrity of an oil and its nutrients. It creates trans-fatty acids and generates free radicals.

### Refining

After extraction, chemicals (bleach, caustic soda, phosphoric acid, butyl hydroxytoluene (BHT)) are used to refine the oil, to lighten the colour and texture, deodorise it and to extend its shelf life by destroying the essential fatty acids, which will go rancid. In this way the nutritional value of the oil, along with its odour and flavour, is lost. Refined oils are produced for cooking, for the food and pharmaceutical sectors, and for products such as paint, varnish, soap, candles, cheaper toiletries and cosmetics and lubricants.

### Oil modification: hydrogenised oils

Hydrogenation is a modification of oils to produce margarine and shortening. Its effect is to destroy the double bonds in the oil and the essential fatty acids, giving it a longer shelf life. This also destroys nutrients and, when used in cooking or processed foods, introduces into the body chemicals known as trans-fatty acids with quite detrimental effects. Foods cooked in hot oil or fat are found to impair cell respiration and inhibit immunity.

### Storage requirements

On extraction, vegetable oils need to be stored in air-tight containers in cool conditions – under nitrogen in wholesale warehouses – and away from exposure to sunlight and moisture. Air (oxygen), heat, water and light all act on the oil to induce deterioration and rancidity. Refining removes the elements most liable to deterioration, but these include the nutritious skin-restructuring elements.

1   What is the difference between a fixed oil and an essential oil?
2   Describe the process of cold pressing.
3   Explain why is it preferable to use a cold-pressed oil for aromatherapy.
4   What makes a vegetable oil nourishing?
5   What are the important storage conditions for vegetable oils?

## Nutrients in vegetable oils

Prominent in vegetable oils are the fat-soluble vitamins, A, D, E and K, and essential fatty acids. Note, these will not be present in refined or modified oil products.

### Vitamin E

Also called tocopherol, this is an outstanding anti-oxidant: it acts in the oil and in our bodies to protect from damage to cells – including collagen, elastin and skin cells – by oxidation and free radicals. Wheatgerm oil is particularly rich in vitamin E, which is why wholegrain bread stays fresh longer than white bread (unless preservatives are added). Vitamin E is needed for tissue repair, for normal blood clotting, for strengthening capillary walls. It is protective for the heart, joints, eyes (cataracts) and against cancer. It helps heal scars and burns.

### Vitamin A

This controls the rate at which dead skin cells are shed and replaced by new ones. A shortage causes a sallow, scaly complexion and flaky, dry skin.

### Vitamin D

This vitamin is necessary for the absorption of calcium, and thus for growth of healthy bone, teeth and skin; and for muscle activity.

### Vitamin K

This is needed for normal blood clotting. It is produced in the gut but can also come from plant oils and vegetables.

### Vitamin F

This is another name for essential fatty acids (EFAs). EFAs are one of the basic components of fats and oils, known chemically as lipids.

As the term fatty acid implies, a fat in the form of an alcohol (glycerol) reacts with an acid to produce a type of ester, triglycerol, which is a lipid or fatty acid. Our bodies cannot synthesise EFAs; they must be derived from our foods and so are 'essential' to health.

### *The function of essential fatty acids*

Contrary to popular belief oils and fats are healthy – if they are of nutrient quality. The body does not produce them on its own. Every cell needs essential fatty acids to carry out its functions. The body breaks

> **REMEMBER**
> Oils contain fat-soluble vitamins: A, D, E, B-complex.

down the EFAs to provide energy, to rebuild and produce new cells, and to synthesise prostaglandins, the hormone-like regulators of many vital processes, particularly anti-inflammatory processes and platelet formation. Needed in large amounts in the brain, EFAs help the transmission of nerve impulses and normal development and functioning of the brain. A deficiency shows as impaired learning and poor recall of information. They have also been found to be low in people with depression. Essential fatty acids are also able to reduce the adhesiveness of fatty deposits (LDL or low density lipo-proteins) in the walls of arteries.

### Prostaglandins

Prostaglandins are immune regulating substances. There are two main types.

- Type E1 prevents thrombosis, lowers blood pressure, helps keep blood vessels dilated, slows production of cholesterol, facilitates insulin metabolism and reduces inflammation. GLA (gamma-linoleic acid) is a precursor of E1 prostaglandins.
- Type E2 is associated with inflammatory processes – arthritis, ulcerative colitis, eczema – and with muscle weakness and lack of control, as in multiple sclerois. It is thus linked to auto-immune conditions.

Some people seem not to produce enough of Type E1 prostaglandins because of a lack of gamma-linoleic fatty acid, GLA, which is crucial to its bio-synthesis. Factors that will inhibit the production of GLA include: stress, low mineral and vitamin intake, and certain disease processes, as well as a diet high in saturated fats, processed oils and alcohol.

### Omega fatty acids

Functionally EFAs can be grouped into Omega 3 and Omega 6 types.

- Omega 3s are high in linolenic acid and are found especially in fish oils and in walnut, flaxseed and rapeseed oil.
- Omega 6s contain linoleic acid, which is converted into gamma-linoleic acid. Linoleic acid supports cell membranes. Omega 6 EFAs are found especially in corn, safflower, sunflower, borage, evening primrose and olive oil.

Symptoms of Omega3-type fatty acids or linolenic acid deficiency include: skin problems like eczema, hair loss, excessive sweating with thirst, lowered immunity to infections, poor wound healing, sterility in males, miscarriage, osteo-arthritis, heat and circulatory problems, and growth retardation.

Symptoms of Omega 6/gamma-linoleic acid deficiency include: premenstrual syndrome (PMS), eczema, psoriasis, heart and vascular disease, rheumatoid arthritis, multiple sclerosis. It is found in evening primrose and borage oil.

Symptoms of linolenic acid deficiency include: growth retardation, muscular weakness or lack of coordination, tingling of limbs, vision disturbance and behavioural changes.

## Chemistry and types of fatty acids

Chemically a fatty acid is a long (10–24 carbon atoms), hydrocarbon chain with glycerol (an alcohol) molecule at its beginning end and a carboxyl acid group (–COOH) at the other end.

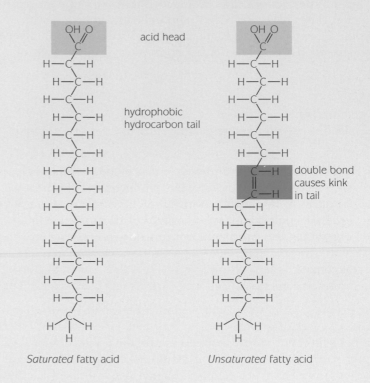

**Fig. 8.1** *Types of fatty acid molecules*

Chemically there are two types of EFAs: saturated and unsaturated, depending on the type of covalent bond.

- Saturated fats have single bonds (C–C) and the maximum number of hydrogen atoms possible has already been attached, so the chain is 'saturated' with hydrogen. This makes them very stable, i.e. less liable to go rancid and solid at room temperature, because the carbon atoms are not free to react with any available atoms. Fats, such as butter and coconut oil, have carbon chains based on stearic, palmitic and myrstic acids. Some saturated fat is needed by the body for energy storage and insulation, but with today's lifestyle and diet, most people consume too much saturated fat, which then raises low density cholesterol level and increases the risk of cardiovascular disease.
- Unsaturated fats are liquid at room temperature and have mostly unsaturated units in their chain. They have one or more double bonds (C=C). The chain has not filled all its potential places of bonding with hydrogen, so the carbon atom bends back and bonds with itself, creating the double bond. At such points on the chain there is flexibility and 'weakness' in the sense that the carbon atom can break off and bond – react – with available oxygen atoms. This 'weakness' of the double bonds gives both positive and negative qualities. They can absorb other molecules and thus transport them, i.e. into the skin. Taken internally, they are easily broken

down and their energy released. They can help the digestive breakdown of triglycerols (or triacylglycerides), i.e. they help lower LDL cholesterol. However, they are less stable than saturated fats, therefore vulnerable to oxidative breakdown and rancidity.

## Phytosterols

**Phytosterols** are plant saponins and chemically related to human steroids and sex hormones. They include sterol, beta sitosterol, sitosterol, campesterol, squalene. They can strengthen skin cell membrane integrity and moisturise. Inside the body they lower HDL and increase LDL cholesterols.

## Phospholipids

These are an important subgroup of the triglyceride lipids needed for cell membrane integrity (triglyceride = 3 molecules of fatty acids linked to 1 of glycerol). The most prominent of these is lecithin. Phospholipids emulsify fats, i.e. keep them in solution with water. Internally, this emulsifying property inhibits the plaquing of cholesterol in the walls of arteries. Externally, phospholipids benefit sensitive and oily skin. They are used in formulations for high quality creams and cleansers.

## Other components

Nutrients such as minerals and proteins are present in trace amounts in oils. It is not known if they are metabolised by the skin.

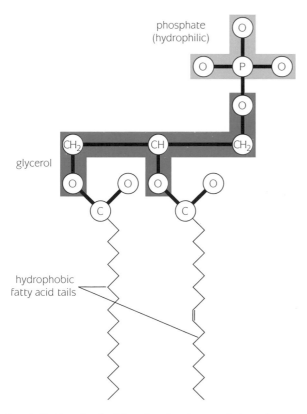

**Fig. 8.2** *A phospholipid molecule. Note the phosphate and glycerol group forms an electrically charged polar end, making it hydrophilic, while the fatty acids form a hydrophobic end. This gives it dual properties – partly water soluble and partly non-mixing with water – called amphipatic. In cell walls phospholipids help form the structure and prevent in-flow of water-soluble molecules. The hydrophilic end faces outward, the hydrophobic end faces inward*

1 Explain the term essential fatty acid.
2 What is the main difference, in terms of the chemical structure of EFAs, between a saturated and an unsaturated fat? What are the implications of this for its shelf life?
3 What are prostaglandins?
4 Which EFA is needed for the synthesis of prostaglandins and is sometimes missing in some people?
5 Which are the fat-soluble vitamins?

## Using carrier oils

### General carrier oils used 100% in blending

These oils are economic to use, provide good lubrication in massage and nourish the skin.

### *Almond, sweet* **Prunus amygdalis var. dulcis**

A native of Central Asia, the almond tree is cultivated widely in the Middle East, the Mediterranean countries, America and India.

Character: pale yellow, mild odour like marzipan.

Constituents: vitamin D, E; trace minerals; mono-unsaturated oleic acid, 8–28%; polyunsaturated linoleic acid (26%); small amounts of saturated fats.

Good for: all skin types. Itching, soreness, dryness, scaling, inflammation, eczema, chapping, irritation, sun exposure.

Properties: emollient, protective, nourishing; low rancidity.

Comment: an excellent massage oil for aromatherapy.

### *Coconut* **Cocos nucifera**

A native of South Asia and the East Indies, the coconut palm is now also cultivated in the West Indies, South America and Africa.

Character: white or clear, solid at room temperature, unless highly refined; odourless; heavier texture.

Constituents: notably higher in saturated fat (lauric, caprylic, capric acids) than unsaturated fats.

Good for: all skin types, but may irritate some people with sensitive skin. Used for sun protection, hair care, it moisturises dry skin; makes good lip balm base; useful for massage.

Properties: emollient, protective through its coating quality.

Comments: coconut oil may be used as a base for essential oil perfume formulation. Coprah oil, a liquid at room temperature, is a further refined fraction of the same oil. Perform a patch test for skin sensitive persons.

> **REMEMBER**
>
> Essential fatty acids are found in vegetable oils and are essential for health.

> **REMEMBER**
>
> Do not confused sweet almond vegetable oil with bitter almond essential oil, extracted from *Prunus amygdalis* var. *amara*, which contains prussic acid. Prussic acid converts to cyanide during extraction; cyanide is poisonous. This is the source of almond essence used as a food flavouring, but with the prussic acid removed.

## Corn oil     Zea mays

A native of the Americas and sacred to Native Americans, it is now cultivated widely. The ears of its large green stalks provide a highly nutritious grain-vegetable.

Character: light golden colour; medium texture.

Constituents: rich in linoleic acid, vitamin E (6%) if unrefined, cold pressed.

Good for: all skin types.

Properties: emollient, preservative; medium texture.

Comments: extracted mainly for the food industry; used in cheaper cosmetics; likely to be genetically modified and likely to be highly refined unless stated otherwise on the label. It can be added in small amounts to creams and blends where, like wheatgerm oil, it acts as a preservative.

## Grapeseed oil     Vitis vinifera

A native of the Mediterranean, and the Middle East. Since ancient times grapes have been cultivated as a food and their fruit juice used for wine making.

Character: on cold pressing a dark colour; colourless to greenish if refined; light texture.

Constituents: high in unsaturated fats, but an acceptable oil product is difficult to obtain without much heat and processing, which leaves it denatured.

Good for: all skin types.

Properties: emollient, lubricating; lighter texture.

Comments: a serviceable, cheaper oil; not recommended for quality products or blends. Its availability is a recent by-product of modern juice extraction and the seeds must be highly refined to get an acceptable product.

## Hazelnut oil     Corylus avellana

A native to the Mediterranean; widely grown in Europe, North America, Asia

Constituents: oleic acid (71–80%), linoleic acid (7–18%); rich in vitamins A, B, E.

Character: light with sweet, nutty odour; light, fine texture.

Good for: all skin types, congested, dehydrated skin.

Properties: slightly astringent, very moisturising and softening; excellent penetration without a greasy feel; natural sun filter.

Comments: the nut is also known as filbert, cobnut and noisette; the oil content is 40%, so it yields easily on pressing. Most oil is refined for the cosmetic and food industry; source with care.

## Olive oil     Olea europa

A native of the Near East, its cultivation spread throughout the Mediterranean countries in ancient times; now also cultivated in California. The olive tree is central to the Mediterranean life and diet. It gives food, oil for lamps and for cooking. It is used in health care and medicine. Hippocrates prescribed massage with olive oil.

Character: varies according to the ripeness of the olive on extraction and whether extraction is cold-pressed extra virgin, or heated and further refined; green to light yellow, almost colourless; heavier texture.

Constituents: rich – up to 80% – in mono-unsaturated fatty acids, which resist oxidation, especially oleic acid (60–85%), linoleic acid (9–14%), linolenic acid (1%); anti-oxidants vitamin E and polyphenols.

Good for: all skin types. Skin irritation, bites, stings, dermatitis, chapping, psoriasis, burns.

Properties: emollient, nourishing, skin protective, sun protective.

Comments: taken internally it stimulates bile flow and may be used as liver cleanser. Extra virgin – cold pressed is the best therapeutic and food quality. Unless labelled with these terms, it will be refined, blended and bland. However, when cold pressed, olive oil does retain more odour, which many people may find unacceptable and overpowering to fragrances of essential oils. For these reasons, practitioners may prefer more refined products. Cold pressed, it is one of the best oils for the skin and body.

## Safflower     Carthamus tinctorius

A native of Central Asia, the plant became cultivated in ancient Egypt and the Mediterranean; now widely cultivated also in Africa and California.

Character: pale yellow, traces of red if unrefined; light-medium texture.

Constituents: vitamin E; rich in poly-unsaturated linoleic acid (70–80%), oleic acid (14–15%).

Good for: all skin types.

Properties: emollient, nourishing, natural sun screen.

## Sesame     Sesamum indicum

A native to the Near East, the sesame plant has been cultivated in the eastern Mediterranean, Egypt, China, Indian sub-continent, Africa since ancient times. Sesame seeds are the basis of the sweet halva.

Character: cold pressing of white seeds yields a pale yellow oil; mild odour; light texture.

Constituents: oleic acid (37–42%), linoleic acid (37–47%) plus the lignans sesamine and sesamoline with beta sitosterol, all of which give it excellent keeping qualities.

Good for: all skin types, particularly dry.

Properties: emollient, nourishing (re-structuring), protective, a natural sun screen.

> **REMEMBER**
>
> Anti-oxidants are substances, including vitamin E and EFAs, which inhibit oxidation. In a vegetable oil oxidation causes rancidity. In the human body it causes free radical damage to cell walls, compromising their function and accelerating ageing.

Comments: do not obtain oil from roasted seeds, which has a strong odour and loses its therapeutic properties through heating. The genuine oil is stable and excellent for use in skin care; blends well with other oils, up to 20%. It is highly prized in Ayurvedic medicine for its healing and strengthening properties.

## *Sunflower*    **Helianthus annuus**
A native to the Americas, now widely cultivated in western Europe and in Russia and eastern Europe, where it has become a staple similar to olive oil in the Mediterranean. It is related to safflower.

Character: yellow; sweet, nutty odour if unrefined; medium to heavy texture (finer than olive oil).

Constituents: rich in oleic acid (15–25%), linoleic acid (62–70%), whose amounts will vary with the variety and refinement; inulin (an expectorant).

Good for: all skin types; resembles human sebum, natural skin lipids; helps damaged hair, leg ulcers, bruises.

Properties: emollient, skin and hair protective, nourishing; slightly diuretic internally.

Comments: an economic and good general massage oil; cold pressed is preferred. Organic is now available and affordable. It can extend more expensive material in a blend. Good for herbal macerations. In folk tradition it was rubbed it into rheumatic joints.

## *Soybean*    **Glycine max**
A native to China where it has been widely cultivated since very ancient times as a food. It is the basis of tofu, soymilk, miso and tempeh.

Character: pale yellow; light texture.

Contsitutents: rich in lecithin and vitamin E, polyunsaturated EFAs, oleic acid (17–23%), linoleic (50–62%), linolenic (4–10%).

Good for: all skin types.

Properties: emollient, protective, prevents drying.

Comments: it is usually highly refined, being produced mainly for the food and other industries. Its high lecithin content makes it a good base for such ingredients as dispersants, detergents and emulsifiers in cosmetics and food products. Not recommended for extensive use.

## Vegetable oils used 5–10% in a blend
These oils are either too expensive or too heavy in texture to be used 100% as a base for massage. They can be added in small amounts to the main massage oil or to a cream, lotion or gel base to provide further therapeutic properties.

## *Apricot and peach kernel oils*    **Prunus armeniaca and Prunus persica**
Natives of the Near East, their cultivation spread widely around the Mediterranean in ancient times and later to the Americas with European colonisation.

Character: similar to almond oil in appearance, these are light, fine oils.

Constituents: high in vitamins A and E; and oleic (55–75%) and linoleic (13–30%) acids.

Good for: all skin types; mature, dry, sensitive, inflamed skin.

Properties: anti-inflammatory, protective, moisturising.

Comments: both are good oils for facial applications. They are expensive to produce and often almond oil may be substituted for them or used to extend the true kernel oils and make them cheaper. So source with care to obtain genuine oils.

### *Avocado oil*    **Persea americana**
A native to central and southern America, the fruit is pear-like in shape; of the Lauraceae family.

Character: on cold pressing from the dried flesh, it will be slightly brown; on refining it becomes lighter, even green in colour; heavier texture.

Constituents: high in vitamin D and the phytohormone sterol, with lecithin and squaline.

Good for: all skin types; dry, damaged, fragile skin.

Properties: avocado has good penetration properties; it softens, moisturises and protects. Its cell-regenerating properties recommend its use for dry, damaged, fragile skin. The presence of sterol indicates a use for hormonal related skin changes.

### *Borage*    **Borage officinalis**
A native to Europe, it is also known as starflower. It has stunning blue flowers and is cultivated as medicinal herb and source of seed oil.

Character: clear; light texture.

Constituents: highest in GLA (8–25%) of the vegetable oils, plus substantial amounts of linoleic acid (30–40%), oleic acid (15–20%), palmitic acid (9–12%).

Good for: all skin types; ageing, inflamed skin.

Properties: anti-inflammatory.

Comments: its benefits are best obtained by taking it internally, though a capsule can be opened and the oil added to blends.

### *Evening primrose*    **Oenothera biennis**
A native to the United States, this biennial is now naturalised in Britain as a wayside flower.

Character: clear; light texture.

Constituents: second highest in GLA after borage oil (9–11%); high in linoleic acid (65–70%) and oleic acid (8–12%).

Good for: all skin types; dry, inflamed, ageing, damaged skin.

Properties: anti-inflammatory. Add to blends for eczema, psoriasis, dry skin, ageing or damaged skin.

Comments: the oil should also be taken internally for above conditions and PMS symptoms.

### *Jojoba oil*    **Simmondsia chinensis**
A native evergreen shrub of the deserts of California and Mexico (Baja).

Character: termed a 'liquid wax'; odourless and colourless; solidifies on cooling.

Constituents: yields up to 60% of a substance more like a wax because it has mostly wax, not alcohol based esters (triglycerides); high vitamin E content, making it more stable.

Good for: all skin types; ageing and inflamed skin.

Properties: highly skin compatible and used for moisturising, for protection, for inflammatory conditions such as acne, eczema, psoriasis as well as to inhibit ageing. It will combine with sebum, emulsifying it gently to unblock pores.

Comments: a balm-like consistency, useful for lip balms. It can be added to extend the life of a blend.

### *Macadamia nut oil*    **Macadamia ternifolia**
A native of Australia, the tree is now also cultivated in Hawaii.

Character: on cold pressing a pale, light odour; light texture.

Constituents: oleic acid (54–63%) and palmitoleic acid (16–23%), rare in a vegetable oil, which is also found in human sebum. Substantial amounts of saturated fats along with the unsaturated fats give it greater stability.

Good for: all skin types; inhibits skin and cell ageing.

Comments: add to a blend for its therapeutic properties and to inhibit rancidity.

### *Rose hip seed oil*    **Rosa rubiginosa**
A native of the Andes mountains of South America.

Character: on cold pressing, a golden red colour; light texture.

Constituents: trans-retinoleic acid, along with substantial amounts of linoleic and linolenic acids.

Good for: all skin types; especially for regenerating aged or damaged tissue, it is one of the best available oils. Use also for wounds, burns, eczema.

Comments: it is also obtained by solvent extraction. Extracting the seed from the pith is labour-intensive and this along with its shorter keeping time make a quality oil more expensive. Purchase in small amounts. Chilean scientists have done extensive research on this oil.

*Wheatgerm oil*     **Triticum sativum**
It is derived from the germ of the wheat grain.

Character: on hot pressing a deep orange, lightening to yellow if more refined; strong odour; heavier texture.

Constituents: high in anti-oxidant vitamin E; also contains phytosterols, vitamin A and B complex, and lecithin.

Good for: all skin types; dry, ageing or damaged skin. Use it also for tired muscles, e.g. in a sports massage blend.

Properties: highly anti-oxidant, skin protective.

Comments: no cold pressing is used for this oil; solvent or vacuum extraction methods are used.

Due to content of vitamin E, it is often added to blends to extend life, and nourish the skin.

## Macerated herbal oils
Fat-soluble components of medicinal herbs can be extracted when they are macerated (soaked) in vegetable oil, a process also called infusion. This is another way to bring the healing substances of plants to the body through the skin. These oils may be added in small amounts to a blend or used on their own for topical application.

*Arnica*     **Arnica montana**
Swiss mountain climbers found this alpine flowering herb healed their sprains and bruises. It must not, however, be applied to broken skin. It is good for injuries such as strained muscles or tendons, bruising (contusion), swelling and bone fractures. Homoeopathic preparations are also available for external and internal use.

*Calendula*     **Calendula officinalis**
The flowering heads of the 'pot marigold' contain carotenes and carotenoid, which give its characteristic orange and yellow colours. They are precursors of vitamin A and have excellent anti-oxidant properties. Calendula is a vulnerary and anti-inflammatory and is useful for damaged, bruised, wounded, skin; rashes, chapping, eczema, venous inflammation (varicose veins).

*Carrot*     **Daucus carota**
The root is rich in carotenoids and fat-soluble vitamins A, B, D, E. The extracted oil helps rejuvenate the skin. Use it for dry, ageing or damaged skin.

*Meadowsweet*     **Filipendula ulmaria**
This wayside herb has a long history of use as an anti-inflammatory and analgesic. It is one source of salicylic acid, the precursor of aspirin. Use it for arthritic conditions, inflammations and joint pain.

*St John's wort*     **Hypericum perforatum**
Since ancient times in Greece this has been used externally as a vulnerary. The flowers contain a red pigment, which gives the macerated oil its characteristic red hue. It is used for muscle aches, pains, strains

and sprains and for nerve-related pain such as sciatica, neuralgia. It is also good for wounds, haemorrhoids, sores, ulcers. It does increase the photo-sensitivity of skin so care should be taken not to expose the skin to sunlight immediately after its use.

## Other carriers

### Gels
These are produced from plant starches, any long chain polysaccharides such as are found in seaweeds (agar), quince and fungi. They are also produced from synthetic mimics of starches such as carbomer. Gels are highly hydrophyllic (water-attracting), thick and concentrated. They can absorb large amounts of added water, water-based substances or oil. They are clear and non-greasy and make ideal carriers where it is important to avoid heaviness and greasiness, for example, for a light application. They can be used to aid dispersal. Aloe vera has a natural gel in its leaves extracted by peeling the leaf and removing the gel. Unless preservatives are added, aloe gell must be used fresh but will keep for a few days in the cool (fridge).

### Cream bases
These are formed by the careful mixing of water, oil and wax. A quality **cream base** will have superior spreading qualities, i.e. be light to the touch, smooth and quickly absorbed. A cream base should be hypo-allergenic and non-perfumed.

### Lotions
These are formed by diluting a cream base with water, or hydrolat to create a thinner, lighter product.

### Cleansers
The best cleansers are derived from vegetable oils such as coconut or olive. They are used for shampoos and liquid soaps, providing another vehicle for applying essential oil. They are indicated for conditions of the hair or scalp or where a condition such as eczema is present in the scalp.

### Foods and herbs
These can also be used for face masks and poultices (Chapter 9) to which essential oils may be added. They can be produced by crushing, mashing or powdering. Some may need to have water added to achieve the right consistency of thickness and 'spreadability'. Oatmeal, ground rice, cucumber, potato, tofu, avocado and slippery elm powder are examples.

### Clays
These include Fuller's earth, green clay (French), betonite. They contain montmorillonite. They are detoxifying because they have excellent drawing/absorbent and astringent/toning properties. However, they also can be drying unless used carefully. Use only cosmetic grade clays.

### Honey
Honey is slightly astringent, inhibits bacteria and is healing. It can be used in small amounts in a face mask, poultice or clay pack, and as base for topical applications to wounds, infections and ulcers.

## Progress Check

1   What are the desired properties of an oil intended to be used as base oil 100%?
2   Why are some oils used less in a blend?
3   Why is it important to know the therapeutic properties of carriers?
4   What are the properties of clay?
5   What are the ingredients present in a good base cream?

*Making a simple cream base or Galen's cold cream*
Ingredients:

40 g/ml almond oil
10 g beeswax, grated or shredded
40 g/ml rose hydrolat
10 drops essential oil of choice

1   Place vegetable oil in a stainless steel or pyrex bowl and add beeswax. Place water or hydrolat in another bowl and place both bowls in a large shallow pan of warm water over a gentle heat.
2   Stir the oil and beeswax until well blended and melted.
3   Turn off heat.
4   Start adding the warm water to the oil–beeswax mixture a teaspoon or two at a time while beating with a rotary whisk. Continue to add water gradually while beating. It is like making a mayonnaise. When the water has been incorporated, the whole will form a firm, set cream.

5    When all the water has been incorporated stop beating at once. If using an electric mixer be sure to set it at the lowest speed. Over-beating can make the cream separate.

6    Add the essential oils. Divide up and bottle in jars and keep in a cool place or fridge. Or, alternatively, dispense the cream into different jars and store. Add and incorporate different essential oils to different jars as needed.

The cream will keep for several weeks in the cool. But if making larger batches, store in the fridge and dispense into smaller containers as needed. Other materials can be incorporated into the cream such as coco butter, or an enriching oil like wheatgerm. Adjust the amounts of beeswax or vegetable oil in this case.

## Key Terms

You need to know what these words mean. Go back through the chapter or check in the glossary to find out.

- carrier
- cold pressing
- cream base
- essential fatty acids
- fixed oil
- gel
- heat extraction
- Langerhans cells
- lotion
- phospholipids
- phytosterols
- solvent extraction

After reading this chapter you will be able to:

- understand how to create and prepare therapeutic blends of essential oils
- know the different carriers and material used in applying essential oils
- be able to choose the best application of essential oils for an intended purpose.

One important advantage of aromatherapy is that there are several ways in which essential oils may be introduced into the body. These are based on the pathways discussed in Chapter 2 and it would be a good idea to review that chapter now. Flexibility in application means that a therapist can choose the most appropriate method or methods for each client and also vary the methods used over time as needed. It is possible to effectively 'surround' the patient with aromatic essences by different applications, which helps to maximise their healing potential.

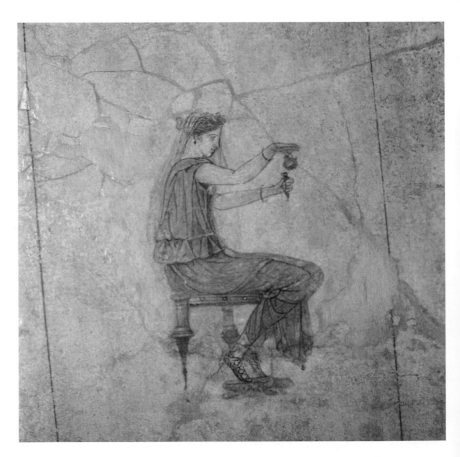

**Fig. 9.1** *Wall painting from the Villa Farnesina, Rome, c.50 BC. A girl pours scent into a small vase*

# Blending: an art and a science

Preparing essential oils for a therapeutic purpose is a very good example of the holistic approach to healing. The aromatherapist uses precise technical skill in dealing with the material substances. When choosing the essential oils, application route and carrier, the aromatherapist applies knowledge of the therapeutic properties of essential oils and relevant carrier substances. Knowledge of human biology and physiology is applied in understanding and assessing the patient's condition and constitutional type, in understanding how an essential oil is affected by the body. In addition the practitioner calls on his or her intuition and insights gained from clinical experience.

## Selecting the oils for the individual patient

Choosing oils will be based on the therapeutic strategy you have worked out for the patient or client after conducting the consultation and assessments, as taught by your tutor (perhaps using reflexology, muscle testing or a traditional medical model as guides).

The aim is to create a blend of essential oils to match the energetic balance and therapeutic needs of the patient. The blend aims to be a holistic one so you will include essential oils for:

- the important presenting symptom(s)
- the physical body and the mental–emotional or psychological, perhaps even the spiritual aspects of the patient, if these need attention
- the inherent constitutional balance or any imbalance you feel underlies the current condition, presenting symptoms.

Your tutor will be instructing you in the best method he or she has found for creating a blend. It is best to practise using only one to three essential oils in a blend at first for learning purposes. Use a format such as one suggested in Chapter 3 (pages 69–70) to record your selection.

The method of selecting essential oils for a patient:

1   Decide on the primary, secondary and, if indicated, a third condition of the patient that needs treatment. Then, for each condition, research and choose two or three relevant essential oils, using the therapeutic reference, the essential profiles and the aromatic biogram. Try to choose at least one from the **base, middle** and **top note** groups (see page 163). Write all these down. Take into account the chemistry and properties as well as the overall character of the essences and any precautions in their use, including whether the patient has an aversion to a particular scent.
2   Check your list and see if one essential oil is good for both primary and secondary conditions. Choose that essential oil as a preference and write it down.

3    Check the list again and see if another essential oil is good for both the secondary and tertiary conditions

4    Select a third essential oil from your list of possibles to cover a remaining condition, constitutional or energetic imbalance or psychological state not addressed by the first two selections. Try to make your blend holistic.

5    Review your list and make any adjustments.

6    Decide a method of application and a carrier material. For massage, choose the most appropriate carrier oil or oils.

7    Prepare the blend using the appropriate dilution (see page 166).

8    Check if the scent is satisfactory. More importantly, present the blend to the patient for acceptance. A good idea is to rub a tiny bit on to the skin of the patient's hand and request he or she smell it. Alternately, present the selected essential oils for the patient to scent before blending. If the patient is not pleased by the blend/selection, you can alter it, perhaps by adding a drop of lavender. If you have to alter it, again present it for acceptance. It is of course very important that the blend be attractive to the patient.

> **REMEMBER**
>
> A blend of essential oils is a synergistic new therapeutic entity, 'as if you had created a new essential oil' (Tisserand, 1977).

## Some considerations for blending

An essential oil can address one imbalance with one of its properties and another with another property. When blending, this versatility is put to good use. For example, both basil and ginger can help with sluggish digestion, while basil could also help with an anxious mood, and ginger with a generally sluggish circulation. Using both in a blend creates a synergy as they re-enforce or support each other in treating the digestion, while extending the blend to address two other aspects.

Sometimes, on the other hand, it may be a question of having to choose between two oils with the same property because one better matches the patient's needs or constitutional type in its other respects. This is where your own intuition and assessment of the patient's primary needs is your guide. There is a range of possibilities and two aromatherapists will not necessarily choose the same blend for the same patient – a phenomenon that underscores the uniqueness of each therapeutic encounter.

Another reason to choose an essential oil is because while suiting the therapeutic needs its fragrance contributes to the pleasing scent, for example, by enhancing, balancing or harmonising the different essences chosen. A harmonious fragrance that is attractive to the patient plays an important role through its effect on the mind and moods, promoting a sense of well-being that makes the body more open to other effects.

Finally it is entirely possible that just one essential oil is sufficient to address the needs of the patient. Do not feel you must blend several essential oils, if one answers the need.

## Fragrance notes

Another factor that can guide your selection is the concept of **fragrance notes** used by perfumers. It was devised by the Frenchman S. Piesse in the 19th century, when he grouped essential oils according to their different evaporation rates to obtain a quantitative measurement. He then related these to the range of notes in a musical scale. These categories can provide a useful guideline when learning about essential oils. You may find that different authors you refer to disagree slightly on the category for a given essential oil, one calling it a top note and one a middle note. This reflects the individuality inherent in the essential oils and in the practitioner. The top and base notes are a more sure contrast. You will in time get a feel for which note best describes an essence.

Relative to itself any essential oil can have all three notes, since its molecules themselves evaporate at different rates. However, rose, jasmine, frankincense, cypress and ylang ylang are considered to be the essences that most embody this phenomenon.

Bear in mind that in a particular blend a middle note may act as the top or base note, if a top or base note, respectively, is not included. Each category is relative to the others.

### Top notes
Their molecules evaporate at the fastest rate so they are first to stimulate olfaction. They give the very important first impression of a blend. If a drop is placed on blotting paper, the scent will not last as long as middle or base notes, only up to 24 hours. They can be sharp (lemon, thyme) or sweet (cinnamon, clove). Generally they impress as light, uplifting and refreshing. They may form a smaller proportion of a blend. Because they penetrate or act more quickly, they are considered to help relieve acute conditions, shock or pain.

In energetic terms they are opening and releasing.

Examples: basil, rosemary, bergamot, eucalyptus, lavender, lemon, petitgrain, cinnamon, clove.

### Middle note
The molecules evaporate at a slightly slower rate than the top notes. The scent of a drop placed on blotting paper lasts two or three days and so they are thought to give body to a blend and to link the top and base notes. They can enhance a blend by balancing other notes. Some consider that they act primarily on the digestion – notice many are the traditional culinary herbs – or the general metabolism.

In energetic terms they are centring.

Examples: chamomile, lavender, marjoram, peppermint, rosemary, black pepper.

### Base notes
The molecules evaporate at a slower rate and are thus used in perfumery to 'fix' a blend, to slow the evaporation of other notes. A base scent lasts up to one week. Some base notes may not be detected until a few minutes or moments after a bottle is opened (sandalwood). Their scent tends to develop over time. Others have a scent that is intense and can overpower in a blend. If so, it should comprise a smaller proportion of a blend. Base notes impart the lasting impression to a fragrance. They have a deepness and roundness to them, and are said to draw the blend down deep into the body.

In energetic terms they are grounding and can be used for relaxing or stabilising a nervous, erratic or spacy state.

Examples: benzoin, cedarwood, sandalwood, jasmine, rose, ylang ylang, neroli.

### Odour intensity

Another point to bear in mind when blending is that each oil has its own **odour intensity**. This is partly related to its evaporation rate and partly to other factors. It is just a fact of its personality, its nature and how this is perceived by an individual. Usually the more volatile top notes are the more intense – tea tree is an example – but not always. Sandalwood is very delicate and demurring. You may have to wait patiently before you can sense it. Rose, chamomile and jasmine are quite intense, yet they are base notes. You can only decide for yourself by practising olfaction on several oils and comparing them. Use odour intensity designations as a guide but remember the client or patient may react quite individually.

### *Table of odour intensities*
(From *The Art of Aromatherapy* by Robert Tisserand (1977))

Increasing from low to high odour intensity:

4 benzoin, bergamot, cedarwood, cypress, lavender, melissa

5 camphor, clary sage, juniper, marjoram, neroli, patchouli, sandalwood

6 fennel, geranium, hyssop, rosemary, ylang ylang

7 basil, black pepper, frankincense, jasmine, myrrh, peppermint, rose

8 eucalyptus

9 chamomile, cardamom

The main point is that if an odour is intense then it will probably need to be included in smaller amounts or it will overpower others in the blend. In general, add the intense essential oil first in half the amount of the others chosen, then add the others one by one, assessing as you go.

If meant for immediate use, the top notes will predominate on application, but as the oils live together for a while, for example, in a home prescription, the lower notes or less intense fragrance will come through.

### Testing a blend

Having prepared a blend, take a moment to scent it. Stir or swirl the blend together and smell it as a synergy. If preparing it for a client, rub a small amount to her inner wrist to let it react with her skin chemistry and stimulate her smell sense. Observe her reaction. If she is unhappy with it you can then rebalance it by adding more of one essential oil. Lavender can be used to harmonise a blend as it has the capacity to link other notes happily.

### Compatible blends of essential oils

Experience has shown that some essential oils will blend particularly well together. These are known as **compatible blends**. This can also be used as a guide to creating a synergistic blend.

## Essential oil fragrance groups. Essential oils within each group blend well together and also with oils from the starred groups

| Group 1 Flowers | Group 2 Citrus-like | Group 3 Herbs | Group 4 Trees |
|---|---|---|---|
| Chamomile | Bergamot | Basil | Cajeput |
| Geranium | Citronella | Clary sage | Cedarwood |
| Jasmine | Grapefruit | Fennel | Cypress |
| Lavender | Lemon | Hyssop | Eucalyptus |
| Neroli | Lemongrass | Marjoram | Juniper |
| Rose | Mandarin | Peppermint | Niaouli |
| Tagetes | Orange | Rosemary | Petitgrain |
| | Tangerine | Thyme | Pine |
| * 2 & 6 | * 3 & 1 | * 2 & 4 | Rosewood |
| | | | Tea Tree |
| | | | * 3 & 5 |

| + Group 5 Spices | Group 6 Exotics** | Group 7 Resins |
|---|---|---|
| Black pepper | Palmarosa | Benzoin |
| Cardamom | Patchouli | Frankincense |
| Cinnamon | Sandalwood | Myrrh |
| Clove | Vetivert | |
| Coriander | Ylang ylang | |
| Ginger | | |
| * 2 & 7 | * 1 & 7 | * 5 & 6 |

** Exotic is a relative term. To people of Asian or African culture Groups 3 or 4 could be exotics.

## Pre-blended formulations

In a beauty therapy clinic or spa or as a convenience in a clinical setting, practitioners may wish to make available blends, which are generally good for certain conditions that many people suffer from. In general, the same procedures are followed as for individual prescriptions with some exceptions:

1    Assess the purpose of the blend.
2    Choose the essential oils for the purpose, arranging them according to an order of therapeutic value. Remember to check them for suitability and cautions. You may want to differentiate them into types, for example: 'for normal skin', 'for sensitive skin'.
3    Choose the most appropriate carrier or combination of carrier materials.
4    Blend the essential oils and the carrier(s) in separate containers and leave for several hours if possible. Then blend them together, adding the essential oils slowly to the carrier base.
5    Label them with contents, date of preparation, title, your name and batch number if relevant.
6    Keep an exact, dated record of the blend's ingredients and their purpose in the blend.

**REMEMBER**

Margarite Maury greatly emphasised the importance of creating a blend as an individual prescription: matching the right essential oils for each patient at each encounter. This is what we strive to do in clinical aromatherapy. This is the holistic blend that will spark or strengthen the patient's innate healing energy.

## Summary

Here are some considerations to ponder when choosing essential oils, carriers and method of application:

◆ Is the ailment manifesting primarily as physical or as psychological/emotional?
◆ Is it an acute/superficial or a chronic/therefore more complex condition?
◆ Is it primarily a hot or a cold condition? Moist or dry? Local or systemic?
◆ Is the underlying constitutional type or *terrain* basically strong and experiencing only a temporary imbalance, or does it need strengthening or supporting in some aspect?
◆ Which approach needs most emphasis at this stage: cleansing–stimulation–elimination of congestion or toxins? soothing–calming–relaxation? strengthening–nourishing–tonification? (It is possible to combine two or more but the primary one receives more emphasis in a blend.)
◆ Does the blend include a top, middle and base note?
◆ Is the patient particularly sensitive or have other cautionary factors? (Age, frailty, skin sensitivity; upcoming travel arrangements can be disturbing to the system or may expose the patient to novel influences affecting the use of a particular oil.)
◆ Can you link the character of the patient to the character of the essential oil?
◆ Will the patient find the scent of the blend pleasing?

> **REMEMBER**
>
> If the scent of the blend is 'not quite right', or the patient is not happy with it, yet another essential oil can be added to balance, enhance or extend it. Be aware that some essential oils have quite an intense odour and tend to dominate a blend. They may need to be used in smaller proportions. Lavender is often used to harmonise other essential oils.

> **ACTIVITY**
>
> 1 Using the note categories and odour intensities, practise scenting different essential oils in each category. Make notes as you compare and contrast the groups. Do you agree with the placements?
>
> 2 Create a blend with an intense scent such as clary sage. Experiment adding quantities of other essential oils until you have a blend that feels well balanced and pleasant to you.
>
> 3 With a partner, give each other hypothetical patient descriptions and each of you create a blend for the patient the partner describes. Compare and discuss your creations and why you made the choices you did.

> **REMEMBER**
>
> Essential oils can range from light liquids to more viscous substances. Because of this variety, the equivalences for volumes and weights to millilitres will vary, e.g. thicker essential oils produce fewer drops per ml.

## Formulation guidelines and methods of application

The several ways of applying or using essential oil have been discussed in Chapter 2. Here are basic formulation guidelines for each.

### Quantities and dilutions

Following Tisserand, 1977, for blending and formulation purposes 1 ml, 1 cc (cubic centimetre) and 1 g are taken as interchangeable.

Equivalences:

1 ml = 20 drops

5 ml = 1 tsp/100 drops

30 ml = 1 fl oz = 30 g

500 ml = 1 pint

1,000 ml = 1 litre.

## Massage oil

For a massage blend the ratio of essential oil to vegetable oil is $2\frac{1}{2}$%. This rounds out as:

Dilution guide:

1 drop e.o. to 2 ml of carrier oil

6 drops e.o. to 12 ml of carrier oil

25 drops e.o. to 50 ml of carrier oil.

### Facial massage oil

Because facial skin can be more sensitive or develop broken capillaries, practitioners prefer to use a 1–1.25% dilution (decrease amount of essential oil) for facial applications.

In a full body massage the facial blend is usually created separately to allow for a higher dilution. Also, if different essential oils are therapeutically indicated for the face, a separate blend is made. Sometimes just one essential oil is used for the facial, often of the patient's favourite aroma. Alternately at the facial stage of the massage, if the selected essential oils are also appropriate for a facial skin, the blend is further diluted by adding an equal amount of carrier.

## Cream and lotion

A cream is an oil-and-wax based material made lighter by adding water and emulsified to hold its consistency. A lotion is formed by adding more water to this for a lighter material. The advantages are that they are not greasy, do not affect clothing, penetrate quickly and are user friendly. In addition to being used for topical application on a symptom area, they can be formulated by the therapist for home use as a hand, body or facial cream or lotion. This gives another opportunity for a daily systemic dose of healing actives and mood-affecting fragrance, which empowers the patient and greatly enhances treatment.

**REMEMBER**

The dilution of a blend may be increased (amount of essential oil decreased) for sensitive skin or decreased (amount of essential oil increased) for patients of larger build or thicker or congested skin.

**REMEMBER**

An evening foot and lower leg massage can be prescribed for home treatment. This is especially effective for insomnia, shaky leg syndrome, poor circulation, varicose veins, stiff or swollen ankles. Feet should be well massaged for up to 10 minutes, including between and around each toe.

**GOOD PRACTICE**

Avoid using mineral oil as it forms a barrier, preventing absorption of essential oils. Source your cream or lotion base from a good supplier.

It is generally more practical to purchase ready-made unfragranced cream and lotion bases. Here again quality is very important. When sourcing, ask for samples from a few wholesalers. Test each on your skin in different places and observe for ease of spread and penetration, a feel of smoothness and light texture. Bases should be hypo-allergenic. Professional quality bases are meant to be extended with therapeutic actives like essential oils, infused vegetable oils, herbal tinctures and hydrolats.

Dilution guide at 2.5%:

1 drop e.o. to 2 ml/2 g

6 drops e.o. to 12 ml/12 g

25 drops e.o. to 50 ml/50 g.

Method: rub gently into the body.

## Gel bases

A gel is a non-liquid, non-oily medium especially suited for rubbing into muscles and joints, for quick penetration without residue, for making eye care remedies, and for face **masks**. A fresh gel can be made at home using the inner juice of an aloe vera leaf or carrageen powder mixed with some water. These will last a few days if kept in the fridge.

Dilution guide:

1 drop e.o. to 2 ml/2 g

1–6 drops e.o. to 12 ml/12 g

6–25 drops e.o. to 50 ml/50 g.

For a face mask use a higher dilution, i.e. 1%.

For eye problems, using a hydrolat is preferable.

Method: apply to affected part, taking extra care if applying to the eye area.

## Ointments

An **ointment** is traditionally made from an animal fat such as lanolin, or a blend of oil and beeswax. It is heavier than a gel or cream and is intended for local or topical application as a healing salve or balm.

Dilution guide:

30 drops e.o. to 30 ml/g of ointment

(Note: the amount in drops is equal to the amount of base, i.e. twice the usual 2.5% concentration.)

Method: apply direct to affected part or place on a **compress** and apply.

Useful for: cuts, wounds, bruises, abrasions or as a chest rub for respiratory conditions.

Helichrysum is good for a bruise or other injury. The addition of a healing herbal infused oil like calendula or arnica, can augment the blend's effectiveness.

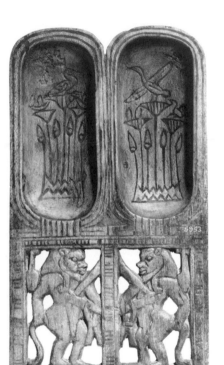

**Fig. 9.2a** *An Egyptian ointment spoon*

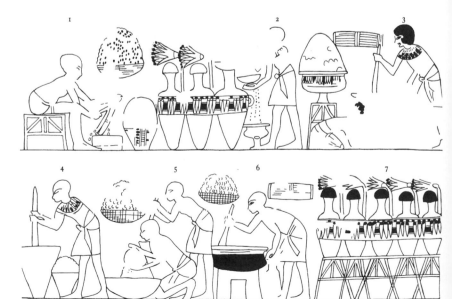

**Fig. 9.2b** *The manufacture of ointments in ancient Egypt*

## Liniments

A **liniment** is an application using spirits or cider vinegar as the carrier. It is non-oily, quickly penetrating and needs only a little rubbing in, if any, since the vinegar itself quickly evaporates. Liniments store for longer periods than oil-based preparations, almost indefinitely.

Dilution guide:

2–5 drops e.o. to every 10 ml of vodka or cider vinegar (1–2.5% dilution).

Method: apply to local area and rub briefly. Spray or drop from a dropper bottle on to the affected area. Use as compress.

Liniments are useful for suppurating skin problems such as herpes and weeping eczema; also for boils and shingles, and hair applications, such as for head lice.

## Mask and poultice

Essential oils can be added to these to enhance and extend their already considerable therapeutic effects.

Dilution guide:

1 drop e.o. for every 2 g of chosen substance, enough to cover the area

Water, warm, tepid or cold depending on the condition.

Method:

For the face mask: first cleanse the face and give a gentle massage with an appropriate essential oil blend. Having mixed the mask ingredients – essential oils last – apply to the face and allow the person to rest for 5–10 minutes. Remove gently with a moist soft sponge or face gauze. Apply some hydrolat, or a little water, then cream or lotion to close the pores and protect the skin.

(Note: if using a commercial mask base, follow instructions of manufacturer.)

For the **poultice**: first add the essential oil to the water. Place the substance chosen as the poultice on a plate and moisten this with the essential oil water, adding more water as necessary to form a cohesive mass. The poultice can either be applied to the local body part directly, or placed on to a piece of cotton gauze or fine cheesecloth cut to a larger size than the target area. It is then covered or wrapped up with more cloth and some plastic to keep it moist, and a hot-water bottle or warmed towel, if heat is needed. Repeat the application according to the condition, for example, if applied to a feverish or inflamed area, change the poultice every few minutes as it dries out; 1–3 times daily in chronic states.

### Compress: a local, external application

A compress takes advantage of the added benefit of water. It can be used in fevers, for local areas of inflammation, congestion or stiffness. It can also be used for internal organs, in which case the compress is placed over an affected part, such as the heart, stomach, intestines, liver, kidneys. As well as being used in the clinic, the treatment can be re-enforced/continued daily by having the patient treat him or herself at home.

Dilution guide:

4–5 drops e.o. in 250 ml of hot or cold water

Method: cut a piece of material – a flannel, gauze or handkerchief – just a little larger than the area treated. Add the essential oils to the water. Dip the cloth just lightly on to the surface of the water to pick up the essential oil, wring out slightly and place on to the affected part. Cover with towel and plastic. Leave for 20 minutes to 2 hours, depending on the case. Repeat as needed: e.g. in acute conditions, every half-hour. In case of inflammation or fever, as the compress dries, replace with a fresh one.

- Hot/warm compress: used for muscle ache, cramps, headaches, sinus blockage, for later treatment of sprain to increase blood circulation. Cover with a towel and perhaps a hot-water bottle or heated gel pack to keep it warm.
- Cold/cool compress: used for initial treatment for sprains, swelling (acute); fatigue; inflammation. Apply to the forehead and feet in fevers. Alternating hot–cold enhances healing by increasing circulation, relieving congestion.

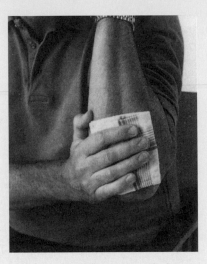

**Fig. 9.3** *Applying a compress*

## Inhalations/vaporisation

This application allows maximum direct penetration of mucous membranes and stimulation of olfactory nerves. **Inhalation** and **vaporisation** are good for respiratory conditions, emotional–psychological balancing and facial skin health.

Dilution guide:

8–10 drops e.o. added to 500–1,000 ml in a bowl of hot water

3–6 drops e.o. added to water in a steamer for a facial steam

2–5 drops e.o. neat on a tissue.

Method: add essential oils to the bowl of water or steamer on a stand in front of you (chair/table/seat). Place a towel over the head and lower head over the bowl, closing the eyes. Inhale calmly for 1 minute. Rest; then repeat several times. Use three or more times a day in acute conditions.

Apply essential oils to a tissue and sniff the tissue frequently during the day.

A warm steam may also be used for vaginal problems, the patient sitting in a suitably adapted seat over the bowl with blankets around to contain the steam.

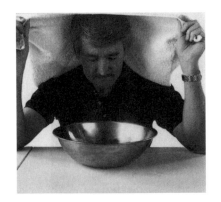

**Fig. 9.4** *An inhalation or facial/respiratory steam*

## Room vapourising

This is used to fill a room with healing aroma. It can be used for respiratory conditions, headache, insomnia or poor sleep, relaxation, improved concentration and mental alertness, hyperactive states or anxiety. It can also be used in rooms in hospices, hospitals or any area to cleanse or counter-balance unpleasant odours.

Dilution guide:

4–6 drops e.o. to a burner, light bulb ring or saucer of water.

Method: place a tablespoon of water in the bowl of a ceramic vaporiser, add essential oils. Light the candle.

(Caution: do not use burners in children's rooms or leave children alone with a burner.)

Add drops of essential oil to a light bulb ring and place over the bulb.

Add drops of essential oil to a saucer of warm water. Renew at intervals.

Use a electrical diffuser as directed by the manufacturer.

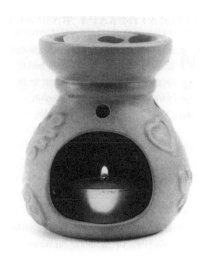

**Fig. 9.5a** *A ceramic burner*

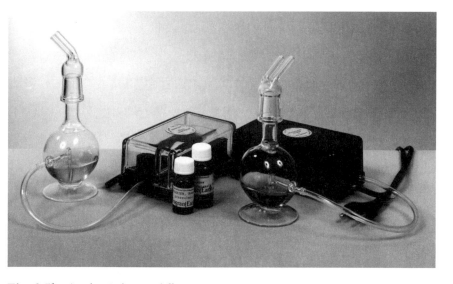

**Fig. 9.5b** *An electrical room diffuser*

## Sprays

A spray bottle can be used to deliver essential oils to an area that cannot be touched, such as a burn, wound or ulcer. This method should only be used after specific training in its administration. Carriers for sprays include spirits (vodka), diluted gels or commercial dispersant. Dilution should be high, e.g. 10 drops in 100 ml.

## Baths

Therapeutic baths are a very ancient form of healing used by many peoples (e.g. Egyptians, Greeks and Romans). Thermal springs are sites of healing. Baths play a central role in naturopathy. Water itself has a strong healing power and is an ideal conductor of the healing properties of natural substances. Do not underestimate the power of this healing technique. Aromatic baths benefit the patient by both the inhalation route and the skin absorption route (penetration is increased many times). Maurice Messegué, the French herbalist who resurrected this form of therapy to great success felt that foot and hand baths were actually more potent than a full bath. The famous 19th-century Father Sebastian Kneipp also used aromatic herbal baths extensively.

A daily aromatic full or foot bath would be excellent as part of a programme for depression, or other mental–emotional conditions. Use uplifting, invigorating essential oils in the morning and relaxing, calming oils in the evening to ensure a good night's sleep. Baths are also good for muscle fatigue and skin conditions.

### Full bath

Dilution guide:

3–12 drops e.o. depending on the size of the bath and the sensitivity of the skin

3 ml/60 drops e.o. to 100 ml carrier for a home preparation, using 10 ml of the blend per bath.

Method: wait until the bath is fully drawn, only then add the essential oils to minimise evaporation before bathing. A good idea, especially for sensitive skin, is to add the essential oils to a teaspoon of fixed oil, milk or vodka first. The essential oils will form a slight film, which will then cling to the body and this along with the warm water aids absorption. Relax in the bath for 15–20 minutes. If possible shower off with a little cold water to invigorate the body. After drying, massage the body lightly with a small amount of massage oil to protect the skin.

(Note: a dispersant bath oil, which enables the oil and water to form an emulsion, is available from some suppliers.)

### Foot or hand bath

Dilution guide:

3 drops e.o. in approximately 2 litres water.

Method: renowned French herbalist Maurice Messegue recommended having therapeutic foot and hand baths morning and evening, soaking the parts up to the wrist or ankle for 8 minutes each time. Generally these are taken in warm water, though hot and cold foot baths may be alternated to increase the beneficial effect and stimulate circulation.

### Sitz baths

A **sitz bath** can be used for conditions of the lower abdomen and genito-urinary organs.

A cold bath lasting for 1–3 minutes is used for inter-menstrual bleeding or excessive menstruation, and is invigorating to the circulation. The room must be warm. A warm bath (about 26°C) for 15 minutes is better for relaxing, relieving pain and treating urinary conditions, gout, haemorrhoids and constipation.

Dilution guide:

6 10 drops e.o. or 5 drops per litre of water.

Method: draw bath water only to cover the hips. A sitz bath is ideally done with two baths/basins designed for the purpose, sometimes one with warm, the other with cold water to generate circulation. At home the effect may be approximated by, if at all possible, sitting sideways in the bath with legs and feet outside the bathtub in another basin.

### Children's baths

For an infant or young child, always dilute the essential oils in a teaspoon of carrier (oil, full-fat milk or dried milk) before adding to the water to prevent irritation if the child puts a hand into his or her mouth or eyes.

Dilution guide:

1 drop e.o. to a baby-bath container of warm water for an infant

2–3 drops e.o. to the amount of water for a toddler in a full bath.

## Douche

This vaginal wash or **douche** is a good method for helping genito-urinary problems such as cystitis, thrush, pruritis (itching).

Dilution guide:

4–6 drops e.o. to 500 ml boiled, body-warm water and 1 tsp cider vinegar/ natural yoghurt. These help restore acid pH to the vaginal environment. Shake well.

Method: fill the douche bag with the aromatic water, and administer as instructed by the manufacturer, ideally lying on the back and retaining for 10–20 minutes. Use once daily for from 3–7 days in acute conditions. Rest a few days. Repeat as needed and monthly for a while to maintain health, in concert with healthy diet.

## Tampon

A mini-tampon can be adapted as a vehicle for aromatherapy to aid genito-urinary problems and haemorrhoids.

Dilution guide:

2–4 drops e.o. to 500 ml of a half-and-half mix of yoghurt, or apple cider vinegar, and spring water.

Method: soak a tampon and insert to vagina (or rectum) in the morning, remove at night, or vice versa. Repeat daily until cleared. You may start with a higher dilution and gradually decrease dilution to the tolerance level.

## Aroma body wrap

This is performed in spas or beauty clinics. It can be done in your treatment room. Try it yourself at home. The warmth of the body will draw the essential oils from the towel and the scent will be inhaled, affecting the entire body via olfaction.

Equipment:

therapy couch (bed/table), head rest

plastic sheeting cut to blanket size

blanket, single bed size

warmed bath sheet towel, smaller towels if needed for feet.

500 ml of hot water in a spray bottle blended with 10–15 drops e.o.

Method: prepare the couch: cover with the blanket, then plastic and then bath towel. Have the client lie down supine, support the head with a cushion. Shake the bottle of essential oil water vigorously and spray the bath towel coming into contact with the skin. Wrap the patient up quickly in towel, plastic and blanket. Leave to rest for 10–15 minutes in a quiet atmosphere.

## Shampoo

This application is good for scalp problems such as dandruff, eczema of the scalp or alopecia.

Dilution guide:

25 drops e.o. to 100 ml unperfumed shampoo base.

Method: shampoo the hair, rinse.

> **REMEMBER**
>
> For those with sensitive skin, infants and young children, essential oils must be diluted before being added to bath water.

## Hair oil treatment

This is useful for head lice, dandruff, alopecia and maintenance of healthy hair.

Dilution guide:

25 drops e.o. to 50 ml carrier oil or

25 drops e.o. to 25 ml aloe vera gel and 25 ml carrier.

Method: apply oil and massage in. Wrap with hot towel creating a skull cap, and allow to soak 20 minutes or, covered with a secured shower cap, leave overnight. Shampoo out the next day, first applying the shampoo neat before rinsing out. Repeat if necessary.

Alternatively put 2 drops of e.o. on the bristles of a brush and brush hair daily to prevent lice or help dandruff. Use rosemary and eucalyptus for adults, tea tree or lavender for children. Use only 1 drop on the brush for under 5s.

## Mouthwash and tooth care

Useful for gingivitis and oral hygiene.

Dilution guide for mouthwash:

3 drops e.o. to 100 ml cool, boiled water or spring water.

Method: rinse the mouth 3 x daily after meals.

Dilution guide for toothpaste:

3 drops e.o. to 100 mg of clay – Fuller's earth, kaolin or green clay. Apply a small amount to a toothbrush.

Method: brush teeth gently after meals.

## Internal/oral use of essential oils

Currently this use is not advised for aromatherapists unless they have undergone further training in aromatic medicine. Unless dispensed by a properly trained person the practice is dangerous. Untrained practitioners will not be insured for prescribing essential oils for internal use. Most professional organisations prohibit internal use by their members. The following is for information only.

Traditionally in France, essential oils have been used internally. In simple home use they are added to honey and perhaps apple cider vinegar and this is mixed into water. Or a drop or two is added to a herbal tea (the important point being to protect the mucous membranes from damage by direct contact). Additionally, many medical practitioners prescribe them, usually after an aromatogram; they will be dispensed in gelules or capsules filled with vegetable oil, or other excipient. They have been used very successfully in this way for acute infections such as bronchitis and gastro-enteritis where their antibacterial, antiviral properties are so important. They have also been used for preventive care, for example, to avoid infections while travelling.

> **REMEMBER**
>
> Giving a client one or more ways of using essential oils at home enhances and extends the effectiveness of the therapy by enabling daily doses of small amounts of essential oils.

**ACTIVITY**

1 Make a cream following the instructions given above and write up your results.
2 Give yourself a douche using essential oils and report on your observations.

3   Practise giving yourself a facial steam using the bowl
    method above and one chosen essential oil. Report on your
    observations of the effect it has on you.
4   Have a foot or hand bath with a chosen essential oil for a
    purpose, for three mornings and evenings, and report on
    your results.
5   Practise using a compress and report your results.

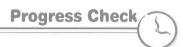

**Progress Check**

1   What are the advantages of a cream and a lotion as carriers?
2   What are the therapeutic benefits of baths?
3   What is the dilution of essential oils for infants and young
    children?
4   In what circumstances would you recommend diluting
    essential oils before adding to the bath?
5   Why is it dangerous to ingest essential oils?
6   For what conditions are inhalations particularly useful? How
    could you use them?
7   When might you use a compress? A liniment?

## Key Terms

You need to know what these words mean. Go back through the
chapter or check in the glossary to find out.

- compatible blends
- compress
- douche
- fragrance notes
- inhalation/vaporisation
- liniment
- mask
- odour intensity
- ointment
- poultice
- sitz bath
- top, middle and base notes

After working through this chapter you will be able to:

◆ relate the properties of essential oils to each of the body's major systems and some conditions affecting them

◆ recall the inter-relationships and integration of the body's organs and functions.

In addition to the information presented thus far about essential oils, their interactions with the body and their therapeutic properties, an awareness of how they can be used to affect imbalances in each of the body's systems is also useful. This chapter can serve as a reference for which essential oils to consider choosing. Even when focusing treatment on a specific area, we need to bear in mind any other areas that may be affecting the local situation and include treatment for these as well. Again, the aim is to trigger or enhance the body's own healing mechanisms and optimise the performance of organ functions.

This chapter is not intended as a substitute for the necessary study of anatomy and physiology and basic pathology required of a professional aromatherapist, study of which is a separate aspect of training beyond the scope of this book. Texts explaining basic pathology of common conditions include:

Balch, James F. and Balch, Phyllis A. (2000) *Prescription for Nutritional Healing*, Avery Publishing, New York.

Ball, John M. D. (1990) *Understanding Disease*, C. W. Daniel, Saffron Walden.

Murray, Michael and Pizorno, Joseph (1990) *Encyclopedia of Natural Medicine*, Little, Brown and Company, New York and London.

Battaglia, Salvatore (1995) *The Complete Guide to Aromatherapy*, The Perfect Potion, Queensland, Australia (includes very good discussions of conditions for different body systems).

The suggestions of essential oils presented here aim to give a broad idea of possible selections. They are not to be exhaustive or prescriptive. When treating a patient, students should research each suggested oil's profile to match the best oil(s) for the individual patient's condition and constitutional type.

## The nervous system

Communication, response, movement.

The nervous system is an important body communication network, mediating between sensations and the reactions to these, and initiating all

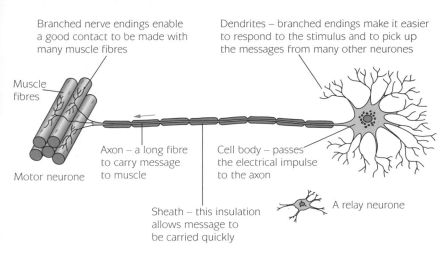

Branched nerve endings enable a good contact to be made with many muscle fibres

Dendrites – branched endings make it easier to respond to the stimulus and to pick up the messages from many other neurones

Muscle fibres

Motor neurone

Axon – a long fibre to carry message to muscle

Cell body – passes the electrical impulse to the axon

Sheath – this insulation allows message to be carried quickly

A relay neurone

**Fig. 10.1a** *Motor neurons carry impulses from the CNS (brain and spinal cord) to muscles and some glands via the sympathetic and parasympathetic systems*

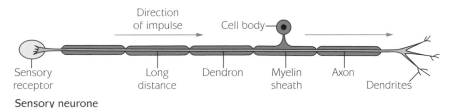

Direction of impulse

Cell body

Sensory receptor

Long distance

Dendron

Myelin sheath

Axon

Dendrites

Sensory neurone

**Fig. 10.1b** *Sensory neurons convey impulses to the CNS from sensory receptors in tissues*

the body's muscular activity, both voluntary and involuntary. The system works in conjunction with the endocrine glands to maintain the body's immunity, homeostasis, and its response to – and recovery from – stress, whether physical, emotional or mental. The nervous system is involved in every bodily function.

The system makes possible the organism's sensitivity to its internal environment and external surroundings, and provides mechanisms for relating to these, adjusting to them, and coordinating a response. In many conditions, the nervous system needs attention, and particularly if stress is a factor the autonomic system, whose two aspects, sympathetic and parasympathetic, may need balancing, calming or strengthening.

Pain is the body's communication that there is something wrong in a bodily part. Pain experienced in one place may in fact be referred from a problem located in another. Physiologically pain is a heightened state of nerve activity. When the cause or imbalance is not resolved, pain becomes part of a chronic pattern, which further weakens and depletes the body's energy. Therefore, when treating pain, it is important to also determine the imbalance that is causing it and to treat that system or part as far as possible.

Energetically the nervous system corresponds primarily to the air element and is prone to imbalance due to excess cold, to blockage or to irritation. Air, which is closely linked to the innate vital force, *vis vitalis*, ideally moves freely and smoothly while at the same time being grounded in regularity and rhythm. When air energy is ungrounded, it may show as: lack of concentration, a spacey feeling, loss of memory or consciousness, poor sleep, or signs of hyperactivity. When air is blocked

REMEMBER

Deep abdominal breathing nourishes vital energy. Essential oils breathed during the practice of deep relaxation help maintain its free and balanced flow.

or congested, this may show as tension, numbness, tingling, spasm, paralysis, pain, arrhythmia. Any trauma significantly influences the nervous system. If a person feels cold either physically or emotionally (isolated, lonely), a nervous system/air energy imbalance is a possible result. Accordingly, balance comes from warming, from clearing obstructions, from soothing and relaxing, and enhancing emotional support.

## Integrative physiology

Postural imbalances in the spine or tight muscles may interfere with optimum transmission of nerve impulses to organs and tissues. Irritations from repetitive strain injuries, or injuries that have not healed can cause chronic pain. Emotions can affect the functions of the nervous system.

## Essential oils for the nervous system

| |
|---|
| Grounding: valerian, benzoin, frankincense, lavender, vetiver |
| Relaxing tension or spasm, relieving stress: lavender, basil, marjoram, petitgrain, bergamot, neroli, rose, chamomile (especially *C. nobile*), clary sage, ginger, jasmine, geranium, sandalwood, vetiver, ylang ylang; In general, ester-rich essential oils for relaxation, ether-rich for muscle spasm or tension |
| Pain (headache, muscular, nerve): chamomile, basil, marjoram, lavender, juniper, eucalyptus, peppermint, juniper |
| Calming the sympathetic nervous system: spikenard, benzoin, lavender, petitgrain, bergamot, ylang ylang, bitter orange |
| Anxiety: basil, bergamot, lavender, jasmine, ylang ylang, neroli, patchouli, rose, marjoram, frankincense, sandalwood, bitter orange |
| Toning the nervous system, relieving mental fatigue: sage, rosemary, peppermint, tropical basil, juniper, clove bud, thyme |
| Depression: as for anxiety, plus geranium, melissa, mandarin, sandalwood |

REMEMBER

Use passive holding or gentle massage techniques to relax the diaphragm, head, feet and/or spinal column whenever the patient has been experiencing pain as part of his or her condition. This will have a deep effect on the whole body.

ACTIVITY

Research and describe the difference between the central and peripheral nervous systems. Draw a diagram of the sympathetic and parasympathetic systems. As you work visualise the anatomy and function of each part.

## The immune system

Preservation of individual vital force.

Believing prevention is better than having to cure, aromatherapy recognises that when the vital force, the constitution and the body's *terrain* are strong, the body can usually overcome disease organisms. The strength and integrity of the immune system is a reflection of the vital force.

Immunity epitomises holism because it involves the whole body and the body's relationship with its environment. Our immunity is provided for both in each and every cell – called cellular immunity – and also in bodily fluids and hormonal processes – called humoural immunity. It has many aspects including hormones, special lymphatic cells, the blood transportation system, nerves, organs like the liver and spleen, and chemicals such as neurotransmitters and neuropeptides. When the body is congested, when it is weakened by repeated stress, when waste is allowed to build up in the body – either physically through poor nutrition and poor elimination, or emotionally or mentally in the form of unwanted or unneeded feelings and attitudes – immunity becomes compromised because the constitutional balance or *terrain* is altered to one in which pathogens can thrive, tissues degenerate and auto-immune conditions manifest (food intolerance, allergies, chronic inflammatory states). Immune integrity needs to be nourished and protected by positive life habits.

The immune system comprises:

- the endocrine glands – pineal, pituitary, thymus, thyroid, parathyroid, adrenal, pancreatic
- the nervous system
- the eliminative, detoxifying organs such as the liver, kidney, skin, lungs
- the lymphatic system
- the spleen
- the skin and mucous membranes
- mechanisms within individual cells for self-protection.

Each of these interacts in the complex functions of the immune system.

Energetically the immune system involves every element and quality and represents their harmonious functioning. When weakened, symptoms usually appear as imbalances of water and fire. Immunity operates in a fluid medium; it mounts fiery defensive mechanisms to counter toxins. Treat imbalances with fluid balancing or circulatory essential oils (diuretic, diaphoretic, circulatory regulators or venous tonics) and disinfecting, blood purifying oils to clear toxins or pathogens provoking inflammation or fever.

> **REMEMBER**
> Stress is known to greatly lower the body's immune function. Consider essential oils to counteract stress when immunity is low.

## Essential oils for the immune system

| |
|---|
| Restoring, strengthening or protective for membranes: eucalyptus, rosemary, pine, sage, thyme, tea tree, peppermint, juniper, myrrh |
| Stress relieving and balancing of psycho-neuro-endocrine function: lavender, basil, marjoram, petitgrain, bergamot, neroli, geranium |
| Enhancing organs of detoxification: lemon, rosemary, juniper, eucalyptus |
| Stimulating elimination of excess mucus: tea tree, niaouli, rosemary, thyme, sage, cajeput |
| Auto-immune/allergic reactions: chamomile (*Matricaria recutita*), lavender, clary sage, geranium |
| Tonifying the spleen: coriander |
| Supporting the fight against infectious pathogens: bergamot, cajeput, cinnamon, eucalyptus, lemon, lemongrass, niaouli, pine, rosemary, sage, tea tree, thyme |
| Reducing fever or inflammation: chamomile, yarrow, ginger, eucalyptus, lemon, peppermint, lavender, sandalwood |

# The endocrine system

Communication, balance and integration.

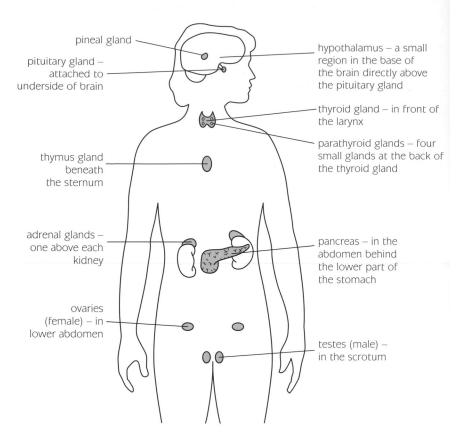

**Fig. 10.2** *The endocrine glands*

The endocrine glands secrete hormones into the bloodstream. Each hormone carries a message to a particular organ or cell, regulating its functions (stimulating or inhibiting a function) and keeping it in tune with the rest of the body. The endocrine glands help maintain homeostasis, the integrating and balancing of functions into one finely-tuned whole.

## Functions of hormones

- In close co-operation with the nervous system, hormones enable inner communication between cells and regulate many physiological functions to maintain homeostasis and balance. Good endocrine function is important for both optimum energy and restful calm.

- As part of the immune system, hormones enable us to both respond to and recover from stress and pathogenic challenges.

- As part of the reproductive system, hormone secretions regulate healthy functioning of the reproductive organs.

## Endocrine glands and hormones

| Gland | Hormone |
|---|---|
| The pineal gland | melatonin, adrenoglomerulotropin |
| The pituitary gland | GH, MSH, TSH, ACTH, ADH FSH, LH, prolactin, oxytocin endorphin |
| The thyroid gland | thyroxin, tri-iodo-thyronine, calcitonin, oxytocin, antidiuretic hormone |
| The para-thyroid glands | parathyroid hormones |
| The thymus gland | thymosin, thymic humoural factor, thymic factor, thymopoetin |
| The islets of Langerhorn (pancreas) | glucagon, insulin |
| The adrenal glands | mineral corticoids, gluco-corticoids, gonado-corticoids (cortex), adrenalin, noradrenalin (medulla) |
| The ovaries | oestrogen, progesterone, relaxin |
| The testes | testosterone, inhibin |

**ACTIVITY**

Research the activity of each endocrine gland and what action each of the above hormones performs.

## Essential oils for the endocrine system

By means of the olfactory-neuro-endocrine pathway, any essential oil whose fragrance is pleasing to an individual can be used to influence endocrine function (see Chapter 2).

Adrenal tonic: geranium, thyme ct. thymol, pine, basil

Calm sympathetic nervous system, regulating adrenals: ylang ylang, lavender, jasmine

Pituitary/endocrine tonic: peppermint

Thyroid balancing: clove bud, marjoram, myrrh

Balance of pancreatic hormones: benzoin

Promote secretion of endorphins: sandalwood, jasmine, ylang ylang, rose, lavender. Any essential oil whose odour is very pleasing and comforting to an individual has this capacity for that person

## Integrative physiology

Endocrine glands need to receive good nerve and blood supply, and optimum nutritional support.

**ACTIVITY**

Review the anatomy and physiology of the endocrine glands. Then visualise the process of olfaction-neuro-endocrine stimulation and the initiation of a cascade of benefits to the system.

# The respiratory system

Rhythm of life, vehicle of consciousness.

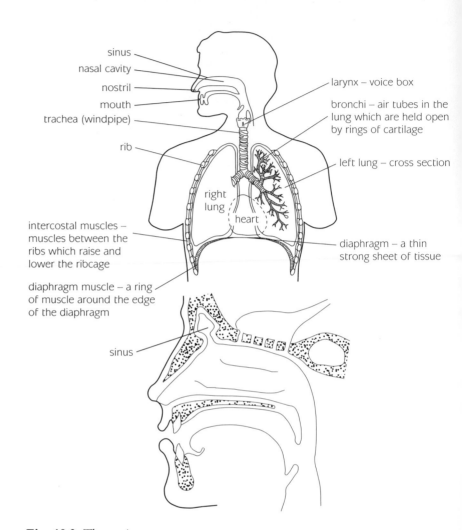

**Fig. 10.3** *The respiratory system*

Without the breath of life we would not live for more than a few minutes, hence breathing is the primary vital function. The respiratory system receives the nourishing vital force as air. Respiration has a dual life-saving function: providing oxygen for the metabolic functions of cells and eliminating their gaseous waste. The lungs nourish and they cleanse. Through the mucous membranes and cilla of its passages, the respiratory system forms a first line of defence against airborne pathogens.

Energetically the respiratory system relates to the air element. This makes it vulnerable to excess dryness and cold, and also to congestion if the mucous membranes are clogged with excessive mucus. Excess mucus is an ideal breeding ground for pathogens. Often the excess is created by an imbalance in the stomach or colon. Balance with warming, stimulating or calming, or antimicrobial essential oils as needed.

## Integrative physiology

- Breathing is a rhythmic activity, closely related to the heart's rhythmic contractions. Blood passes from the heart to the lungs for oxygenation before returning to the general circulation. The depth and rhythm of the breathing is intimately connected to the nervous system, to our emotions and our mental awareness. Breathing is in a sense the physical manifestation of our consciousness. Emotional and mental issues, for example, fear and anxiety, can both influence and reflect breathing. As the yogis of India have demonstrated, we can influence our emotions and our mental states, our response to stress, indeed our entire health by practising deep, rhythmic, calm breathing.
- Breathing influences the lymphatic system and immune systems.
- A poorly functioning digestive system (salivary glands, stomach, small intestine, colon) can influence the respiratory system. Along with poor diet, poor digestion can create dysbiosis in the gastro-intestinal tract, an environment that fosters formation of excess mucus or can trigger the onset of allergies such as asthma.
- Respiration influences olfaction. While olfaction is not neurologically part of the breathing mechanisms, still volatile molecules are airborne to olfactory sensors in the mucous membranes of the nose. If these membranes are congested, olfaction and consequently the limbic brain's responses to it are affected.

## Essential oils for the respiratory system

| |
|---|
| Sinus/lung/mucous membrane congestion: eucalyptus, rosemary, sage, thyme, pine, tea tree, niaouli, cajeput, myrtle, basil, ginger, black pepper |
| Cough: aniseed, peppermint, thyme, sage, pine |
| Promote elimination of toxins: diaphoretics and diuretics to cleanse the blood and lymph; juniper, ginger, black pepper, fennel, rosemary, yarrow |
| Digestive balance, to prevent formation of toxins and excess mucus: carminatives and cholagogues; cardamom, ginger, fennel, chamomile, basil, marjoram, mandarin, lemon, rosemary |
| Counter pathogens in the respiratory system: terpene, ketone or alcohol rich essential oils; tea tree, thyme, niaouli, eucalyptus, pine, sage, thyme |
| Irregular or anxious breathing, asthma: aniseed, cedarwood, frankincense, basil, sandalwood, lavender, myrtle, petitgrain, ylang ylang |

## The lymphatic system

Ocean of life: nourishing, cleansing, protecting.

The lymphatic system is intimately connected with all systems and functions: for example cardio-vascular function, cell metabolism, immunity, nutrition, glandular secretions, bone and nerve.

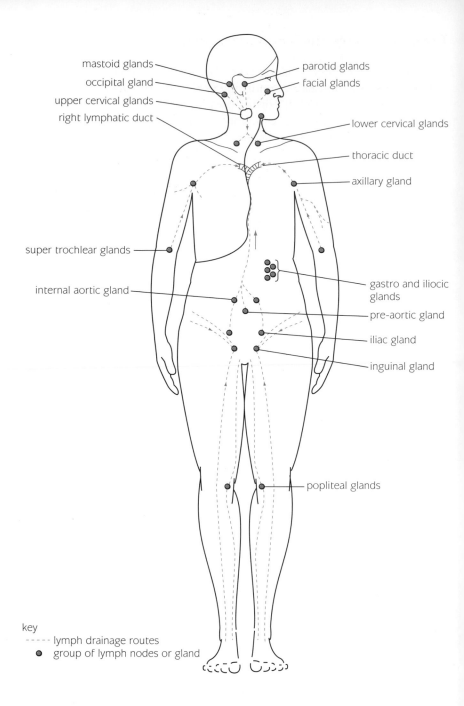

mastoid glands
occipital gland
upper cervical glands
right lymphatic duct
parotid glands
facial glands
lower cervical glands
thoracic duct
axillary gland
super trochlear glands
internal aortic gland
gastro and iliocic glands
pre-aortic gland
iliac gland
inguinal gland
popliteal glands

key
----- lymph drainage routes
● group of lymph nodes or gland

**Fig. 10.4** *The lymphatic system*

Energetically, it is an aspect of the water element and is like an ocean of life-giving fluid in which all our cells are floating and by means of which they receive nourishment and are relieved of their wastes.

## ACTIVITY

Review the anatomy and physiology of the lymph system. Visualise the lymph fluid as a viscous, straw-coloured, honey-like liquid. This fluid is transported through special vessels and to nodes for filtering and removal of pathogens by special lymph-immune cells. Lymph lacteals in the small intestine aid in the absorption of nutrients. The lymph fluid around cells has a role in regulating osmotic pressure and fluid balance. Lymph vessels interconnect with blood capillaries, carrying in nutrients, removing cell waste.

## Essential oils for the lymphatic system

Infections: antimicrobials; tea tree, niaouli, thyme, sage, eucalyptus, pine, lemongrass, palmarosa, cajeput

Fluid retention: warming, fluid circulating stimulants; black pepper, ginger, rosemary, cypress

Fluid retention: diuretics, astringents; juniper, cedarwood, fennel, sandalwood, coriander, geranium, grapefruit

Immune enhancing: chamomile (*Matricaria recutita*), basil, lemon balm/melissa, yarrow, lavender, tea tree, lemon, thyme, bergamot

Lymphatic congestion, swelling: circulation stimulants (above) and astringents: lemon, cedarwood, benzoin, rosemary, sage; soothing inflammation: lavender. Hydrolat gargles for sore throat: lavender, rose, chamomile

**REMEMBER**

Lymph lacteals in the small intestine can become irritated by poorly digested proteins or entero-toxins, which can trigger allergic responses or auto-immune inflammations.

## Essential oils and cellulite

When the body produces too much waste and/or cannot efficiently eliminate it, it sometimes stores it in connective tissue surrounding subcutaneous fat cells. Or the body may try to dilute the toxins by fluid. Due to such water and waste these tissues harden, creating the formation of thicker, congested skin, which shows as pitting when skin is pinched. Hormone factors also influence the collection and storage of wastes in tissue cells.

Essential oils can help reduce cellulite if used as part of a holistic programme to improve the body's functions. Such a programme should include reducing or coping positively with any contributing stress factors, adequate exercise, improving the diet and avoiding stimulants, enhancing blood and lymph circulation by, for example, massage and skin scrubbing, ensuring the liver and the eliminative channels (skin, kidneys, lymph, colon and lungs) are working optimally.

A suggested programme for cellulite is to create several blends and alternate them on a weekly basis. Each blend should be massaged into affected areas by the patient twice daily and the patient should receive aromatherapy massage once a week as part of the health improvement programme.

Essential oils for cellulite: juniper, rosemary, lemon, cypress, grapefruit and fennel.

**REMEMBER**

Massage promotes good lymph circulation. The lymph circulation is partly a cleansing mechanism. Give attention to it at each treatment.

## Integrative physiology

The lymph interacts with: adrenal glands, liver, heart and blood circulation and vessels, immune system, blood cleansing by the liver, kidneys, lungs and skin.

# The urinary system

Waters of life.

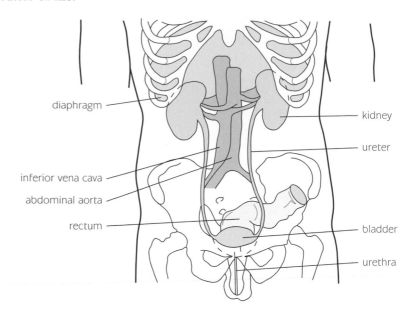

Fig. 10.5 *The urinary system*

The pairing of kidneys reminds us of a pair of balancing scales, symbolising their function of balancing water metabolism and acidity–alkalinity. The kidneys help purify the heat and acidity from the blood and eliminate metabolic waste. Good kidney function supports good cardio-vascular function through purifying the blood and by their influence on blood pressure. The kidneys regulate fluid balance and blood volume via the antidiuretic hormone and the kidney enzyme rennin. The bladder is also involved in the stress response and can react to emotions of fear and anxiety.

Energetically the kidneys and water element symbolise the balance of the water as emotional balance. Kidneys represent the discrimination between what attitudes and emotions are good to conserve and what need rejecting. Since water is inherently cool and heavy, collection of fluid in the lower extremities suggests kidney weakness. Moisture is the vital fluid enabling reproduction and growth. It is a stabilising, life-promoting influence. However, if it becomes damned up to excess (fluid retention, swelling) or depleted to deficiency, it can provoke tension, irritability, worry, fear and anxiety. If isolated from the warmth of love, water can become cold, congested and unable to promote healthy function. The kidneys influence the lower extremities, lower back and legs, the motivation to move through life.

## Essential oils for the urinary system

(Note: do not use juniper in cases of nephritis, or any infection of the kidneys.)

**REMEMBER**

The urinary system is one of the five eliminative channels of the body.

Diuretics: juniper, cedarwood, sandalwood, benzoin, fennel, cypress

Pathogens in urinary system, cystitis, urinary tract infections: coriander, basil, benzoin, bergamot, frankincense, sandalwood, tea tree, geranium, cedarwood, chamomile, palmarosa

Stones: carrot seed, fennel, geranium, hyssop, juniper, lemon

Tonify kidney: cedarwood (*Juniperus virginiana*), clove bud, fennel

**Integrative physiology**
Kidney function interacts with functions of the adrenal glands and heart, lymph fluid and is involved in stress response.

## The digestive system

We are what we eat.

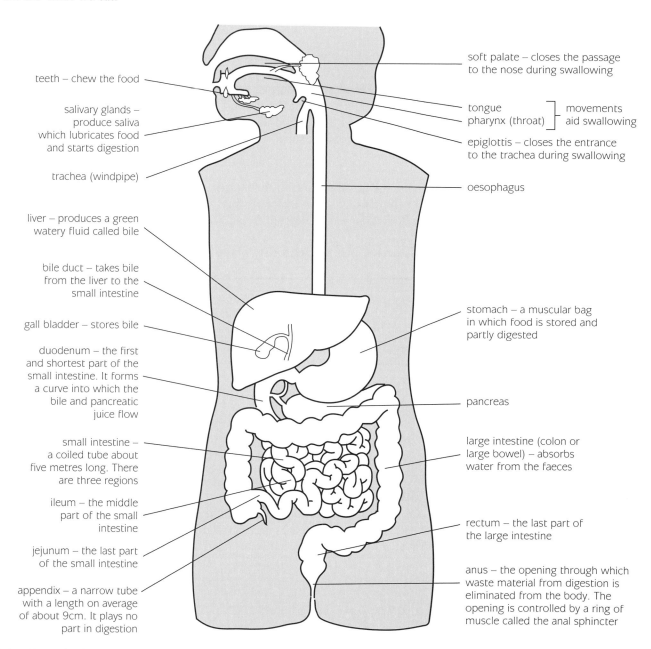

soft palate – closes the passage to the nose during swallowing

teeth – chew the food

salivary glands – produce saliva which lubricates food and starts digestion

trachea (windpipe)

tongue

pharynx (throat) } movements aid swallowing

epiglottis – closes the entrance to the trachea during swallowing

oesophagus

liver – produces a green watery fluid called bile

bile duct – takes bile from the liver to the small intestine

gall bladder – stores bile

duodenum – the first and shortest part of the small intestine. It forms a curve into which the bile and pancreatic juice flow

stomach – a muscular bag in which food is stored and partly digested

pancreas

small intestine – a coiled tube about five metres long. There are three regions

large intestine (colon or large bowel) – absorbs water from the faeces

ileum – the middle part of the small intestine

jejunum – the last part of the small intestine

rectum – the last part of the large intestine

appendix – a narrow tube with a length on average of about 9cm. It plays no part in digestion

anus – the opening through which waste material from digestion is eliminated from the body. The opening is controlled by a ring of muscle called the anal sphincter

**Fig. 10.6** *The digestive system*

The digestive system is a central channel by means of which nutrition is made available to every cell, tissue and organ. While good food and nutrition is important, equally important is whether that food is fully digested and assimilated. If digestion is weak we do not derive the energy we need from food. In addition, incompletely digested residues can accumulate and create a state of dysbiosis in the digestive tract (irritable bowel syndrome (IBS)/leaky gut syndrome/candida), which means the body has to use extra energy to expel or contain the toxins. The toxins can irritate immune tissue in the small intestine and trigger auto-immune responses such as allergies and even auto-immune diseases. The environment in the gut also can influence mood and brain activity through the feedback loop of peptide-hormone communications and the enteric nerve plexi. Many people experience relief from their symptoms simply by adopting a cleansing diet or fast, which simultaneously improves digestion and allows the body to eliminate the toxins from the digestive tract.

Organs such as the stomach, liver, pancreas and gall bladder play important parts in the digestive process, and their healthy functioning is also necessary to good digestion. The stomach and colon are influenced by our state of mind and emotions, as well as by such things as sleep and exercise. Good food, good digestion, good elimination along with mental–emotional balance are all important for a healthy digestive system.

Energetically, digestion in the stomach and small intestines represents the fire element, which transforms food into absorbable nutrients. The colon embodies the earth element, which helps ground us.

### Essential oils for the digestive system

> Poor digestion, flatulence: digestive stimulants and carminatives; mandarin, fennel, coriander, ginger, rosemary, thyme, basil, cinnamon, juniper, cardamom
>
> Sluggish liver: cholagogues and hepatics; lemon, rosemary, lemongrass, grapefruit, immortelle/helichrysum, carrot seed
>
> Calming, relieving tension: antispasmodics; chamomile, lavender, clary sage
>
> Constipation: carminatives and laxatives; fennel, black pepper, ginger, marjoram, rosemary

### Integrative physiology

The quality of digestion is often telling of imbalances in other areas. Digestion is influenced by nervous–endocrine function, breathing rhythm, mental–emotional states and stress.

## The reproductive system

Cycles of life.

This system comprises the male and female reproductive organs and the glands secreting reproductive hormones. Health of the reproductive organs is important for the bringing forth of new life. Their health influences the health of the body as a whole. In a sense our own life is a series of births and deaths, or rites of passage by which we leave one stage to grow into another. At each stage we must let go of some things

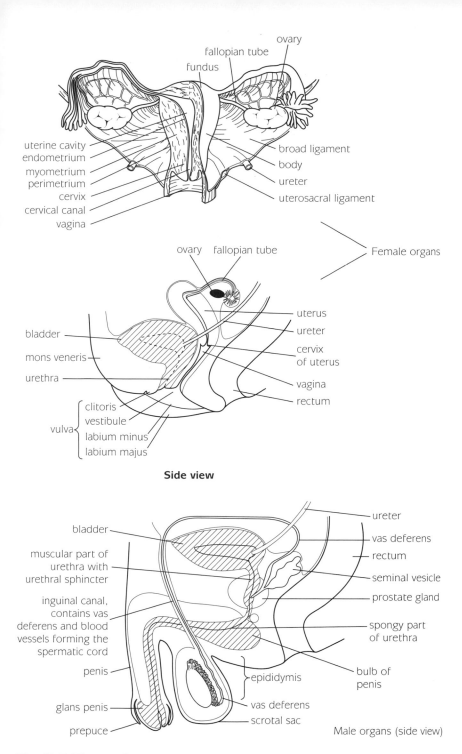

**Fig. 10.7** *The reproductive system*

as we are reborn to new ideas, new possibilities. Life that does not continue to grow and develop fails to thrive. Our sense of identity is linked to our gender and sexuality. A healthy sense of self-esteem is reflected in positive loving relationships, and physically as strong immunity. Even minor problems in the cycles of reproductive organs can influence our overall health, weakening the vital force.

Herbs and essential oils, even foods which by tradition have been known as aphrodisiacs (enhancers of sexual function) can be truly understood as substances that promote the health of the reproductive system and the endocrine glands. When these are strong, our vitality is maintained, not just sexually but at all levels, and ageing is inhibited.

Energetically, the reproductive organs and glands reflect the generative water element and the vital heat. Balance involves maintaining vital fluids, countering damaging heat and dryness. A stressful or unhealthy lifestyle depletes both these aspects of vitality.

### Integrative physiology

Reproductive organs can be influenced by the stress response and neuro-endocrine system, by psychological states, by the lymphatic and immune systems, and by the functions of the urinary system. The liver also plays a role because it cleanses the blood and metabolises hormones. If the liver is congested, this can have an effect on the reproductive organs or their function.

### Essential oils for the reproductive organs
*Female*

Regulating periods: emmenagogues; lavender, juniper, ginger, vetivert, fennel, cypress, clary sage, myrrh

PMS: astringents for fluid retention; geranium, cypress, grapefruit

Nervines for irritability: lavender, ylang ylang, jasmine, basil, spikenard/valerian, chamomile

For painful periods: warming antispasmodics; ginger, marjoram, fennel, lavender, chamomile

Pregnancy: avoid use of essential oils until the last three weeks. Jasmine, lavender, mandarin, ylang ylang, geranium, and sandalwood may be used from that time.

Morning sickness: ginger tea and lavender

Stretchmarks: wheatgerm oil with lavender, rosewood, frankincense, myrrh

Childbirth: jasmine, neroli, rose, lavender, mandarin, clary sage

Lactation: fennel, geranium, lemongrass, jasmine

Post-natal depression: geranium, rose, neroli, jasmine, clary sage, bergamot, ylang ylang

Menopause: hot flushes: rosemary, sage, geranium, lemon, clary sage; water retention, bloating: grapefruit, sage, fennel; disturbed mood: rose, ylang ylang, jasmine, neroli lavender; leuchorrhoea thrush: eucalyptus, tea tree, lavender, lemongrass, myrrh

A useful method for women is to have the selected essential oil blend put on to a small piece of cotton wool that is then placed on the skin over the ovaries or uterus and secured with light surgical tape. It is renewed morning and evening.

*Male*

Prostate swelling: basil, juniper, niaouli

Impotence: peppermint, pine, rose, sandalwood, ylang ylang

# The muscular–skeletal system

Structure of life.

This system is as intimately involved with the workings of the whole as any other. Marrow within bones is necessary for the health of the lymph and thus the entire immune system and healthy bones provide structure for the rest of body and its activities. Voluntary and involuntary muscles activate movement. Muscle tissue is penetrated with nerves, nourished and cleansed with blood and lymph fluid. Muscles need both exercise and rest, and stretching work along with relaxation; nutrition and waste removal. The heart is a muscle organ and has the needs of any other muscle to keep it healthy.

Correct alignment of the spinal vertebrae allows proper nervous communication to other systems and functions. Strength of bone and

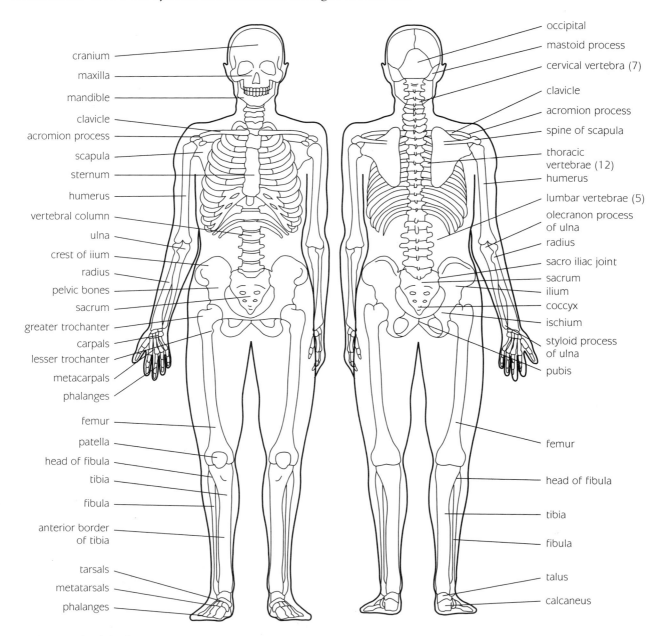

**Fig. 10.8a** *The skeletal system*

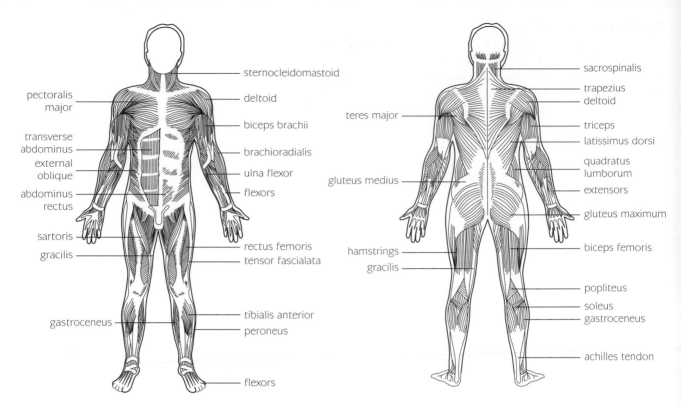

**Fig. 10.8b** *The muscular system*

flexibility of joints is part of good health. Stiffness and rigidity, tension and pain in any joint can affect the whole organism.

Energetically, bones and muscles, ligaments, cartilage and tendons combine the solidity of earth with the lightness of air. Bone is constructed of calcified connective tissue formed as a honeycomb-like structure that creates space within, making it both strong and light. When the air element is constricted or stuck, stiffness in joints can result. The nerves within muscles, aspects of the air element, make it possible for them to initiate movement. Muscles seem particularly susceptible to cold, which inhibits circulation and induces spasm. Blockage of the air element can be reflected in muscular tension or nervous spasm.

### Essential oils for the muscular-skeletal system

Cramp, spasm: warming antispasmodics; basil, ginger, marjoram, lavender, chamomile, yarrow

Muscle tone, sports training: rosemary, juniper, sandalwood, basil, black pepper

Muscle or joint pain: eucalyptus, peppermint, juniper, lavender, yarrow

Muscle sprain/trauma: basil, eucalyptus, immortelle, peppermint, juniper, rosemary, cypress, yarrow

Formation of bone marrow: yarrow

Arthritis pain: lavender, peppermint, eucalyptus, juniper. Support with a cleansing, blood–lymph circulation improving programme.

## Integrative physiology

Muscles are influenced by hormones released by the adrenal glands. They are reliant on the nervous system, blood and blood circulation for healthy function. The urinary system removes metabolic wastes of muscle activity, such as uric acid. The digestive system provides needed nutrients for strength and energy. The endocrine system supplies growth hormones for normal development and growth.

## The cardio-vascular system

River of life.

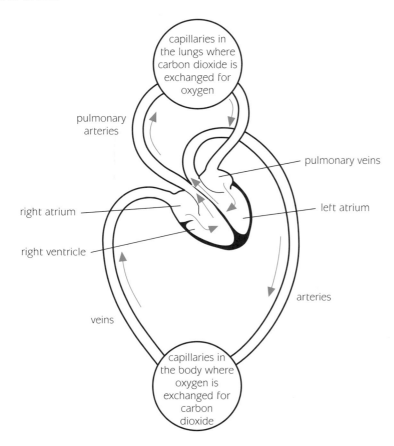

capillaries in the lungs where carbon dioxide is exchanged for oxygen

pulmonary arteries

pulmonary veins

right atrium

left atrium

right ventricle

arteries

veins

capillaries in the body where oxygen is exchanged for carbon dioxide

**Fig. 10.9** *The cardio-vascular system.*

Our blood is literally our river of life, both a transport medium and system that carries oxygen, nutrients, enzymes, neurotransmitters, immune factors to cells and removes metabolic wastes. When blood carries impurities, it naturally will weaken the healthy functioning of cells and tissues. When obstructions such as plaques on vessels walls, or weak vessels impair the flow, the heart muscle must work ever harder to supply blood to the body. The heart and blood symbolise the joy of life, the optimism of spring and the courage to face the challenges of life. The heart, in its rhythmic emptying, filling and giving forth symbolises our loving relationships with others, our openness to receiving and giving love.

Energetically, the blood's warmth reflects fire while its fluidity reflects water.

## Essential oils for the cardio-vascular system

Clean toxins with blood purifiers (diaphoretics, lymphatic and liver cleansers, diuretics and stress relieving essential oils). Ensure good nourishment via the digestive system with digestive stimulants.

| |
|---|
| Hypertension: hypotensives; lavender, melissa, basil, frankincense, neroli, sandalwood, jasmine, ylang ylang |
| Tension/stress affecting blood pressure: regulate nervous system; lavender, sandalwood, bergamot, petitgrain, jasmine, ylang ylang, clary sage, rose, neroli |
| Tonifying the heart: benzoin |
| Varicose veins: venous tonics; cypress, clary sage, lemon, geranium, ginger, patchouli |
| Haemorrhoids: cypress, lavender, myrrh, frankincense, yarrow |
| Oedema: astringents and diuretics; geranium, carrot seed, cypress, clary sage, juniper, cedarwood, fennel |

## Integrative physiology

The blood supplies nutrients, removes wastes in all body parts; blood vessels and the heart contain muscle tissue; the blood circulates to the lungs for oxygenation and waste release. The liver and kidneys purify blood and influence blood pressure. Hormones are circulated via the blood. The lymph system is interconnected with the blood circulation.

# The skin

The living surface.

The skin or integumentary system is not just a covering but a vital organ in its own right and the largest in the body. It mediates between our outer and inner environments. The health of the skin reflects the health of interior organs and systems. It plays a role in immunity. Always take into account health of other organs when assessing skin problems.

## Essential oils for the skin

(Note: essential oils for stress can have a role in treatment of skin conditions.)

| |
|---|
| Inflammations, including acne, boils, infections: tea tree, lavender, patchouli |
| Allergies, including eczema: German chamomile (*Matricaria recutita*), lavender, yarrow, neroli, bergamot |
| Viral infections of the skin: cajeput, niaouli, tea tree, eucalyptus, chamomile, yarrow |
| Healing and toning (including stretchmarks): rosewood, jasmine, Texas cedar (*Juniperus mexicana*), neroli, lavender |
| Detoxification and elimination: grapefruit, juniper, geranium, ginger, yarrow, cypress |

Rejuvenating mature skin, inhibiting ageing: frankincense, myrrh, neroli, jasmine, patchouli, rose, sandalwood, carrot seed, rosewood, immortelle

Dry, damaged, chapped skin: rose otto, chamomile (*Matricaria recutita*), neroli, rosewood, sandalwood, jasmine, ylang ylang

Excess oily: citronella, lemongrass, lemon, cypress, juniper

Sensitive skin (tends to be dry/pale/finely textured/low in natural lubrication): lavender, neroli, immortelle, yarrow, chamomile (*Matricaria recutita*)

Combination skin: geranium, lavender, neroli, palmarosa, sandalwood

## Integrative physiology

Skin function is influenced by the functions of the kidneys, liver, lungs, adrenal glands (stress response), neuro-endocrine system, immune system, blood and lymph. The digestive system makes possible the nourishment of skin cells.

**REMEMBER**

The skin benefits from the use of essential oil hydrolats.

**ACTIVITY**

Research each topic and make notes to extend the information given. For example, study the essential oils in Chapter 11 and add more detail to the list of essential oils for skin problems.

The following essential oils are included within this chapter:

| | | | | |
|---|---|---|---|---|
| ◆ Basil | *Ocimum basilicum* | | ◆ Lime | *Citrus aurantifolium* |
| ◆ Benzoin | *Styrax benzoin* | | ◆ Mandarin | *Citrus nobilis/C.reticulata* |
| ◆ Bergamot | *Citrus bergamia* | | ◆ Marjoram | *Oreganum marjorana* |
| ◆ Black pepper | *Piper nigrum* | | ◆ May chang | *Litsea cubeba* |
| ◆ Cajeput | *Melaleuca leucadendron* | | ◆ Melissa | *Melissa officinalis* |
| ◆ Cardamom | *Elettaria cardomomum* | | ◆ Myrrh | *Comiphora myrrha* |
| ◆ Carrot | *Daucus carota* | | ◆ Myrtle | *Myrtus communis* |
| ◆ Cedarwood | *Cedrus atlantica* | | ◆ Niaouli | *Melaleuca viridiflora* |
| ◆ Cedarwood | *Juniperus mexicana* | | ◆ Orange bitter | *Citrus aurantium* |
| ◆ Cedarwood | *Juniperus virginiana* | | ◆ Palmarosa | *Cymbopogon martini* |
| ◆ German chamomile | *Matricaria recutita* | | ◆ Patchouli | *Pogostemon cablin* |
| ◆ Roman chamomile | *Chamaemelum nobile* | | ◆ Peppermint | *Mentha x piperita* |
| ◆ Citronella | *Cymbopogan nardus* | | ◆ Pine | *Pinus sylvestris* |
| ◆ Clary sage | *Salvia scleria* | | ◆ Rose, cabbage | *Rosa x centifolia* |
| ◆ Clove | *Eugenia caryophyllata* | | ◆ Rose, damask | *Rosa x damascene* |
| ◆ Cypress | *Cupressus sempervivens* | | ◆ Rosemary | *Rosemarinus officinalis* |
| ◆ Eucalyptus | *Eucalyptus globulus* | | ◆ Sage | *Salvia officinalis* |
| ◆ Fennel | *Foeniculum vulgare* | | ◆ Sandalwood | *Santalum album* |
| ◆ Frankincense | *Boswellia carteri* | | ◆ Spanish sage | *Salvia lavandulaefolia* |
| ◆ Geranium | *Pelargonium graveolens* | | ◆ Spearmint | *Mentha spicata* |
| ◆ Ginger | *Zingiber officinalis* | | ◆ Tea tree | *Melaleuca alterniflora* |
| ◆ Grapefruit | *Citrus y paradisi* | | ◆ Thyme | *Thymus vulgaris* |
| ◆ Hyssop | *Hyssop officinalis* | | ◆ Valerian | *Valeriana officinalis* |
| ◆ Jasmine | *Jasminum officinale* | | ◆ Vetiver | *Vetiveria zinzanoides* |
| ◆ Lavender | *Lavandula angustifolia* | | ◆ Yarrow | *Achillea millefolium* |
| ◆ Lemon | *Citrus limonum* | | ◆ Ylang ylang | *Cananga odorata* |
| ◆ Lemongrass | *Cymbopogan citratus* | | | |

The information presented on chemical constituents represents a composite approximation of amounts in each essential oil. It is based on information found in Rosemary Caddy's *Essential Oils in Colour: Caddy Classic Profiles,* Salvatore Battaglia's *The Complete Guide to Aromatherapy*, Julia Lawless's *The Encyclopedia of Essential Oils*, Shirley and Len Price's *Aromatherapy for Health Professionals*, Malcolm Stuart's *Encyclopedia of Herbs and Herbal Medicine, Herbalgram 58* and Mrs Grieve's *A Modern Herbal.* Constituents of essential oils vary from year to year, and according to distillation, climate and other factors. When buying essential oils the aromatherapist should request data from the supplier on constituents for the source/batch being offered for each essential oil purchased.

I have not tried to be exhaustive, but rather to offer thorough information, while leaving plenty of scope for tutors to present the nuances of essential oils and enhance students' learning with their own knowledge and experience.

## Note on uses

Unless otherwise stated, information on usage includes the historical uses of the plant in herbal medicine. Only relatively recently have essential oils been used in aromatherapy practice to an extent significant enough to establish uses exclusive to aromatherapy. While aromatherapy use may not always be identical to herbal medicine use, it usually is identical because it is usually the aromatic components of a plant that give an aromatic herbal medicine its main therapeutic properties. What is generally lost in distillation are the effects of any glycosides, carbohydrates and waxes that may be present.

The uses given also include those for conditions normally considered as requiring medical diagnosis for the reason that herbal medicine/essential oils have historically been used in the treatment of most of these, before the establishment of modern medical categories. For such conditions, students are advised to use essential oils only in concert with the patient receiving medical attention, and as an adjunctive, supportive therapy, and as directed by their tutor.

A particular feature of this section is that the energy of each essential oil is given. I have also attempted to bring together in this one volume, along with the energy, the humoural, dosa or meridian designations according to Greek–European/Unani traditional medicine, then Ayurvedic medicine and then Chinese medicine, respectively. I have based this on my studies with Michael Tierra, David Frawley, Vasant Lad, Daniel Penoel, on the work of Drs Light and Bryan Miller, and Gabriel Mojay, and on my own research and experience. The classifications are not absolutes and are to some extent theoretical. It remains for them to be proven thoroughly by the empirical experience of practitioners. I invite aromatherapists to engage in this task. I offer them here in the hope that this will help ground aromatherapy more closely to the traditions of herbal medicine, enable practitioners to select oils according to constitutional considerations and be useful to those trained in traditional medical systems.

# Basil

**Name** Basil

**Latin name** *Ocimum basilicum*, 'basil' comes from the Greek for king or royal, and 'okimum' is the ancient Greek name for this plant.

**Family** Lamiaceae/Labiateae

**Synonyms** French basil, sweet basil, European basil, linalool type.

**Other species** *Ocimum basilicum* chemotype tropical basil/Réunion basil/Comoran basil/exotic basil contains higher amounts of phenols and phenolic ethers.

*Ocimum canum* (East Africa, India, South America); *Ocimum gratissumum* (India, Morocco, Egypt, South Africa, Brazil, Indonesia); *Ocimum sanctum* 'Tulsi' (India), *Ocimum minimum* 'bush basil' (Chile).

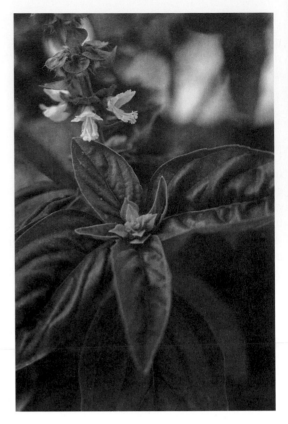

*Basil*

**Description** A multi-branched tender annual herb, 30–60 cm; square stems bearing dark green, ovate serrate or entire leaves and clusters of 2-lipped white or purplish-white flowers on terminal racemes (spikes). The whole plant is aromatic.

**Habitat/distribution** Native to the Middle East, and to Iran and southern India; naturalised in parts of Africa; Okimum was used by Hippocrates and is discussed by Theophrastus, Dioscorides and Pliny. Some authorities say it was introduced to Europe in the 16th century.

**History** 'Okimum' is discussed by Dioscorides as a laxative, digestive, galactagogue and used for eye problems, rheum (running mucus) and – significantly – for melancholy. The Romans used it in cooking. It was likewise valued by Unani physicians. Culpeper, finding other authorities disagree about it, recommends it only for bites, as it draws the poison, and as a parturient. Gerard, following ancient use, recommends it for taking away sorrows. Dr Valnet recommends it for epilepsy and paralysis. In India, *O. sanctum* is considered sacred to the gods Vishnu and Krishna and is planted before homes for protection and purification. Medicinally its juice is used to counter snake poison, for skin and respiratory disorders, and it is also used to open the heart, induce mental clarity and to calm anxiety.

**Cultivation** Widely cultivated commercially in central and southern Europe, North Africa, Asia and subtropical America as a culinary herb. Propagated from seed.

**Part used** Flowering herb

**Extraction/yield/adulterations** Steam distillation of essential oil.

**Characteristics** Colourless or pale yellow, liquid; a light, sweet–spicy odour reminiscent of clove or anise. Top note.

- 💧 **Skin:** insect bites.
- 💧 **Digestive:** weak digestion, stomach upsets, flatulence, dyspepsia; threadworms; sluggish liver.
- 💧 **Respiratory:** congestion, asthma, cold, flu.
- 💧 **Immune:** fever; convalescence.
- 💧 **Circulatory:** hypertension.
- 💧 **Endocrine:** exhaustion/weak adrenal cortex.
- 💧 **Muscular–skeletal:** cramp, strain, sprain.
- 💧 **Genito-urinary:** amenorrhoea, dysmenorrhoea, cramps; galactagogue; cystitis.
- 💧 **Nervous:** weakness, exhaustion; anxiety, mental confusion, melancholy, depression, mental fatigue, insomnia, nervous headaches; hypertension.
- 💧 **Mental–emotional:** uplifting and refreshing; promotes calm, mental clarity; alleviates anxiety; promotes courage.

**Basil**

*Ocimum basilicum*

**Energy** Warming, drying, uplifting, calming. Clears phlegm and blood, calms and uplifts melancholy, cools choler, strengthens pneuma. Tridosic: calms vata, reduces kapha and pitta, strengthens agni. Clears wind, cold, phlegm and stagnation (lungs, stomach, lower warmer/kidneys, uterus), regulates triple warmer, regulates qi, tonifies kidney yang. According to Tisserand basil has a simultaneous warming and cooling energy similar to but distinct from peppermint.

**Chemical constituents** Features alcohols as linalool, citronellol, geraniol, terpinen-4-ol, α-terpineol 40–50%; phenols/phenol ethers as methyl chavicol, eugenol, methyl eugenol (20–25%); monoterpenes as limonene, camphene, α-pinene, β-pinene, γ-terpinene, ρ-cymene, *cis*-ocimene; oxides as 1.8-cineol 4%; esters as linalyl acetate, fenchyl acetate, methyl cinnamate 3%; sesquiterpenes as β-caryophellene 1%. (NB: the presence of esters is thought to quench the effects of phenols.)

**Therapeutic actions** Calming nervine, nervine tonic, anxiolytic, antispasmodic, analgesic; diaphoretic, refreshing, febrifuge; emmenagogue; digestive tonic, carminative, liver stimulant; anticatarrhal, expectorant; mild circulatory stimulant, hypotensive, cardio tonic; anti-inflammatory; antiviral, antifungal, antimicrobial; adrenal cortex tonic.

**Blends with** rosemary, lavender, clary sage, frankincense, fennel, black pepper, myrrh.

**Other uses** Use fresh basil freely in cooking to improve digestion and assimilation. Apply a poultice of leaves to insect bites. Used as a commercial flavouring and perfume agent.

 **Safety** Non-toxic, non-irritant but possible sensitisation in some individuals. Avoid in pregnancy. The chemotype with a high linalool, low methyl chavicol and eugenol content is safe.

# Benzoin

**Name** Benzoin

**Latin name** *Styrax benzoin*

**Family** Styracaceae

**Synonyms** Gum benzoin, gum benjamin.

**Other species** None

**Description** A tropical tree, to 7 m tall; leaves simple, elliptic, entire or slightly toothed, pale green; flowers white, several, in drooping clusters on pedicels; fruit hard shelled.

**Habitat/distribution** Native to south-east Asia, Sumatra. It occurs wild in mixed forests near rivers.

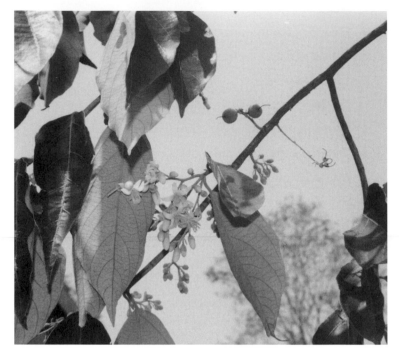

*Benzoin*

**History** Ibn Batuta, who found it on his visit to Sumatra in *c.* 1325, named it 'Luban Jawi' or Javan frankincense. Over time this became 'banjawi' then 'benjamin' and finally benzoin. Importation to Europe began in the 1580s. In the 1800's compound and simple tinctures were sold over-the-counter for antisepsis and it was added as preservative for medicines and cosmetics, a use which continues today. It is used in the Russian Orthodox church for incense.

**Cultivation** Benzoin is cultivated in several countries. From seed the tree is quick growing. Incisions are made in the trunk only after 7 years; the gum exudes for 12–20 years, (after which the tree is felled).

**Part used** A white oleoresin exudate of 7–10 to 20-year-old trees. A liquid resin forms within the cambium layer of the bark only when it is injured; then oleoresin ducts form and secrete the liquid, which becomes a gum when it hardens on exposure to air. The crude gum is dark red-brown, or reddish yellow, streaked with white internally.

**Extraction/adulterations** Solvent extraction of the crude benzoin produces a resinoid, or 'resin absolute'. Extraction is from the gum of two varieties of tree, each of a slightly different character: Malaysian, Sumatran and Javan trees produce 'Sumatra benzoin', which is traded as grey-brown, brittle lumps with red streaks; Vietnamese, Laotion, Thai, Cambodian and Chinese trees produce 'Siam benzoin', which is traded as oranage-brown pebbles or tears. Benzoin resinoid is very viscous and therefore is often supplied dissolved in ethyl glycol or – and this is preferable for aromatherapy – dissolved in wood alcohol. Benzoin resinoid is sometimes a mix of extractions from the two trees. Check with suppliers for provenance.

- **Skin:** wounds, cuts, chapped, inflamed or irritated skin; psoriasis, eczema; oral hygiene.
- **Digestive:** flatulence.
- **Respiratory:** cough, bronchitis, catarrhal congestion.
- **Immune:** fevers, flu.
- **Circulatory:** poor circulation; cordial – 'warms, gladdens the heart'.
- **Muscular–skeletal:** arthritis, gout.
- **Urinary:** cystitis, gout.
- **Nervous:** depression, tension, stress.
- **Mental–emotional:** depression, loneliness, grief. Comforts, warms. Uplifts, brings clarity and calm.

**Benzoin**
*Styrax benzoin*

**Characteristics** Sumatra benzoin: a viscous mass; a strong storax or almond-like odour in the finest grade. Base note.

Siam benzoin: a viscous mass; sweet, balsamic, vanilla odour. Base note.

The mixed resinoid is an orange-brown very viscous mass; intense, sweet, vanilla odour.

**Energy** Warming, drying. Clears phlegm, cools choler, clears blood; both revives and calms melancholy. Reduces kapha, cools pitta, calms vata. Tonifies yang, spleen and lung qi; clears cold, stagnation from lower warmer.

**Chemical constituents** Features acids as benzoic and cinnamic acids 70%; esters of the acids as coniferyl benzoate, coniferyl cinnamate 70%; aromatic aldehydes as cinnamate and benzaldehyde, vanillin.

Siam benzoin has less or no cinnamic acid, more benzoic acid and more coniferyl acetate ester.

**Therapeutic actions** antiseptic; styptic, vulnerary; expectorant, mucolytic; anti-inflammatory; carminative, cordial, deodorant, diuretic; nervine sedative; circulatory stimulant, tonic.

**Blends with** sandalwood, jasmine, frankincense, myrrh, cypress, juniper, coriander, lemon, rose.

**Other uses** Benzoin is an ingredient in Friar's Balsam and other proprietary remedies; a fixative and fragrance in pot pourris, soaps, toiletries, cosmetics, perfumes; a flavouring for food products and beverages because of its vanilla aroma.

**Safety/precautions** Non-toxic, non-irritating, possible sensitising in some individuals (based on reports of irritation after using a proprietary 'compound tincture' comprising benzoin and several other ingredients).

# Bergamot

**Name** Bergamot

**Latin name** *Citrus bergamia*

**Family** Rutaceae

**Synonyms** *Citrus aurantium* ssp. *bergamia*

**Other species** Do not confuse *C. bergamia* with the garden mint bee balm or bergamot *Monarda didyma*.

**Description** A small tree up to *c.* 4.5 m; leaves smooth, oval; fruit small, round, ripening from green to yellow and very like a small orange.

**Habitat/distribution** Native to tropical Asia, bergamot is cultivated extensively in the Calabria region of southern Italy and along the Ivory Coast of Africa.

**History** It takes its name from Bergamo in northern Italy where it was first popularised and sold in the 16th century. It is widely used in Italian traditional medicine for fever and worms. More recently, Italian research has highlighted its healing properties for skin, mouth, respiratory and urinary conditions.

**Cultivation** It is grafted to the bitter orange root stock, *Citrus aurantium* var. *bigarade*.

**Part used** Fruit peel

**Extraction/adulterations** Expression

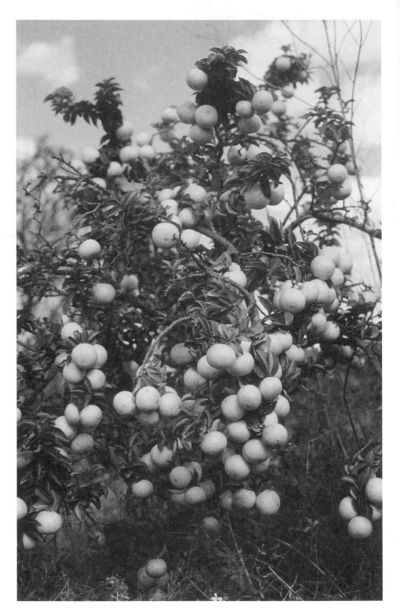

*Bergamot*

## USES

- **Skin:** inflammations, acne, excess oil, boils, cold sores, eczema, psoriasis, insect bites/repellants, wounds, ulcers; deodorising.

- **Oral hygiene:** halitosis, mouth infections.

- **Digestive:** flatulence, loss of appetite, anorexia, colic, dyspepsia; sluggish bile.

- **Respiratory:** cold, flu.

- **Immune/lymph:** cold sores, chicken pox, shingles, sore throats, tonsillitis, fever, infectious diseases. Rovesti recommends it to allay the side-effects and symptoms of uterine cancer (Tisserand, 1977).

- **Genito-urinary:** cystitis, leucorrhoea, pruritis, thrush, gonococcal infections.

- **Nervous:** anxiety, depression, stress.

- **Mental–emotional:** uplifting and refreshing; anxiety, depression, low self-esteem.

**Characteristics** A light green-yellow liquid, which on age becomes brownish-olive; light, delicate citrus-like scent with slightly floral/sweet/balsamic character. Top note.

**Energy** Calms and uplifts melancholy, stimulates bile, cools choler. Reduces kapha and pitta, calms vata, stimulates and balances agni. Regulates and strengthens liver and stomach qi; clears damp and wind heat.

**Chemical constituents** It comprises up to 300 components featuring esters as linalyl acetate 40%; monoterpenes as limonene, α-terpinene, β-pinene, γ-terpinene 33%; alcohols as geraniol, linalool 18%; lactones and fourocoumarins, e.g. bergaptene 5%; sesquiterpenes as β-bisabolene 0.5%.

**Therapeutic actions** anthelmintic/vermifuge, parasiticide; antiseptic (respiratory, genito-urinary), antiviral, bactericidal, antifungal; nervine antispasmodic, analgesic, antidepressive; digestive tonic, carminative, laxative, stomachic; diuretic; rubefacient, vulnerary.

**Blends with** lavender, neroli, petitgrain, jasmine, cypress, geranium, lemon, chamomile, juniper, coriander.

**Other uses** It is extensively used as a scent for cosmetics, eau de cologne, perfumes, suntan lotions; and as a flavouring for teas (Earl Grey), beverages, foods.

**Safety/precautions** Bergaptene can be phototoxic. Exercise care in dermal application: do not expose skin to sunlight; use high dilution, e.g. less than 1%; or use bergaptene-free e.o. Otherwise, it is non-toxic, non-irritant.

# Black pepper

**Name** Black pepper

**Latin name** *Piper nigrum*, Latin from the Sanskrit *pippali*; *nigrum* Latin for black.

**Family** Piperaceae

**Synonyms** None

**Other species** Do not confuse *P. nigrum* with cayenne or paprika from Capsicum species. Both black and the related long pepper, *P. longum*, are used in Ayurvedic medicine.

**Description** A perennial, woody vine, up to 5 m; leaves glossy, heart-shaped; flowers small, white; fruit a berry (drupe) ripening from red to black.

**Habitat/distribution** Native to India, introduced to Thailand, Indo-China, Malaya. The best pepper comes from the Malabar coast of western India. It is now widely cultivated in both the East and West Indies, in Indonesia, China and Brazil. It requires shade and high humidity.

**History** It has a long history of use in southern and south-east Asia and in Ayurvedic and Unani medicine. It was also widely traded in ancient times and has been used in the West by Hippocratic, Roman and European physicians for medicinal and culinary purposes. It was so highly prized that it was once used as a ransom and in the 15th century tenants could pay 'pepper rents' to their landlords. Venice was the trading centre for pepper in the Middle Ages. The European quest for direct trade routes for spices like pepper directly led to the 'discovery' of the Americas and the colonial era.

**Cultivation** Wild. Cultivated commercially, frequently inter-planted with coffee in plantations.

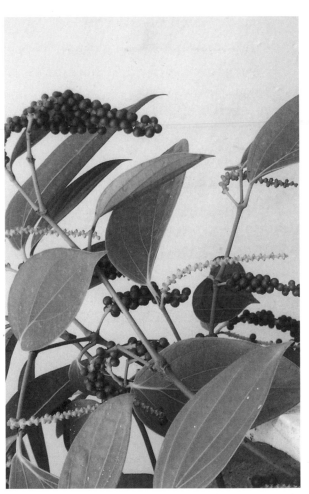

*Black pepper*

- **Skin:** chilblains, feeling cold, Raynaud's syndrome.
- **Digestive:** dyspepsia, flatulence, weak digestion, colic, constipation, diarrhoea, loss of appetite, anorexia, nausea; toxins in the digestive tract.
- **Respiratory:** cold, flu, congestion, excess mucus.
- **Immune system:** bacterial, viral infections, fevers.
- **Circulation:** poor circulation, chill, bruising, Raynaud's syndrome, anaemia.
- **Muscular–skeletal:** aches and pains, arthritis, neuralgia, poor tone, stiffness, strain, sprains.
- **Nervous:** pain, neuralgia.
- **Mental–emotional:** grounding and yet also helps disperse congested, stuck feelings.

**Black pepper**
*Piper nigrum*

**Part used** Unripe berries (peppercorns), dried and crushed.

**Extraction/adulteration** Steam distillation, producing a light or a heavy oil by either low or high boiling fractions respectively. An oleoresin is also produced by solvent extraction for the flavouring industry.

**Characteristics** Light to pale olive colour liquid; a dry, woody, warm and spicy odour. Base note.

**Energy** Warming, drying; tonifying, stimulating. Clears phlegm, warms blood and melancholy; aids digestion. Reduces kapha, grounds, warms and moves vata, but can be too drying in excess; strengthens agni. Clears damp and cold; tonifies spleen qi; moves qi.

**Chemical constituents** Features sesquiterpenes 20–30%, and monterpenes, 70–80% as bisabolene, β-carylphylene and thujene, pinene, camphene, sabinene, terpinine, myrcene, limonene, phellandrene; small amounts of ketones, phenols, alcohols, other.

**Therapeutic actions** Antimicrobial, antiseptic; digestive aperitif, stomachic, carminative, laxative; diaphoretic, diuretic; circulatory stimulant, rubifacient; nervine analgesic, antispasmodic; tonic.

**Blends with** frankincense, sandalwood, lavender, rosemary, marjoram and many spicy, floral or citrus essential oils.

**Other uses** Use in cooking and recommend its free use to your clients. It is included in perfumes for spicy, oriental note. The oleoresin is used as a flavouring in food and alcoholic beverages.

 **Safety/precautions** Non-toxic, non-sensitising. Pepper is a rubifacient so exercise caution: use in low dosage to avoid irritation.

# Cajeput

**Name** Cajeput from the Malaysian *kayu-puti,* 'white wood'

**Latin name** *Melaleuca leucadendron.* The genus name from the Greek *melan* black and *leuco* white, because one species has these colours. Species name is from Greek for 'white tree'.

**Family** Myrtaceae, bottle brush group

**Synonyms** Punk tree, white wood, paperbark tree, white tea tree, swamp tea tree

**Other species** *M. alternifolia,* tea tree, *M. viridifolia,* niaoli. Cajeput is related to eucalyptus and clove spp.

**Description** A large tree with spongy, shiny, peeling bark; pendulous branches bearing oblong, tapering, strongly-veined leaves; flowers borne on terminal spikes, creamy white, small with numerous stamens, the flowers themselves terminate in a tuft of leaves; fruit a brown capsule.

**Habitat/distribution** Native to Australasia, south-east Asia, tropics where it grows wild. Cajeput likes swamps.

**History** It has a long history of traditional use in its native habitat (see **Other uses**). Cajeput was introduced to Europeans in the 17th century and popularised by the Germans in the early 18th century.

**Cultivation** Wild and cultivated from cuttings, in plantations.

**Part used** Fresh leaves and twigs.

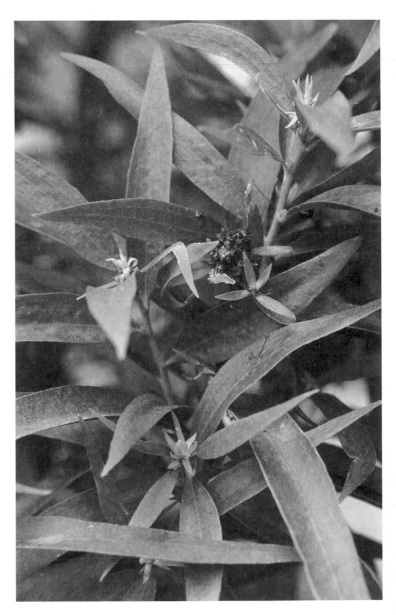

*Cajeput*

- **Skin:** infestations, bites; oily skin, spots.
- **Digestive:** flatulence, worms, toxins.
- **Respiratory:** cold, flu, cough, catarrh, sinus congestion or sinusitis; bronchitis, asthma.
- **Immune-lymph:** sore throats, viral infections, fevers.
- **Circulation:** stimulant, quickens the pulse.
- **Muscular–skeletal:** muscle ache, pain, sprain; arthritis, rheumatism.
- **Genito-urinary:** bacterial infections (cystitis, UTI).
- **Nervous:** neuralgia, spasm, cramp.
- **Mental:** induce mental clarity, invigorate faculties; fainting.

**Cajeput**
*Melaleuca leucadendron*

**Extraction/adulterations** Steam distillation.

**Characteristics** A pale, yellow-green liquid (the green derives from traces of copper); camphorous–medicinal, highly penetrating odour with a slightly fruity note, compared to eucalyptus (Lawless, 1992). Top note.

**Energy** Warming, dispersing, drying, draining. Stimulating, invigorating. Clears phlegm, cools choler and blood. Reduces kapha, cools pitta, stimulates agni. Clears wind–cold and phlegm, stimulates qi (lungs and generally), removes stagnation; tonfies spleen yang.

**Chemical constituents** Features 1.8 cineol 14–65%, terpenes 45%; alcohols 5%; esters.

**Therapeutic actions** Antimicrobial, antiseptic, insecticide; nervine analgesic, antispasmodic; digestive carminative, anthelmintic; diaphoretic, febrifuge, expectorant.

**Blends with** niaouli, tea tree, eucalyptus; ginger, black pepper; spike lavender; camphor; thyme, sage, rosemary; pine, peppermint.

**Other uses** A tea is made from the leaves and twigs and used medicinally (colds, fever, cholera, infections, skin diseases, toothache). An insect repellant and anthelmintic is made from leaves and essential oil. It is used as a fragrance for soaps, detergents, perfumes; occasionally for foods and beverages.

**Safety/precautions** Non-toxic, non-irritant. It may sensitise some individuals' skin if used in high concentrations.

# Cardamom

**Name** Cardamom

**Latin name** *Elettaria cardomomum*

**Family** Zingiberaceae

**Synonyms** *E. cardomomum* var. *cardomomum*; cardomon, cardamomi, cardomum, Mysore cardamom.

**Other species** *Amomum cardamomum* of India and China. Wild: *E. cardamomum* var. *major* and numerous related local species.

**Description** A perennial; rhizome fleshy, thick; bearing 8–20 smooth, erect green stems to 2.7 m; leaves alternate, oblong or lanceolate, sheathed; yellow flowers arise from near the stem base on a peduncle and are arranged in a panicle; fruit is an ovoid, 3-celled red-brown capsule with many tiny black seeds.

**Habitat/distribution** Native to southern and western India, cardamom thrives in shady mountain rain forests, and moist, wooded hillsides. It grows wild in Burma. It has been introduced in other tropical countries.

**History** Cardamom has a long history of use in India and other Asian countries for cooking and medicine. Ayurveda uses it to strengthen digestion or agni and to

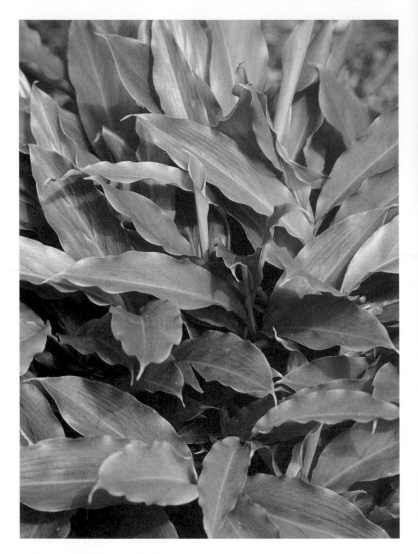

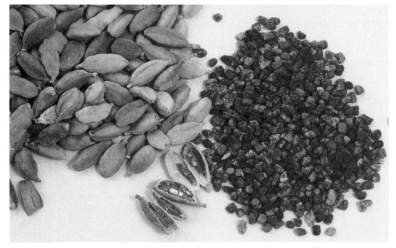

*Cardamom seeds*

## USES

- **Digestive:** dyspepsia, colic, cramp, flatulence, halitosis, heartburn, nausea, vomiting; lack of appetite, anorexia.
- **Respiratory/immune:** colds, mucous congestion/phlegm, coughs, bronchitis.
- **Nervous:** spasm, cramp; mental fatigue, nervous strain.
- **Mental–emotional:** calming to the mind, bringing clarity, dispersing heaviness, confusion.

promote satva, clarity and calm. In traditional Chinese medicine it is a qi tonic. It was also used by Hippocratic physicians (5th century BC) and it passed into European and Unani medicine as warming carminative/digestive and decongestant.

**Cultivation** Wild. Cultivated in Asia and the Americas.

**Part used** Dried ripe fruit: the seed pod and seeds.

**Extraction/adulterations** Steam distillation; an oleoresin in small quantities is also produced.

**Characteristics** A colourless to pale yellow liquid; warming, sweet-spicy odour with hint of woody or balsamic note. Middle note.

**Energy** Warming. Clears phlegm, calms melancholy, warms blood, increases choler and digestive fire. Reduces excess kapha and vata, kindles agni, satvic; may increase pitta in excess. Circulates qi, tonifies and warms spleen yang and lung qi; dispels cold, damp, phlegm.

**Chemical constituents** Features esters as terpinyl acetate, linalyl acetate up to 50%; oxides as 1–8 cineol up to 50%; terpenes as limonene, sabinene, pinene; alcohols as linalool, citronellol, nerol; sesquiterpenes as zingiberene.

**Therapeutic actions** Antiseptic; sialagogue, digestive tonic, stomachic, carminative; nervine antispasmodic and tonic; stimulant decongestant.

**Blends with** rose, orange, bergamot, neroli, cumin, cinnamon, clove, ylang ylang, cedarwood.

**Other uses** In India cardamom is a common ingredient in spice *masalas* (mixtures) for tea and cooking; it is popular in sweets and desserts made with milk and it counteracts the mucous forming properties of milk; it is a flavouring and odorant for medicines, toiletries, cosmetics. Arabs add it to coffee; it may counteract the caffeine. Perfumers use it in oriental scents.

 **Safety/precautions** Non-toxic, non-irritant, non-sensitising.

# Carrot

**Name** Carrot seed

**Latin name** *Daucus carota* ssp. *carota. Daucus* is the Greek and *carota* is the Latin for this plant.

**Family** Apiaceae/Umbelliferae

**Synonyms** Wild carrot, Queen Anne's lace, birdsnest, beesnest.

**Other species** *D. carota* ssp. *sativa*; the edible carrot also produces an essential oil from leaf, flower, root and seed.

**Description** Annual or biennial (depending on location); single white root; stem hairy, branched; leaves bipinnate, finely cut; flowers white, concave umbels, like lace with usually one umbel dark, purplish in the centre.

**Habitat/distribution** Native to Europe, western Asia, N. Africa; prefers dry, stony, sandy or seaside location; naturalised and cultivated widely.

**History** Carrot was used by Hippocratic physicians; Dioscorides commends the seeds, decocted or in a pessary to 'move the menstrum', for painful urine and pleurisy, as a diuretic and an aid to conception; for bites of venomous insects. Culpeper adds to this a use for wind and abdominal fullness, dropsy, colic, kidney stone. Carrot is also used in Ayurvedic medicine.

**Cultivation** Wild.

**Part distilled** Seeds/dried fruit.

**Extraction/adulterations** Steam distillation.

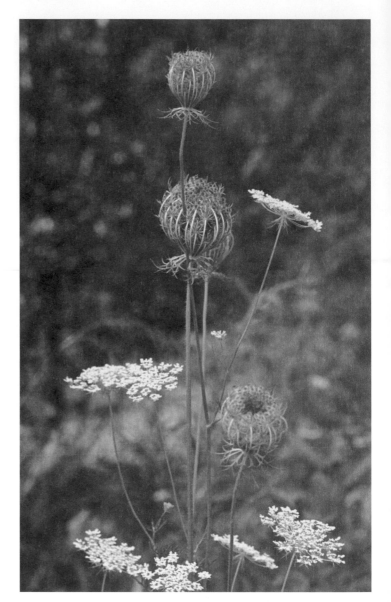

*Carrot*

## USES

- **Skin:** dermatitis, eczema, psoriasis, rashes, bites and stings; rejuvenating and toning for aged or damaged skin, blood vessels; inhibits wrinkles.
- **Digestive:** weak digestion, flatulence, dyspepsia, liver congestion and jaundice; anaemia, anorexia.
- **Circulation/lymph:** blood purifying, mild stimulant, oedema.
- **Endocrine:** regulator of thyroid; tonic.
- **Muscular–skeletal:** arthritis, gout, aches and pains.
- **Genito-urinary:** difficulty conceiving, amenorrhoea, dysmenorrhoea, PMS, glandular imbalance; diuretic, alterative; stones, cystitis.
- **Nervous/Mental–emotional:** antispasmodic, calming anxiety.

**Chemical characteristics** A yellow or amber liquid; warm, dry, woody or earthy odour. Middle note.

**Energy** Warming, drying; tonic, balancing. Clears phlegm. Reduces kapha, improves agni. Tonifies spleen and kidney.

**Chemical constituents** Features alcohols as carotol, daucol, linalool, geraniol, 26%; esters as geranyl acetate, 3%; sesquiterpenes as daucene, bisabolene, elemene, caryophyllene, 16%; monoterpenes as limonene, α-pinene, β-pinene; acids; phenol as asarone.

**Therapeutic actions** Antiseptic, anthelmintic; carminative; emmenagogue; nervine antispasmodic for smooth muscles; vasodilatory; hepatic stimulant; tonic; blood purifying; aids conception.

**Blends with** cedarwood, fennel, cypress, rosemary, mandarin, sandalwood, geranium, citrus and spicy essential oils.

**Other uses** Carrot root vegetable can be used medicinally (raw, juiced) for kidney and liver complaints, indigestion, acid stomach, weak vision and for purifying the blood in chronic conditions; soup for diarrhoea, stomach problems; as a poultice for skin ulcers. The essential oil is a fragrance for soaps, detergents, cosmetic, perfumes, flavourings.

**Safety/precautions** Non-toxic, non-irritating, non-sensitising.

**Name** Cedarwood: the common name 'cedarwood' is used for oils from at least three botanical sources. The first, *Cedrus atlantica* syn. *atlas* is from the family Pinaceae. The next two, *Juniperus mexicana* and *J. virginiana,* are from the family Cupressaeare. Be clear which you require when purchasing. Essential oil of Atlas/Atlantic cedar is quite different from that of the two Juniperus species. Prickly cedar, *J. oxycedrus*, yields oil of cade.

Atlas cedar, Atlantic cedar

**Latin name** *Cedrus atlantica*

**Family** Pinaceae

**Synonyms** Atlantic cedar, Moroccan cedar, African cedar, satinwood. The essential oil known as libanol.

**Other species** Closely related to cedar of Lebanon, *C. libani*, which is native to Palestine and Cyprus, and to the Himalyan deodar, *C. deodorata.* The extracted essential oils of these are very similar.

**Description** Majestic evergreen tree, to 40 m high; wood hard and fragrant.

**Habitat/distribution** Native to the Atlas mountains of Algeria and Morocco.

**History** Natural exudations of *C. libani* and *C. deodar* have been used since ancient times as the wood is full of aromatic substance. The cedars of Lebanon were used to build the fragrant temple at Jerusalem and for embalming, and for cosmetics by the Egyptians. It may have been an ingredient in mithradat, a famous poison antidote in Roman times – Dioscorides

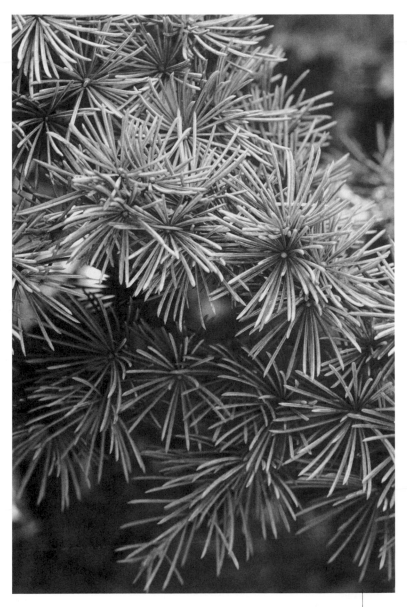

*Cedarwood, Cedrus atlantica*

## USES

- **Skin:** acne, dermatitis/eczema, fungal infections, dandruff, scalp problems excess oiliness, alopecia, eruptions, ulcers.
- **Respiratory:** bronchitis (especially chronic), phlegm, cough, colds, catarrh.
- **Muscular–skeletal:** arthritis, aches and pains, stiffness.
- **Genito-urinary:** urinary tract and vaginal infections, cystitis, pruritis.
- **Nervous:** stress, tension, exhaustion.

discusses 'Kedros' but this is considered to be a juniper. Deodar bark, wood and leaves are used in Ayurveda, Tibetan and Unani medicine for fevers, skin conditions, diarrhoea, ulcers, inflammations, kidney stones. Cedars have been used in incense in ancient Egypt, Rome and are in use today in India and Tibet. *C. deodorata* is classed as hot in the 2nd degree, drying in the 2nd degree in Unani medicine.

**Cultivation** Wild.

**Part used** Wood, stumps, sawdust.

**Extraction/adulterations** Steam distillation. A resinoid and an absolute are sometimes produced.

**Characteristics** The colours range from yellow, through orange to amber of this viscous essential oil; warm, woody/woody-balsamic odour with a note of camphor, a hint of sweetness. Base note. The scent is attractive and acceptable to men.

**Energy** Warming, drying. Clears phlegm, purifies blood. Reduces kapha, warms vata. Tonifies qi and yang, clears damp.

**Chemical constituents** Features sesquiterpenes as caryophyllene, cedrene, thujospsene, cadinene, 50%; alcohols as atlantol, cedrol 29%; ketones as atlantone, 19%.

**Therapeutic actions** Antiseptic, antibacterial, fungicidal, astringent, expectorant, mucolytic; nervine sedative; circulatory stimulant; tonic, aphrodisiac; diuretic; antiseborrhoeic.

**Blends with** rosewood, bergamot, cypress, jasmine, juniper, neroli, clary sage, vetiver, rosemary, ylang ylang.

**Other uses** Fragrance and fixative in cosmetics and toiletries; household products, soaps, detergents.

 **Safety/precautions** Non-toxic, non-irritating. Avoid in pregnancy.

**Name** Cedarwood, Texas cedar, Mexican cedar

**Latin name** *Juniperus mexicana* syn. *J. ashei*

**Family** Cupressaceae

**Synonyms** Mountain cedar, Mexican cedar, Texas cedar, rock cedar, Mexican juniper.

**Other species** *J. virginiana* of North America, *J. procera* of East Africa.

**Description** A small evergreen up to 7 m high; needles stiff, trunk and branches irregular shaped, crooked, twisted. The wood cracks easily so it is not used for timber.

**Habitat/distribution** Alpine areas of the south-western United States, Mexico, central America.

**History** Traditionally used by Native Americans for skin rashes; arthritis, rheumatism.

**Cultivation** Trees are cultivated, principally in Texas.

**Part used** Heartwood, shavings.

**Extraction/adulterations** The tree is felled for the essential oil obtained by steam distillation of heartwood and shavings. A crude and a rectified essential oil is produced.

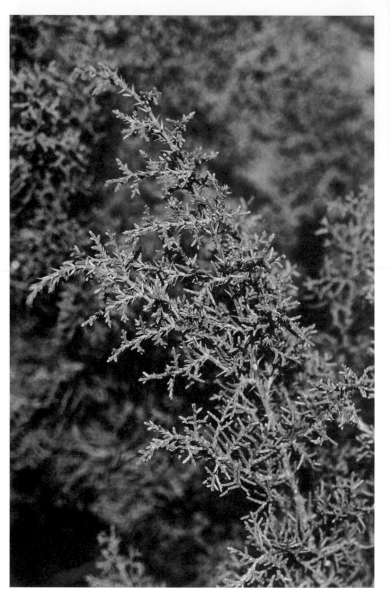

*Cedarwood, Juniperus mexicana*

## USES

- See *J. virginiana* (page 216).

**Characteristics** Crude: orange to brownish; viscous; woody, sweet, tar-like odour. Base note. Rectified: colourless to pale yellow; liquid; sweet balsamic odour harsher than *J. virginiana*. Base note.

**Energy** Warming, draining, drying. Clears phlegm, cools choler, calms melancholy, purifies blood. Reduces kapha, cools pitta, calms vata. Tonifies qi and yang of spleen and kidney; clears damp.

**Chemical constituents** Features sesquiterpenes as cedrene, thujopsene, sabinene, 60%; alcohols as cedrol, widdrol, 35%.

**Therapeutic actions** See *J. virginiana*.

**Blends with** patchouli, pine, vetiver.

**Other uses** See *J. virginiana*.

**Safety/precautions** Relatively non-toxic; can cause local irritation, possible sensitisation in some. It is generally safer than *C. atlantica* due to its lack of ketones. On ingestion it is abortifacient: avoid in pregnancy.

# Cedarwood

**Name** Cedarwood, Virginia cedar

**Latin name** *Juniperus virginiana*

**Family** Cupressaceae

**Synonyms** Red cedar, eastern red cedar, southern red cedar, Bedford cedarwood (oil).

**Other species** *J. mexicana*, European *J. sabina* (known as savin, traditionally used for animals), East African *J. procera*.

**Description** An evergreen, coniferous tree to 33 m high; slender/narrow and pointed in shape; very dense as scale-like, opposite leaves adhere to branchlets; flowers greenish-yellow; brown-purple berries 2-seeded on pedicles; trunk diameter can reach 1.5 m and is reddish; wood is reddish and streaked with red hues.

**Habitat/distribution** Eastern North America; widely distributed and wild in southern states.

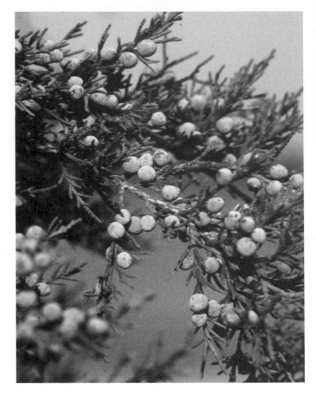

*Cedarwood, Juniperus virginiana*

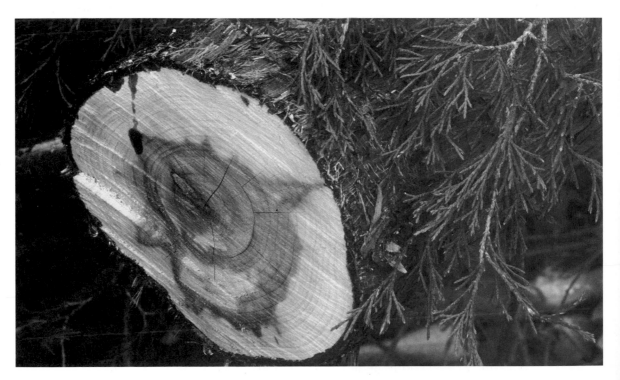

*Cedarwood, Juniperus virginiana*

## USES

- **Skin:** acne, dermatitis/eczema, dandruff and scalp problems, psoriasis, greasy hair, excess oiliness.
- **Respiratory:** bronchitis, catarrh, cough, sinusitis.
- **Muscular–skeletal:** aches and pains, stiffness, arthritis, rheumatism.
- **Genito-urinary:** cystitis, leucorrhoea.
- **Nervous:** stress, tension.
- **Mental–emotion:** uplifting and strengthening; calming.
- **Insect repellant:** combine with citronella.

**History** Traditionally cedar was used by Native Americans as a decoction of leaves, bark twigs or fruit for respiratory infections with excess catarrh, amenorrhoea, arthritis, rheumatism, skin rashes, warts, pyelitis and kidney infections, gonorrhoea; as an insect and vermin repellant. Once used commercially as an insecticide.

**Cultivation** Cedar is cultivated commercially for its timber; cedarwood is used as a lining for clothes closets and chests; off-cuts are used to fashion boxes, decorative souvenirs.

**Part used** Sawdust and shavings; occasionally heartwood of trees 25 years old.

**Extraction/adulterations** Steam distillation.

**Characteristics** A pale yellow or orange, oily liquid; mild, sweet-balsamic, dry odour. Base note.

**Energy** Warming, draining, drying. Clears phlegm, cools choler, calms melancholy, purifies blood. Reduces kapha, cools pitta, calms vata. Tonifies qi and yang of spleen and kidney; clears damp.

**Chemical constituents** Sesquiterpenes as cadinene, cedrene, thujopsene, cuparene, 60%; alcohols as cedrol, cedrenol, widdrol, γ-eudesmol, 30%.

**Therapeutic actions** Abortifacient (internally); antiseborrhoeic; antiseptic; astringent; diuretic; emmenagogue; expectorant; sedative, antispasmodic; circulatory stimulant.

**Blends with** sandalwood, juniper, cypress, vetiver, patchouli, benzoin, rose, pine.

**Other uses** In household insect repellants, and room sprays; fragrance for soaps, toiletries, cosmetics, perfumes, household cleansers; insect-repellant lining for clothes containers. Industrially used as a starting material for cedrene.

**Safety/precautions** Relatively non-irritant though some individuals may react with some local, acute irritation and sensitisation. On ingestion it is abortifacient. Avoid in pregnancy. Generally safer than *C. atlantica*.

**Name** Chamomile species, German chamomile

**Latin name** *Matricaria recutita*, synonym *Chamomilla recutita*, previously *M. chamomilla*. From the Latin *mater*, mother or *matrix*, womb – indicating a traditional use for female complaints; and the Greek *kamai*, ground and *melon*, apple = 'ground apple' because of its apple-like fragrance.

**Family** Asteraceae (Compositae).

**Synonyms** German chamomile, Hungarian chamomile, blue chamomile, scented mayweed and sweet false chamomile – because botanically it is not considered a true chamomile (see Grieve, 1984 and Stuart, 1989).

**Other species** See Roman chamomile.

**Description** An annual herb; stem hollow, round, branched, procumbent or upright, bearing pale green, bipinnate leaves, sharply incised and sessile; flowers on single stems are a composite of yellow, hollow, conicle disks with white rays, which tend to bend back (reflex) and feature the raised disk. The flowers are aromatic but bitter.

**Habitat/distribution** Native to Europe, northern Asia and northern India; fields, roadsides, gardens; naturalised in North America.

**History** A chamomile is mentioned in Egyptian sources and in Dioscorides. German chamomile is part of the pharmacopoeia of Unani medicine. The herb, and to a lesser extent the essential oil, has been clinically researched in recent decades and is included in the pharmacopoeias of 26 countries.

**Cultivation** Wild, especially in southern Europe. Cultivated widely in temperate regions.

**Part used** Flower heads; up to 1.9% yield.

**Extraction/adulterations** Steam distillation. An absolute is produced in small quantities and is of deeper blue, more tenacious fragrance with greater fixative properties.

**Characteristics** Very dark blue turning green on age; a viscous, sticky liquid; strong, sweet-herbaceous scent. Middle note.

**Energy** Cooling, moistening; calming, balancing. Clears phlegm, cools choler, calms melancholy, purifies blood. Reduces kapha, cools pitta, calms vata; strengthens agni. Clears wind-heat; moves and circulates qi (liver qi); tonifies spleen yang.

**Chemical constituents** Features a high percentage of alcohols as $\alpha$-bisabolol, 35% and sesquiterpenes as chamazulene, farnesene, 20%; oxides as $\alpha$-bisabolol oxide; ethers as *cis*-spiro ether, en-yn-dicycloether.

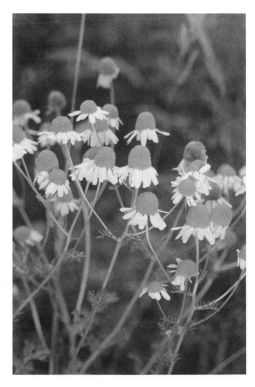

*Chamomile German*

## USES

- **Skin:** acne, allergies, cuts, wounds, chilblains, dermatitis/eczema, thread veins, rashes, inflammations, sensitive skin, burns, boils; hair care; teething in infants (high dilutions, 1%, apply to cheek).

- **Digestive:** dyspepsia, colic, nausea, indigestion, colitis, diarrhoea (including in children), liver congestion, gallstones, jaundice.

- **Respiratory:** colds, flu, fever.

- **Immune/lymph:** infections, fevers, earache.

- **Circulatory:** hypertension, blood vessel dilation.

- **Muscular–skeletal:** arthritis, inflammation, pain, swelling, strains and sprains.

- **Genito-urinary:** vaginal thrush, delayed menses, dysmenorroea, menorrhagia, PMS, fluid retention, depression; essential oil alleviates labour pains; menopause.

- **Nervous:** pain (especially dull), neuralgia, insomnia, headache, migraine, tension, stress, irritability, anxiety, depression.

- **Mental–emotional:** mental or emotional upset, irritability; depression.

- **Other:** chamomile herb has been investigated and found to relieve chemotherapy and radiation-induced mucositis (*ABC Clinical Guide to Herbs*, 2003).

**Therapeutic actions** Anti-inflammatory (greater than *C. nobilis* due to alcohols, sesquiterpenes), antispasmodic due to ethers; nervine antispasmodic, analgesic, muscle relaxant and anxiolytic; antibacterial, antifungal; diaphoretic-febrifuge, stimulates leucocytosis; vasoconstrictor; digestive carminative, antispasmodic, cholagogue, hepatic, stomachic, vermifuge; emmenagogue; vulnerary, cicatrisant; insect repellant.

**Blends with** geranium, lavender, patchouli, benzoin, rose, neroli, bergamot, marjoram, lemon, ylang ylang, jasmine, clary sage.

**Other uses** The herb tea is used for gastric disorders as its bitter principle promotes bile and gastric secretions, increases appetite and tones; large doses are emetic. The tea is diaphoretic for colds, fevers; especially good for children's upsets as it is soothing and calming to stomach and nerves. Use as a vaginal douche, a gargle for mouth ulcers, as vulnerary wash or poultice for haemorrhoids, wounds, skin conditions. It is used a flavouring in alcoholic drinks and as an anti-allergenic ingredient in cosmetics. The tea is used to lighten blond hair.

**Comments** This chamomile has been the focus of much clinical research. The scent can be overpowering for some people, so obtain acceptance from the patient. Use the essential oil as a compress over affected parts when using for internal conditions (e.g. colitis, pain, indigestion) and re-enforce with drinking of the tea.

**Safety/precautions** Non-irritant, non-toxic; non-sensitising; it may cause dermatitis in some individuals; conduct skin test.

# Chamomile

**Name** Chamomile species, Roman chamomile

**Latin name** *Chamaemelum nobile*, formerly *Anthemis nobile*. From the Greek *kamai melon*, ground apple.

**Family name** Asteraceae (Compositae)

**Synonyms** Wild chamomile, English chamomile, Manzanilla (Spanish for little apple).

**Other species** There are several species in Europe, four are native to Britain: *Anthemis matricaria,* stinking mayweed; *A. cotula, A. ravens*. In North Africa Moroccan chamomile grows and is cultivated: *Ormensis multicolis* syn. *Ormensis mixta*.

**Description** A perennial herb, rhizome short, multi-branched, creeping; stems 8–36 cm long, decumbent or ascending, branched, hairy; leaves arranged in spirals, sessile, oblong, pinnate; flowers solitary, disks yellow, covered in scales, tubular, hermaphrodite; rays white, spreading, female (the disk is not as conical as *M. recutita* and is solid); fruit a compressed achene with three stripes. A double-flowered variety was developed in England, and once preferred for preparations.

**Habitat/distribution** Native to the Mediterranean countries, Europe. Cultivated commercially in central Europe and now in other temperate countries. Prefers dry, sandy soil, but can be found in roadsides, waste places, pastures and grassy places.

**History** A chamomile is found used by the Egyptians and is discussed in Dioscoride's herbal. Roman chamomile was one of nine herbs held sacred by the Saxons and was recommended by Culpeper, Parkinson and Turner. It was used for digestion, sprains, jaundice and ague (malarial fever). It is milder and has a much more pleasant flavour than German chamomile. It is known as the 'plant's physician' because it keeps its companion plants in good health. It was introduced to Germany from Spain in the 16th century. This is the chamomile found marketed as a herbal tea.

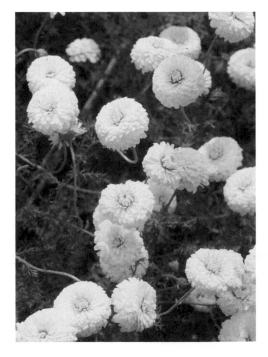

**Cultivation** Wild. Propagated by seed, and by 'sets' or runners of old plants. Much cultivated for ornament, medicine and as a scented lawn.

**Part used** Flowers.

**Extraction/adulterations** Steam distillation.

**Characteristics** A pale blue liquid, turning yellow as it ages; warm, fruity scent. Middle note.

**Energy** Cooling, balancing. Clears phlegm, cools choler, calms melancholy, purifies blood. Reduces kapha and vata, cools pitta; stimulates agni; promotes satva. Moves and circulates qi, tonifies spleen yang; clears wind and heat.

*Chamomile Roman (double flowered)*

## USES

- **Skin:** dermatitis, eczema, irritation, wounds, abrasions, bruises; acne; conjunctivitis; psoriasis, scarring; dilated capillaries (strengthens).

- **Digestive:** nausea, morning sickness, colic, diarrhoea, flatulence, weak appetite, anorexia, loss of appetite in the elderly.

- **Respiratory:** nervous asthma, colds.

- **Muscular–skeletal:** muscle spasms, muscle pain (back); swollen, stiff and/or painful joints.

- **Urinary:** cystitis, urinary tract infections, gout.

- **Reproductive:** delayed menses, PMS, dysmenorrhoea, menopause.

- **Nervous:** migraine and headaches; neuritis, neuralgia; anxiety, depression, paranoia; insomnia; shock, trauma.

- **Mental–emotional:** worry, anxiety, depression, irritability, tension, stress, hyperactivity. Calms and uplifts, clears mental paralysis (mental 'antispasmodic').

**Chemical constituents** Features esters as angelates, tiglates, butyrates, propionates 75%; oxides as 1.8-cineole 5%; monoterpenes as α-terpene, sabinene 5%; alcohols as farnesol, nerolidol, α-terpineol, trans-pinocarveol 5%; ketones as pinocarvone 3%; sesquiterpenes as chamazulene, caryophyllene 3%; aldehydes 2%; traces of lactones and coumarins, and acids.

**Therapeutic actions** Antibacterial, antiseptic; appetite stimulant, digestive tonic and antispasmodic, cholagogue; circulatory vasoconstrictive, mildly diuretic; nervine antispasmodic, calming, sedative; anti-inflammatory, diaphoretic, febrifuge; emmenagogue.

**Blends with** lavender, bergamot, clary sage, geranium, lemon, neroli, petitgrain, rose, sandalwood, jasmine, ylang ylang.

**Other uses** Used to flavour a light sherry in Spain and in traditional beer making. It is used in food and flavouring industries and in cosmetics, toiletries and perfumes.

**Comment** Roman chamomile and German chamomile share the same properties and effects but Roman chamomile (*C. nobile*) is considered by some to be better when an antispasmodic effect is needed and German chamomile when an anti-inflammatory effected is desired. Roman chamomile is higher in esters. According to Grieves (1930s) and (Stuart 1989) it is the traditional chamomile of European herbal medicine, *M. recutita* not being botanically a true chamomile. German chamomile has come to more prominence in recent decades and more research has been conducted on its properties and applications. It contains a bitter principle, which is missing from or milder in Roman chamomile. Use the flowers as a poultice or wash for skin abrasions and irritations. The tea can be used as a gargle and hair rinse.

**Safety/precautions** Non-toxic, non-irritating, non-sensitising; it may cause an allergic reaction (rare) in some individuals; conduct skin test.

# Citronella

**Name** Citronella

**Latin name** *Cymbopogan nardus*

**Family** Graminaceae

**Synonyms** *Andropogon nardus*, *A. citratus.*

**Other species** *C. flexuosus, C. citratus.* Other species grow wild in Pakistan and India. *C. winterianus*, the Java or Maha Pengiri citronella, is cultivated in Java, Vietnam, central America, Africa and other tropical countries to produce a commercial essential oil because the yield is twice as great as that of *C. nardus.*

**Description** A perennial grass; leaves linear, fragrant; flowers in terminal spikes.

**Habitat/distribution** Native to Sri Lanka; widely cultivated in tropical southern India, Sri Lanka.

**History** It has traditional use in Indian and Sri Lankan folk medicine as an infusion for digestive upsets, diarrhoea, vomiting, nausea, fevers, malarial dropsy, dysmenorrhoea. The essential oil is added to coconut oil and applied for pain of arthritis, neuralgia, sprains and for ringworm.

**Cultivation** Wild and commercial plantation.

**Part used** Fresh, partly dried or dried grass.

**Extraction/adulterations** Steam distillation. The component citral is used for adulteration of more costly oils, such as verbena or melissa. Be careful when purchasing.

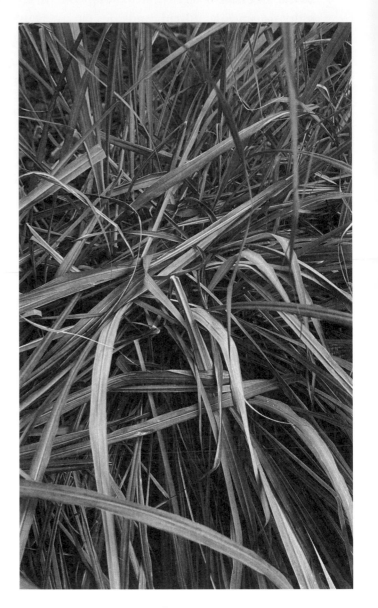

*Citronella*

## USES

- **Skin:** excessive perspiration and oily skin; insect repellant (tradition of use blended with *J. virginiana*); cellulite.
- **Digestive:** stomach upsets, nausea, vomiting, cramp, colic.
- **Immune:** colds, flu, fevers; ringworm, athlete's foot, fungal infections of nails; fleas, insects, pests.
- **Muscular–skeletal:** pain of arthritis, neuralgia, sprain, strain; tired legs; muscle fatigue from exercise.
- **Reproductive:** dysmenorrhoea; stimulate milk flow.
- **Nervous system:** cramp, fatigue; anxiety; headaches, migraine.
- **Mental–emotional:** uplifting, calming for depression, anxiety.

**Characteristics** A yellow-brown liquid; strong, fresh, sweet lemon odour. Top note. Java citronella, a colourless to pale yellow oil with a more woody-sweet odour, is preferred for perfumes.

**Energy** Cooling, moistening. Cools choler, purifies blood, calms melancholy. Reduces pitta, reduces kapha, calms vata; strengthens agni. Tonifies spleen and stomach, regulates qi, clears damp, stagnation.

**Chemical constituents** Features alcohols as geraniol, citronellol, 55–60%; the aldehyde citronellal 7–15%; esters as geranyl acetate; monoterpenes as limonene, camphene. Java oil contains 85% alcohols, 15% aldehydes.

**Therapeutic actions** Antiseptic, bactericidal, fungicidal; nervine antispasmodic; stomachic, vermifuge; diaphoretic, diuretic; galactagogue; tonic; insecticidal.

**Blends with** citrus oils, cedarwood, eucalyptus, tea tree, geranium, lavender, peppermint, rosemary, sage, thyme.

**Other uses** Flavouring for foods and sweets. It is used to scent soaps, toiletries, shampoos, cosmetics. Industrially it is used to isolate citral, which itself can be converted into other substances and isomers with different scents and properties.

**Safety/precautions** Non-toxic, non irritating; may cause sensitisation in some individuals. Avoid in pregnancy.

# Clary sage

**Name** Clary sage

**Latin name** *Salvia scleria* From the Latin *salvere* to save, or to be in good health, and *clarus*, clear.

**Family** Lamiaceae/Labiateae

**Synonyms** Clary, clary wort, clarry, clear eye, see bright, muscatel.

**Other species** Related to garden sage, *S. officinalis*; Spanish sage, *S. lavandulaefolia*; meadow clary, *S. pretense,* and to *S. dioscoridis*.

**Description** A large member of the Lamiaceae; a biennial, or annual herb up to 130 cm (depending on location); stem erect, square; leaves hairy, large, ovate, simple, paired, aromatic, and wrinkled; flowers numerous, lipped, whorled on terminal spikes, interspersed with bracts and both are variegated white, pink, purple; seeds are tiny, black.

**Habitat/distribution** Native to southern Europe, eastern Mediterranean; introduced to Britain in 1562. Prefers dry, sandy, soil; grows to 1000 meters altitude.

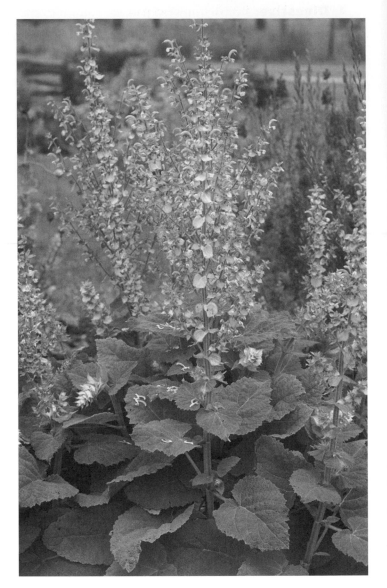

*Clary sage*

**History** Probably used since ancient times in Greek medicine. Hippocrates and Dioscorides mention sages. Gerard reports it naturalised and growing from Holborn to Chelsea. The leaves as well seeds have been used medicinally. Culpeper says that the young leaves are eaten, and are good for the kidneys and weak backs. The mucilage of the seeds he commends for eye problems. The medieval Germans developed its use as a flavouring for Rhenish wine, producing Muscatel. In France it has been used as a perfume fixative.

**Cultivation** Wild. Cultivated widely (USA, Russia, Morocco, Central Europe) from seed in spring.

## USES

- **Skin:** acne, boils, inflammations, excess oil; dandruff, hair loss, oily hair; ageing skin: wrinkles, puffiness.
- **Digestive:** flatulence, dyspepsia.
- **Respiratory:** asthma (calming), congestion, phlegm; cough, whooping cough.
- **Circulatory:** high blood pressure, varicose veins, phlebitis.
- **Reproductive:** uterine tonic, leucorrhea, amenorrhea, menopausal symptoms (hot flushes), parturient, post-natal depression; impotence, frigidity.
- **Nervous:** anxiety, depression, panic attacks; tension, stress, headache, migraine; weakness, convalescence.
- **Mental-Emotional:** uplifting, euphoric, invigorating; Culpeper associated it with the Moon, suggesting its benefits for female imbalances.

**Part used** Flowering tops, leaves.

**Extraction/adulterations** Steam distillation

**Characteristics** A colourless to pale yellow-green liquid; sweet, nutty herbaceous odour, which can be too strong for some individuals. Top note.

**Constituents** Features esters as linalyl acetate, geranyl acetate, neryl acetate70%; alcohols as linalool, sclareol, α-terpineol, α-bisabolol, 20%; sesquiterpenes as caryophyllene, germacrene, bourbonene, 4%; monoterpenes, oxides, acids, lactones, coumarins, ketones, aldehydes.

**Energy** Cooling, moistening. Calms melancholy, purifies blood, clears phlegm, cools choler. Calms vata, reduces pitta, reduces kapha. Tonifies qi of lungs, spleen, stomach; moves qi.

**Therapeutic actions** Anticonvulsive, nervine antidepressant, antispasmodic, sedative and tonic; hypotensive; emmenagogue, aphrodisiac, uterine tonic; carminative, stomachic; regulates sebum; deodorant, febrifuge; antiseptic, antibacterial; antifungal; astringent.

**Blends with** juniper, geranium, cardamom, sandalwood, cedarwood, jasmine, citrus oils, lemongrass.

**Other uses** A fragrance and fixative for soaps, cosmetics, perfumes; a flavouring for drinks and wines.

A seed placed under the eyelid provokes secretions, which help remove foreign particles. (Culpeper). Seeds themselves are mucilaginous when soaked in water. The mucilage, strained, is soothing for irritations and inflammations applied externally.

**Safety/precautions** Avoid in pregnancy, in conditions of hormone-related cancers and after consumption of alcohol.

# Clove

**Name** Clove

**Latin name** *Eugenia caryophyllata* syn. *Syzygium aromaticum*

**Family** Myrtaceae

**Synonyms** *E. aromatica, E. caryophyllata, E. caryophyllus.*

**Other species** None.

**Description** A small, evergreen tree; trunk dividing into large branches; bark smooth, greyish; leaves large, entire, oblong-lanceolate, paired, bright green, fragrant; flowers in bunches at the end of branches. The whole tree is aromatic.

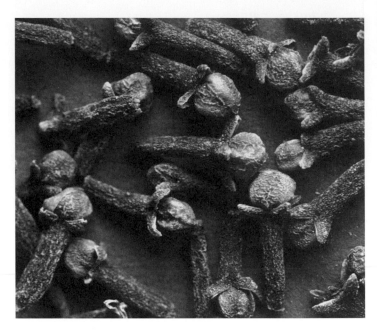

*Clove*

**Habitat/distribution** Native to the Molucca islands of Indonesia, particularly the island of Rum. Grown in Indonesia, Philippines, Madagascar.

**History** Cloves were traditional used by islanders as a carminative and stimulating, anesthetising medicine. Indonesian cigarettes are flavoured with clove. In the 16th and 17th centuries European countries, particularly Britain and Holland, competed fiercely and fought several wars to control the trade and sources of cloves, at that time a most highly valued commodity – considered the most aromatic and stimulating of all spices. At the end of the last of these wars, the island of Manhatten was traded by the Dutch to the British in return for Rum. When the Dutch destroyed all the trees on Ternate island, the islanders were susceptible to previously unknown epidemics. Oranges studded with cloves were originally used to prevent contagion and infection. Clove essence was used by Arab physicians in an ophthalmic ointment and an aqueous solution was used in Russia to treat corneal leucomas and scarring. It has been used in hospitals in surgical dressings (France). Clove oil has traditionally been used for toothache.

**Cultivation** Wild. Cultivated mainly in Indonesia, Réunion, Madagascar for essential oil production. Long, green buds appear at the start of the rainy season. When the calyces, containing the embryo seeds, turn red, they are beaten from the trees and gathered before the seeds can mature.

**Part used** Flower bud, dried; leaves, stalks or stems.

**Extraction/adulterations** Water distillation of buds and leaves; steam distillation of the stalks. A concrete, absolute and oleo resin are also produced. The oil can be adulterated with essential oil of the pimento.

## USES

- **Skin:** acne, athlete's foot, ringworm, impetigo, wounds, burns, cuts, ulcers, bruises; toothache, antiseptic mouthwash.
- **Digestive:** indigestion, dyspepsia, colic, cramp, nausea, enteritis, dysentery.
- **Respiratory:** cough, colds, flu, infections, catarrhal congestion, bronchitis, sinusitis, asthma, tuberculosis.
- **Immune:** herpes, chlorosis, Hodgkin's disease.
- **Circulatory:** hypotension, Raynaud's disease.
- **Endocrine:** imbalance of thyroid function.
- **Muscular–skeletal:** sprains, strains, arthritis, rheumatic pain; muscle tonic (including uterus).
- **Nervine:** neuralgia, spasm.
- **Mental–emotional:** memory loss, Alzheimer's.

**Characteristics** A pale yellow liquid; sweet, spicy odour with a fruity note. Base note.

**Energy** Warming, drying. Clears phlegm, purifies blood, calms melancholy, can increase choler. Reduces kapha and vata, increases pitta (avoid in presence of inflammation, high pitta, hypertension); strengthens agni. Tonifies spleen, stomach and kidney yang; clears wind, cold and damp.

**Chemical constituents** Features phenols, phenol ethers as eugenol, isoeugenol, aceteugenol 90%; sesquiterpenes as β-caryophyllene, humulene 6%; oxides as caryopyllene oxide, humulene oxide 1%; esters, trace; remainders 3%.

**Therapeutic actions** Anti-infectious, antiviral, antimicrobial (against fungi, gram positive and gram negative bacteria), antibiotic; digestive aperitif, sialagogue, stomachic, carminative, spasmolytic; expectorant, mucolytic; vermifuge, anthelmintic; counter-irritant; nervine analgesic–anaesthetic, tonic; circulatory stimulant.

**Blends with** lavender, clary sage, rose, ylang ylang, jasmine, bergamot.

**Other uses** Used in insect repellants (dermal, and placed in linen). Dental preparations. Fragrance in toothpaste, soap, toiletries cosmetics, perfumes.

 **Safety/precautions** Can cause skin and mucous membrane irritation. Possible sensitisation in some people. Use in high dilution/low dosage (less than 1%) and in moderation.

# Cypress

**Name** Cypress

**Latin name** *Cupressus sempervivens*, named for Kyparissos, a youth beloved of Apollo who changed him into this tree, and from the Latin, 'living forever'.

**Family** Cupressaceae

**Synonyms** Italian cypress, Mediterranean cypress.

**Other species** *C. sempervivens* var. *horizontalis*, rare now in Greece and Crete, has more horizontal branches. Many species worldwide are also distilled, e.g. *C. lusitanica* in Kenya.

**Description** 'An exclamation point on a happy landscape' (Paul Vasseur quoted in Valnet, 1982), cypress is a tall evergreen tree, with slender branches and an elegant, slender conical shape.

**Habitat/distribution** Native from eastern Mediterranean to India. Dry, sunny habitat.

**History** Cypress was used by ancient Assyrians and has been part of southern European traditional medicine. It was sacred to the Greeks; its timber was used to build temples, sanctuaries and sarcophagi. It was valuable and used for dowries; even now it is planted at the birth of a daughter. Because it is evergreen, Egyptians, Greeks and Romans also associated it with death and rebirth and planted it in cemeteries. It is used in Ayurvedic medicine and the Chinese eat the nuts, and use them for liver, respiratory and sweating disorders.

**Cultivation** Wild and cultivated in France, Spain, Morocco.

**Part used** Leaves/needles and twigs and fruit – 'cypress nuts'.

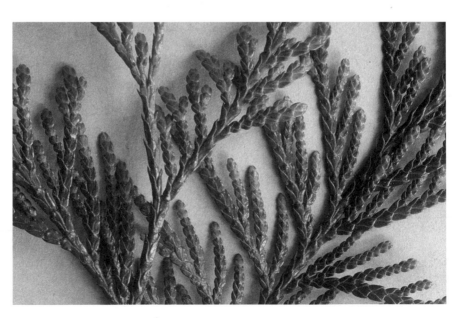

*Cypress*

- **Skin:** excessive odour and sweating of feet (take foot baths), excessive oiliness, bleeding gums, wounds, insect and flea repellant; aftershave.
- **Respiratory:** whooping cough, spasmodic cough, asthma, spitting blood, flu, bronchitis.
- **Immune/lymph:** flu, loss of voice, fevers.
- **Circulatory:** haemorrhoids, varicose veins, cellulite, oedema, poor circulation.
- **Endocrine:** strengthen glandular function, regulate menses. (Cypress essential oil is a homologue of the ovarian hormone oestrogen according to Valnet.)
- **Muscular–skeletal:** arthritis, aches and pains, muscle spasm.
- **Urinary:** bed wetting, incontinence.
- **Reproductive:** irregular cycle, dysmenorrhoea, metrorrahagia.
- **Nervous:** stress, tension; asthma.
- **Mental–emotional:** grounding, gives strength.

**Extraction/adulterations** Steam distillation of the needles, twigs and occasionally the fruit/'nut' or cone. Use only essential oil from *C. sempervirens*.

**Characteristics** A pale yellow or olive-green liquid; sweet-balsamic or woody odour. Base note.

**Energy** Warming, drying. Clears phlegm, calms melancholy, purifies blood. Increases kapha, pitta, calms vata. Moves blood and regulates qi, clears heat and stagnation (kidney and bladder).

**Chemical constituents** Features terpenes as α-pinene, β-pinene, ρ-cymene, camphene, limonene, Δ3-carene 75%; alcohols as cedrol, α-terpineol, borneol, sabinol, manool 10%; esters as α-terpenyl acetate, terpinen-4-yl acetate 5%; sesquiterpenes as cedrene, cadinene 3%; oxides 1.8-cineole, manoyl oxide 1%.

**Therapeutic actions** Antiseptic; astringent, styptic, tonic; nervine antispasmodic (including respiratory muscles) and tonic; hepatic, vasoconstrictive; diaphoretic, diuretic, antirheumatic; deodorant (external, foot odour); counters sweating (external application); glandular balance, especially ovaries.

**Blends with** cedarwood, pine, lemon, bergamot, mandarin, juniper, sandalwood, benzoin, clary sage, lavender, marjoram, cardamom. Useful in blends for men.

**Other uses** Fragrance in colognes, aftershaves, perfumes; ingredient in some pharmaceuticals.

 **Safety/precautions** Non-toxic, non-irritating, non-sensitising.

# Eucalyptus

**Name** Eucalyptus blue gum

**Latin name** *Eucalyptus globulus* var. *globulus* from Greek *eucalyptos* 'well covered', since in bud the sepals and petals fuse to form a cap; *globulus*, 'little globe', describes the shape of the fruit.

**Family** Myrtaceae

**Synonyms** Gum tree, southern blue gum, Tasmanian blue gum, fever tree, stringy bark.

**Other species** The genus comprises 700 species of trees, 500 yielding an essential oil. *E. radiata* combines high proportions of alcohols and cineole for a synergy effective on respiratory and throat conditions. Aldehydes give it significant anti-inflammatory properties combined with a calming effect. It may be substituted for *E. globulus*; which is preferable for children (Price and Price) as its fragrance is sweeter and softer. *E. smithii* is higher in terpenes which synergise with significant amounts of alcohols for stronger anti-infectious, bactericidal and antiviral effects without skin irritation. The terpenes have a quenching effect. *E. citriodora* is high in alcohols with significant amounts of esters and aldehydes (citronella above 50%) giving it anti-inflammatory, non-irritating and calming properties combined with antibactieral, antiviral effects. *E. dives,* with piperitone, is used to make menthol. *E. polybractea* is also cineole-rich.

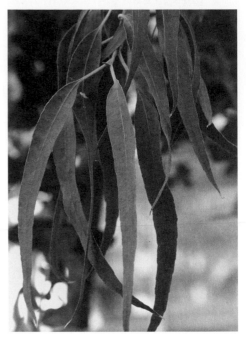

*Eucalyptus blue gum*

**Description** A tree growing to 70 m; trunk smooth, grey or bluish with bark that peels; leaves opposite, lanceolate, leathery with numerous oil-containing glands; the flower bud formed as a lid, which is literally thrown off on blooming; the round fruit a woody receptacle with numerous, minute seeds. The tree grows rapidly.

**Habitat/distribution** Native to Australia and Tasmania; introduced to other semi-tropical and temperate areas world wide. The trees exude so much volatile oil that they may self-ignite during drought and high temperatures.

**History** It has been used by Aborigines for millennia. In the 1870s the German botanist Baron Ferdinand von Müller studied and celebrated its properties. European settlers developed it as a source of timber, oil, shade and learned from the Aborigines such uses as smoking dried leaves for respiratory conditions and infusing them for typhoid, malarial and other fevers, aching joints, dysentery, ringworm, tuberculosis. It has been planted as an ornamental; to encourage draining of marshes and malarial habitats; for timber and as a source for perfumes, fragrances, flavours – i.e. the oils rich in citronellal (*E. citriodora*). Oils rich in terpenes are also used in mining and Valnet cites its use in burn treatment dressings and in facial coverings to prevent spread of infectious fevers.

**Cultivation** Wild; ornamental and commercial cultivation.

**Part used** Leaves, fresh or partially dried, and twigs.

**Extraction/adulterations** Steam distillation.

## USES

- **Skin:** acne, boils, burns, cuts, infections, wounds; herpes cold sores, chicken pox and shingles; athlete's foot; insect infestations; insect repellant.
- **Digestive:** stimulates secretions, hypoglycaemia, diabetes, gall stones (internally).
- **Respiratory:** colds, catarrh, sinus congestion, cough, flu, pneumonia; bronchitis, asthma.
- **Immune/lymph:** tonsillitis, laryngitis, fevers (diphtheria, scarlet fever).
- **Circulation:** toxins in blood, poor circulation (stimulates blood and lymph flow); haemorrhage.
- **Muscular–skeletal:** osteo-arthritis, aches and pains, strain and sprain, rheumatoid arthritis.
- **Genito-urinary:** cystitis, leucorrhoea, gonorrhoea, thrush.
- **Nervous:** weakness, debility, headache, neuralgia, nerve inflammations in shingles.
- **Mental–emotional:** brings clarity, dispels confusion, invigorates, refreshes.

**Characteristics** A colourless to pale yellow, light liquid, which yellows on ageing; strong camphorous or medicinal odour with a woody undertone. Top note.

**Energy** Warming, drying, draining. Clears phlegm, cools choler, purifies blood. Reduces kapha, vata, pitta; can increase pitta in excess. Moves qi, clears damp and phlegm; tonifies wei qi and spleen qi.

**Chemical constituents** Features oxides as 1.8 cineole 75%; terpenes as α-pinene, limonene, ρ-cymene, phillandrene 10%; alcohols as globulol, *trans* pinocarveol 6%; sesquiterpenes as armadendrene 4%; esters as α-terpinyl acetate 1.0%; ketone pinocarvone 1.0%; acids, aldehydes. (NB: The high proportion of oxides with significant amounts of alcohols, sesquiterpenes and esters make *E. globulus* a gentle yet powerful antibacterial, antiviral, anti-inflammatory and mucolytic agent.)

**Therapeutic actions** Antibacterial, antiviral, antiseptic; nervine analgesic; expectorant, mucolytic, decongestant; diaphoretic, febrifuge, alterative; diuretic; vulnerary, cicatrisant; hypoglycaemic (internally); paraciticide, vermifuge; stimulant of blood and immune system; styptic. (NB: 1.8-cineole is immunomodulant, stimulating a reduction in inflammatory reactions, such as swelling of mucous membranes, while countering infective agents.)

**Blends with** thyme, rosemary, sage, marjoram, lavender, pine, lemon, cedarwood, juniper, lemon, lemongrass, tea tree (e.g. for athlete's foot).

**Other uses** Pharmaceutical and proprietary preparations for liniments, inhalants, cough syrups, ointments; toothpastes, mouthwashes; fragrance for soaps, detergents, toiletries; food flavouring.

 **Safety/precautions** Non-toxic, non-irritating, non-sensitising. Taken internally eucalyptus can be toxic: ingesting as little as 3.5 ml has been fatal. Incompatible with homoeopathic treatment.

# Fennel

**Name** Fennel

**Latin name** *Foeniculum vulgare*, from the Latin *foenum* hay and *vulgare* common.

**Family** Apiaceae/Umbelliferae

**Synonyms** *F. officinale, F. capillaceum, Anethum foeniculum,* Fenkel.

**Other species** There are many cultivated and wild varieties. Fennel is related to the Florentine and Sicilian vegetables *F. axoricum* and *F. piperitum,* and also to bitter fennel, *F. vulgare* var. *amarga* and sweet fennel, *F. vulgara* var. *dulce.*

**Description** Perennial or hardy annual, graceful herb, 1–1.5 m high; stem erect, stout, hairless, glaucous, branched; leaves are feathery, much divided, dark green; yellow-golden flowers in flat umbels; seeds tiny, brown. The young shoot is succulent and edible. The whole plant is aromatic.

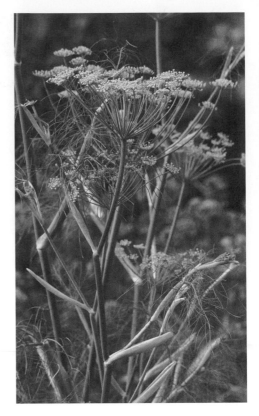

*Fennel*

**Habitat/distribution** Native to southern Europe, it is widely distributed eastwards to the Indian subcontinent; naturalised in British isles. It is cultivated in temperate Europe and Russia, Middle East and India.

**History** Used since ancient times in Mediterranean, Egyptian and Eastern cuisine, rituals and medicine, fennel was prescribed by Hippocrates for jaundice. Pliny recommends it for sharpening eyesight, a tradition that lived on in folk medicine until recently. It was also known in ancient Greece to aid weight loss or fluid retention. (Its Greek name is *marathron*, to grow thin.) Greek athletes at Olympic games and Roman soldiers both used it to maintain strength.

In the Middle Ages it served to ward off witches and evil. Culpeper classes it hot in the 3rd degree and recommends it as a galactagogue, diuretic, parturient, carminative. He used it for obstructions of spleen, lungs, gall bladder; for stones and gout; for wounds and bruising; as an antidote to poisons, bites.

**Cultivation** Wild and cultivated.

**Part used** Seeds, crushed.

**Extraction/adulterations** Steam distillation.

**Characteristics** Colourless to pale yellow, liquid; sweet, aniseed or licorice-type odour. Top to middle note.

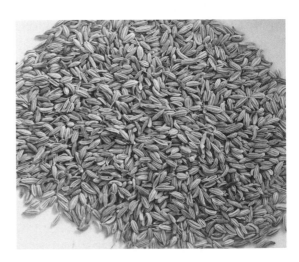

*Fennel seeds*

## USES

- **Skin:** boils, swellings, bruises, oily skin, wrinkles, inhibit ageing.

- **Digestive:** weak digestion, flatulence, constipation, colic, dyspepsia, colitis, nausea; anorexia, obesity.

- **Respiratory:** phlegm, congestion (chest, sinus), colds, asthma, bronchitis, rapid breathing, whooping cough.

- **Circulation/lymph:** fluid retention, cellulite and toxins, cellulitis; oedema; obesity; angina, palpitations, Raynaud's.

- **Muscular–skeletal:** arthritis (via its alterative, blood purifying effects and improvement of kidney function).

- **Urinary:** fluid retention, cystitis, infections, stones, retention of urine, gout.

- **Reproductive:** amenorrhoea, irregular cycle; assist childbirth, stimulate milk; menopause symptoms.

- **Nervous:** digestive cramp, spasm; paralysis.

- **Mental–emotional:** balancing, helps one to let go of unnecessary attachments. When using the essential oil, also recommend the patient drink freely of the decoction of the seeds.

**Energy** Warming, drying. Clears phlegm, cools choler, calms melancholy. Tridosic, balances kapha, pitta and vata; strengthens agni. Tonifies spleen, stomach, kidney-yin qi, moves qi.

**Chemical constituents** Features phenols, phenol ethers as trans-anethole, methyl chavicol (estragol) 62%; terpenes as α-pinene, α-thujene, γ-terpinene, limonene, myrcene, phellandrene 24%; ketones as fenchone 5%; oxides as 1.8-cineole 3%; alcohols as fenchol 3%; acids, lactones and coumarins.

**Therapeutic actions** Antimicrobial, antiseptic, bactericidal anti-inflammatory; diuretic; diaphoretic (mild); carminative, aperitif, laxative; nervine antispasmodic and analgesic; alterative; emmenagogue, oestrogen-like (may stimulate production of oestrogen by adrenal glands during menopause; benefits connective tissue); galactagogue; tonic to spleen, liver, stomach, nerves; vermifuge.

**Blends with** geranium, lavender, rose, sandalwood.

**Other uses** Pharmaceutical products such as lozenges, cough drops, carminatives and laxatives; flavouring in foods and beverages; fragrance for soaps, toiletries, perfumes, room sprays.

 **Safety/precautions** Non-irritating, relatively non-toxic, though narcotic in large doses. Avoid in pregnancy, for children under 6 and in epilepsy. Avoid distilled bitter fennel, which is high in ketones.

# Frankincense

**Name** Frankincense (from the French frank or 'real' incense)

**Latin name** *Boswellia carteri*

**Family** Burseraceae

**Synonyms** 'Gum', its old name was 'olibanum' from the Roman designation of Lebanon.

**Other species** An Indian variety *Boswellia serrata*.

**Description** A small tree or shrub; oblong, serrated leaves alternate towards the tops of branches, unequally pinnate with leaflets in 10 pairs with odd one opposite; flowers white or pink in racemes shorter than leaves; fruit capsular and 3-angular, 3-valved and 3-celled with a single seed in each cell.

**Habitat/distribution** Forests in the Arabian peninsula, Somalia, Ethiopia (Horn of Africa); China, India.

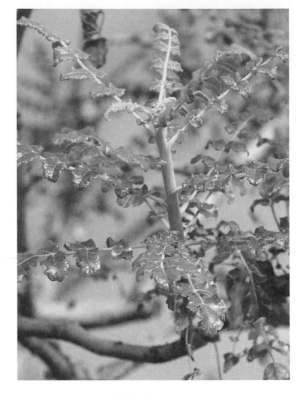

*Frankincense*

**History** It has been used by the most ancient cultures of the Mediterranean and Near East: Egypt, Sumer, Assyria, Babylon, Persia, Greece, Palestine, Rome. Uses include sacramental/ritual purposes, for cosmetics and perfumes and for medicines. Egyptians used it for embalming. It was held to be as precious as gold. Khol is traditionally made of charred frankincense. Pagan, Catholic, Greek and Russion Orthodox churches burn frankincense to induce an atmosphere conducive to spiritual contemplation and connection with the divine. Frankincense calms the breathing and the mind. Its purifying and preservative properties are equally formidable. It is recorded in Dioscorides' herbal for skin conditions, haemorrhage, pneumonia.

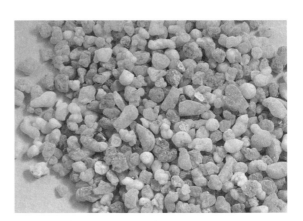

*Frankincense tears*

**Cultivation** Wild on soilless rocks. Young trees produce the best gum after a deep, longitudinal incision is made in the trunk, repeatedly over the 3-month dry season. A strip of bark is removed below to help catch the exudation. The milky resin exudes and hardens to a gum on exposure to air forming large, clear, yellow 'tears'. Any resin that has run to the ground is also collected, but is inferior.

## USES

- **Skin:** blemishes, wounds, scars, ulcers, infections; ageing skin, wrinkles.
- **Digestive:** flatulence, nervous stomach.
- **Respiratory:** deepen and calm breathing; asthma, bronchitis and other infections, catarrh, cough.
- **Immune/lymph:** laryngitis, colds, flu, pneumonia; cancer, strengthen immunity.
- **Genito-urinary:** cystitis, leucorrhoea, dysmenorrhoeal, metrorrhagia. Safe in pregnancy.
- **Nervous:** insomnia, anxiety, paranoia, depressions, obsessions, irritability.
- **Mental–emotional:** calming, euphoric, strengthening. Helps to break unwanted links, assist spiritual development.

**Part used** Oleo gum resin, 'tears'.

**Extraction/adulterations** Steam distillation. The gum is produced in Arabia and the Horn of Africa (Ethiopia, Somalia), China and India and distilled in Europe and India. An absolute is produced as a fixative.

**Characteristics** A pale yellow to greenish liquid; a dry, fresh, penetrating and slightly camphorous or terpene-like odour. Base note.

**Energy** Warming, drying. Clears phlegm, cools choler, purifies blood, calms melancholy. Tridosic: reduces kapha, cools pitta, calms vata; satvic; regulates and improves prana. Moves qi, tonifies qi and yang, dries damp.

**Chemical constituents** Features terpenes as α-pinene, β-pinene, α-terpinene, dipentene, ρ-cymene, thujene, myrcene, phellandrene, limonene 40%; esters as ocytyl and borneol acetate; alcohols octanol, linalool; ketone as incensole.

**Therapeutic actions** Nervine calmative, sedative, euphoric, analgesic, antispasmodic; anti-inflammatory, antiseptic, vulnerary, cicatrisant; digestive carminative and tonic; expectorant, mucolytic; diuretic, emmenagogue; preservative.

**Blends with** sandalwood, lavender, rose, benzoin, bergamot, camphor, basil, vetiver, geranium. 'It modifies the sweetness of citrus blends in an intriguing way' (Lawless, 1992).

**Other uses** Incense; fixative and fragrance component in perfumes, cosmetic, soaps, especially for men. Pharmaceutical ingredient in throat pastilles; flavouring in minute amounts for foods and beverages.

**Safety/precautions** Non-toxic, non-irritating, non-sensitising.

# Geranium

**Name** Geranium

**Latin name** *Pelargonium graveolens* from the Greek *pelargos*, a young stork, because the fruit's shape recalls that of a stork's bill. For the same reason the name geranium is taken from the Greek *geranos*, a crane.

**Family** Geraniaceae

**Synonyms** Rose geranium, pelargonium. Several cultivars exist with scent ranging from lemon to apple.

**Other species** *P. capitatum, P. radens, P. odorantissimum* are also distilled for commercial essences. A large genus, over 700 species; many cultivated for ornamental and commercial purposes.

**Description** A perennial, bushy aromatic herb up to 1 m; longer stems become more woody; leaves petiole, hairy, 5–7 lobed, circular to ovate, margins dentate; flowers pink, unscented, sessile on dense umbels. The whole plant is aromatic.

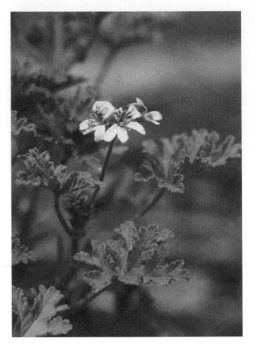

*Geranium*

**Habitat/distribution** Native to South Africa, introduced and cultivated widely (Algeria, Morocco, Madagascar, Réunion, Russia, China, Egypt, Guinea). Geranium prefers dry, well-drained loam, full sun. Almost all scented geraniums are native to southern Africa.
(NB: Réunion and now Madagascar produce an oil with the appellation 'Bourbon', which has a slightly different aroma due to the volcanic soil there.)

**History** It has been used in traditional African medicine. The roots of certain species are used for diarrhoea. Introduced first to Britain in 1632, geraniums became popular in 1840s when their potential for perfumery was recognised by the French. Oil of geranium became an essential ingredient of perfumes for men, and is used as a substitute for rose oil. Pelargoniums are related to the European storkbill and American cranesbill (*G. robertanium*, herb robert and *G. maculatum*), familiar perennial wildflowers used in herbal medicine, primarily for their astringent and vulnerary effects (Culpeper). This use is consistent with the properties of African pelargonium.

**Cultivation** Wild; as a houseplant/tender perennial garden plant; commercially in warmer regions: the south-western Mediterranean, particularly Morocco; central and southern Africa (Zimbabwe). Geranium is propagated from cuttings.

**Part used** Aerial parts: leaves, stalks and flowers.

**Extraction/adulterations** Steam distillation. An absolute is produced in Morocco. It is often used to adulterate and thus 'stretch' rose essential oil. Buyer beware.

**Characteristics** A pale or olive green liquid; a sweet rose-like odour with a hint of mint or 'greenness'. Middle note.

- **Skin:** acne, excess sebum, dehydration, bruises, wounds, burns, dermatitis/ eczema, haemorrhoids, broken capillaries, infestation, fungal infections, ringworm; herpes, shingles, dandruff; oral infections, thrush, gingivitis.

- **Digestive:** diarrhoea, flatulence, gastic ulcer, gastro-enteritis, dyspepsia, colitis, jaundice, diabetes.

- **Circulation/lymph:** bleeding, varicose veins, poor circulation, heavy legs, weak vessels; cellulite, fluid retention, oedema, Raynaud's; tonsillitis; cleanses blood.

- **Endocrine:** strengthens adrenal cortex, regulates hormone function.

- **Muscular–skeletal:** injuries, fractures, swellings, stiffness, pain.

- **Urinary:** cystitis, stone.

- **Reproductive:** breast engorgement, vaginal thrush, painful periods, PMS, uterine haemorrhage.

- **Nervous:** facial neuralgia, anxiety, nervousness, restlessness, Raynaud's, depression.

- **Mental–emotional:** integrates mind and body, balances extremes.

# Geranium
*Pelargonium graveolens*

**Energy** Cooling, combines moistening and astringent properties: balancing, amphoteric. Balances blood, calms melancholy, cools choler. Reduces kapha and pitta, calms vata, balances prana. Tonifies spleen, kidney yin and qi; clears damp, phlegm, heat.

**Chemical constituents** Features alcohols as citronellol, geraniol, linalool 64%; esters as citronellyl formate, geranyl formate 15%; aldehydes as citral 5%; sesquiterpenes as guaiazulene, β-caryophyllene 4%; oxides as *cis*-rose oxide 2%; terpenes as phellandrene, limonene, α-pinene 2%; ketones as menthone 7%.

**Therapeutic actions** Hormone regulator/balancer, tonic to adrenal cortex; astringent, vasoconstrictive, styptic, anticoagulant, vulnerary; bactericidal, antiseptic, antifungal; diuretic; lymphatic stimulant; liver and kidney tonic, litholytic; carminative, aperitif, stomachic; febrifuge, anti-inflammatory; nervine analgesic, antidepressant; vermifuge. Antidiabetic, possibly anticancer effects (Valnet, 1982).

**Blends with** lavender, bergamot and other citrus oils, sandalwood, jasmine, rose, juniper, patchouli.

**Other uses** An ingredient in insect repellants along with bergamot, lemongrass and lemon; fragrance in many toiletries, perfumes, soaps; flavouring in foods and beverages. Fresh leaves can be added to cakes before baking and to fruit dishes.

 **Safety/precautions** Non-toxic, non-irritating, non-sensitising generally, though possible contact dermatitis in some individuals.

# Ginger

**Name** Ginger

**Latin name** *Zingiber officinalis*

**Family name** Zingiberaceae

**Synonyms** None

**Other species** Many varieties of ginger are found in its native habitat. Several varieties are cultivated commercially: Jamaican/white African, Cochin (a region of India). Other genera in the family are zeodary root – *Curcuma zeodaria*, turmeric – *C. longa*, and galangal or Chinese ginger – *Alpinia officinarum*.

**Description** A perennial creeper with a thick, tuberous rhizome; erect annual stem 60–120 cm; leaves lanceolate to linear-lanceolate, 15–30 cm; flowers on radial stalks (direct from the root) ending in spikes, white or yellow. All parts are aromatic, but the rhizome particularly so.

**Habitat/distribution** Native to south and south-east Asia, it has been introduced to tropical countries. Ginger grows at up to 1,500 m altitude. It prefers rich, well-drained loam.

**History** Ginger has been used for millennia. It was valued by ancient Greeks, who imported it from the east, and was highly valued in the Middle Ages. It is important in Chinese, Ayurvedic and Far Eastern medical systems. The Spanish introduced its cultivation to the West Indies. Distilled ginger water has been used for cataracts. Ginger root is one of the most versatile of medicines and should always be kept on hand.

**Cultivation** From cuttings of the rhizome. It may be grown indoors in temperate climates from purchased culinary rhizomes, which show a green bud. Keep moist and in a sunny window.

**Part used** Rhizome, unpeeled, dried.

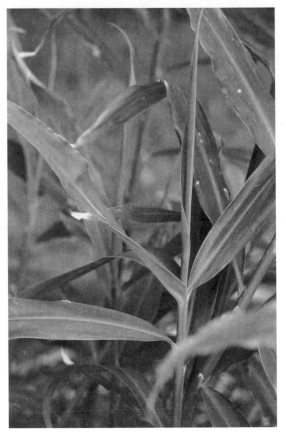

*Ginger*

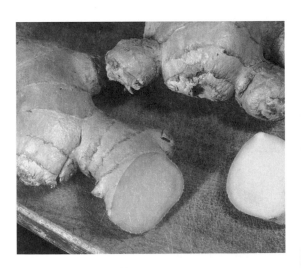

*Ginger root*

## USES

- **Skin:** may be placed as a compress over areas of pain, stiffness.
- **Digestive:** weak digestion, nausea, diarrhoea, constipation, flatulence, dyspepsia, hangover, cramp.
- **Respiratory:** colds, catarrh, sinus congestion, flu, coughs, bronchitis.
- **Immune:** fevers, flu, inflammations.
- **Circulation:** poor circulation, stasis, varicose veins; angina; disperses clots.
- **Muscular–skeletal:** aches and pains, osteo-arthritis, rheumatoid arthritis, sprains, strains, muscle spasms, fatigue.
- **Reproductive:** impotence.
- **Nervous:** spasms, cramps, neuralgia, pain; debility, exhaustion.
- **Mental–emotional:** balancing, warming, cordial.

**Extraction/adulterations** Steam distillation. An absolute and oleo resin are produced for perfumery.

**Characteristics** A pale amber, yellow or greenish liquid, which darkens with age; fresh, pungent, spicy 'green' odour. Top note.

**Energy** Warming, drying. Hot and dry in 2nd degree, it clears phlegm, warms and grounds melancholy, purifies blood. Reduces kapha, warms and reduces vata, increases pitta and stimulates agni. It disperses wind, cold, damp; tonifies yang and kidney yang; moves and tonifes qi.

**Chemical constituents** Features sesquiterpenes as β-sesquiphellandrene, zingiberene, *ar*-curcumene 55%; terpenes as α-pinene, β-pinene, camphene, limonene, phellandrene 20%; alcohols as citronellol, linalool, borneol, gingerol 10%; aldehydes as geranial, neral, citronellal 5%; esters as geranyl acetate 2%; ketones as gingerone; oxide 1,8, cineole 1.3%.

**Therapeutic actions** Digestive stimulant, stomachic, aperitif, carminative, laxative; antispasmodic; anti-inflammatory, febrifuge; diaphoretic; analgesic; rubifacient; antitussive, expectorant; cephalic; aphrodisiac, antiseptic, bactericidal.

**Blends with** citrus oils, sandalwood, vetiver, patchouli, frankincense, cedarwood, juniper, coriander.

**Other uses** The oleoresin is used in pharmaceutical preparations for constipation, flatulence; as fragrance it is found in soaps, toiletries, cosmetics, perfumes – especially oriental scents, men's scents; flavouring for food, beverages.

 **Safety/precautions** Non-toxic, non-irritant in normal doses; slightly phototoxic, may cause sensitisation in some individuals; use in low doses.

# Grapefruit

**Name** Grapefruit

**Latin name** *Citrus x paradisi*, a recent hybrid of *C. maxima* and *C. sinensis*.

**Family** Rutaceae

**Synonyms** *C. racemosa*, *C. maxima* var. *racemose*, *C. grandis*, the shaddock fruit.

**Other species** Grapefruit is a recent hybrid of *C. maxima* and *C. sinensis*; there are many cultivars.

**Description** A small tree, evergreen, 10 m; leaves ovate, glossy; fruit large, yellow, appearing in bunch-like groups, hence, possibly, the naming after grapes; shares qualities with other citrus species.

**Habitat/distribution** Native to tropical Asia. Grapefruit is cultivated commercially in California, Florida, Cyprus, Israel for its fruit.

**History** Introduced to the West Indies in the 18th century and once known as shaddock fruit, its smaller ancestor.

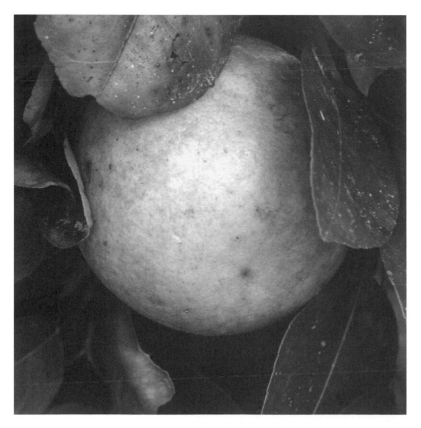

*Grapefruit*

## USES

- **Skin:** acne, congested, oily skin, aged, damaged skin; promotes hair growth.
- **Digestive:** weak digestion, poor appetite, anorexia.
- **Immune:** chills, cold, flu.
- **Circulation/lymph:** fluid retention, cellulite.
- **Muscular–skeletal:** fatigue; use before exercise to prepare muscles.
- **Nervous:** headache, stress, exhaustion, depression.
- **Mental–emotional:** sadness, dejection; balancing, uplifting ('takes one to paradise').

**Cultivation** Commercially for its fruit. The essential oil is produced from the peel after crushing for juice.

**Part used** Peel of fruit.

**Extraction/adulterations** Expression of the fruit peel. The fruit is thick and the essential oil is deep in the peel beneath a thick albedo, making expression difficult. Some essential oil sold is distilled from the pulp after juice is expressed, though this yields an inferior oil with a different profile. Check extraction method with supplier.

**Characteristics** A yellow or greenish, light liquid; fresh, sharp citrus aroma. Top note.

**Energy** Cooling, drying. Clears phlegm, cools choler, calms melancholy. Reduces kapha, calms, reduces vata, strengthens agni; satvic. Moves qi; clears stagnation in the digestive tract; tonifies spleen, clears damp-heat.

**Chemical constituents** Features monoterpenes as limonene as much as 96%. Aldehydes as citronellal, citral, sinensal 1.5%; esters as geranyl acetate 0.5%; alcohols as paradisol, geraniol 1%; ketones, lactones and coumarins as auraptene, limettin; sesquiterpenes as cadidene.

**Therapeutic actions** Antiseptic, bactericidal; astringent; alterative, diuretic; tonic, lymphatic stimulant; digestive tonic, carminative, aperitif.

**Blends** with citrus oils, palmarosa, rosemary, lavender, cardamom, geranium, cypress.

**Other uses** Fragrance for soaps, toiletries, cosmetic, perfumes; flavouring for foods, desserts, beverages.

**Safety/precautions** Non-toxic, non-irritating, non-sensitising. Possibly phototoxic: avoid exposure to sunlight after topical application as it contains traces of bergaptene. Avoid in pregnancy and epilepsy.

# Hyssop

**Name** Hyssop

**Latin name** *Hyssopus officinalis* from the Hebrew *ezoph*, its Biblical name, through the Greek *hussopos*. Significantly the name is almost identical in all European languages. It is not certain that the *hussopos* of the Greeks is the same as that of the Old Testament, which was probably marjoram.

**Family** Lamiaceae/Labiatae.

**Synonyms** None

**Other species** The genus consists of this single species though there are varieties and subspecies, e.g. *Hyssopus officinalis* var. *decumbens*.

**Description** A perennial subshrub, stems erect, branched, 20–26 cm, with fine hairs at the tips; leaves linear to oblong, sessile, opposite; flowers blue in one-sided whorls, in leaf axils.

**Habitat/distribution** Native to central, southern Europe, the eastern Mediterranean, the Near East and western Asia.

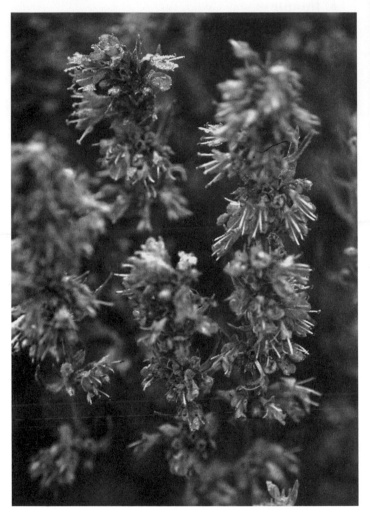

*Hyssop*

**History** Used by Near Eastern and early Mediterranean peoples, hyssop has a long association with both the sacred and with breathing conditions, affirming the traditional link between breath and spirit. Hippocratic physicans employed it for pleurisy and bronchitis, and Galen records it as a fumigant for quinsy and inflammations of the throat. Renaissance physicians of the Salerno medical school, following Dioscorides, prepared it in honey for pulmonary conditions and to remove phlegm. It was known in Britain by the 13th century. Cistercian monks valued the honey from the flowers. Turner and Culpeper used it for ringing in the ears; Turner writes 'The vapor of Hisop driveth away the winde that is in the ears, if they be holden over it' (Grieve, 1984). Culpeper funnelled the fumes of a decoction. It was a strewing herb in large houses and establishments. Traditionally also used for digestion and in aperitifs. Hyssop had also been used for lung conditions, bruising and pains of rheumatism. It continues in herbal *pharmacopoeiae*.

## USES

- **Skin:** Bruises, cuts, wounds, dermatitis/eczema, inflammation, infections; infestations.
- **Digestive:** flatulence, weak digestion, indigestion, colic.
- **Respiratory:** colds, coughs, congestion, catarrh, flu; bronchitis, chronic bronchitis; asthma, whooping cough.
- **Circulation/lymph:** low blood pressure; swellings.
- **Nervous:** multiple sclerosis; anxiety, fatigue, tension, stress.
- **Mental–emotional:** induces calm and clarity, clears confusion; releases unwanted/negative emotions.

**Cultivation** Wild, garden escape; introduced to North America by colonials. It is cultivated commercially in Europe (France, Balkans and Hungary), Russia and India.

**Part used** Aerial parts in flower, leaves and flowering tops.

**Extraction/adulterations** Steam distillation.

**Characteristics** A colourless to pale yellow liquid; strong, sweet-medicinal odour. Middle note.

**Energy** Warming, dispersing. Clears phlegm, cools choler, purifies blood. Reduces kapha, calms vata, increases pitta, strengthens agni. Clears cold, damp, wind; tonifies lung and spleen qi, moves blood.

**Chemical constituents** Features ketones as pinocamphone, isopinocamphone, camphor 46%; terpenes as β-pinene, camphene, limonene, myrcene, *cis*-ocimene; alcohols as borneol, geraniol, linlool 8%; sesquiterpenes as caryophyllene, cadinene 8%; phenols as methyl chavicol 4%; esters as bornyl acetate, methyl myrtenate 2%; oxides as 1.8-cineole, caryophyllene oxide 0.8%.

**Therapeutic actions** Antiseptic, bactericidal, antiviral; cephalic, expectorant; carminative, stomachic; diaphoretic, diuretic, febrifuge; emmenagogue; vulnerary; circulatory stimulant; nervine antispasmodic, sedative, mild analgesic; vermifuge.

**Blends with** eucalyptus, myrtle, lavender, citrus oils, rosemary, sage, juniper, clary sage, geranium.

**Other uses** Fragrance in soaps, toiletries, cosmetics, perfume, especially eau-de-cologne; flavouring for foods and beverages, particularly the liqueur Chartreuse.

**Safety/precautions** Its significant proportion of ketones makes hyssop an oil to use with due caution. Avoid in pregnancy and in conditions of epilepsy and high blood pressure.

# Jasmine

**Name** Jasmine

**Latin name** *Jasminum officinale/J. grandiflorum* from the Persian name for the plant, *yasmin*.

**Family** Oleaceae

**Synonyms** Jasmin, jessamine, poet's jessamine, common white jasmine.

**Other species** Over 150 species exist; many are cultivated in gardens. *J. grandiflorum* (Spanish jasmine) is native to the western Himalyas. *J. sambac* is cultivated in India, Burma, Ceylon and China. These and other species are used in Unani and Ayurvedic medicine and an otto is distilled. *J. sambac* is used in Chinese medicine and to flavour tea.

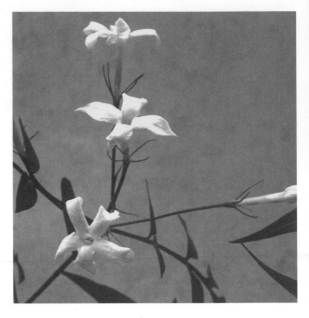

*Jasmine*

**Description** A vigorous climber, though needing support, to over 6 m; leaves opposite, pinnate; leaflets in three pairs with an odd one; flowers white, fragrant especially after sundown. *J. grandiflorum* has stouter branches, and much larger flowers than *J. officinale* and is preferred for production of perfumes and essential oil and absolute.

**Habitat/distribution** Native to Persia, north-west India-Pakistan; widely cultivated in gardens. *J. grandiflorum* was introduced to Europe in the 16th century, possibly earlier to Spain by the Moors.

**History** Used from prehistoric times in its native lands, the 'king' of flowers has a long association with love and love-making. All parts of jasmine have been used in traditional eastern medicine: the fruits are narcotic, the whole plant is diuretic, emmenagogue.

**Cultivation** In France, Italy, Morocco, Algeria, Turkey, Egypt, China, and India. *J. grandiflorum* is grafted on to roots of *J. officinale*, which is an erect bush, thus obtaining a lower growing plant that needs no support and can be planted in rows sheltered from wind and cold. Blossoms come in the second year and flower from July to October. It is harvested mainly in August and September, the flowers collected just after sunrise.

**Part used** Flowers.

**Extraction/adulterations** Traditionally extraction has been by the enfleurage method because the flowers are capable of continuing to emit their fragrance in repeated macerations. The flowers can be removed from the olive oil or purified lard and replaced with fresh ones; more scent is absorbed. The time-consuming, labour-intensive method is little used today in favour of solvent extraction. However, the modern yield is lower because the solvent kills the flowers at once, stopping the process of scent formation. Today the jasmine is usually available as an absolute obtained by solvent extraction of the concrete. An essential oil is then obtained by

## USES

- **Skin:** dry or oily skin, irritation, sensitive skin, stretch marks.
- **Digestion:** upsets of nervous origin, anorexia.
- **Respiratory:** colds, coughs, bronchial spasm, asthma.
- **Muscular–skeletal:** sprains, muscular spasm.
- **Reproductive:** dysmenorrhoea, PMS, labour pains, stimulate milk, post-partum depression, uterine disorders, vaginal infections; low sperm count.
- **Nervous:** anxiety, paranoia; stress, tension, listlessness, exhaustion.
- **Mental–emotional:** euphoric and very balancing; depression, sadness/grief, indifference, apathy; feelings of disconnection; lack of confidence, self-esteem.

steam distillation of the absolute. Thus, strictly speaking the jasmine available to aromatherapists is an absolute. Sometimes an essential oil is obtained by $CO_2$ extraction.

**Characteristics** Absolute: a dark, orange-brown, viscous liquid; highly intense, rich, sweet, floral odour. Base note. Jasmine is popularly more a feminine scent but this should not exclude its use for male patients when indicated. The odour is very intense and only a tiny amount is needed. For this reason many aromatherapists find it convenient and cost effective to purchase jasmine already diluted in some vegetable oil, for example, at 10% dilution.

**Energy** Cooling, moistening, balancing. Cools choler and blood, soothes and revives melancholy. Reduces, calms vata, cools pitta; satvic; excess use may increase vata. Moves blood and qi, purges fire, clears damp and cold; tonifies kidney yang.

**Chemical constituents** A complex essence with over 100 constituents. Features: esters as benzyl acetate, linalyl acetate, benzyl benzoate, methyl jasmonate, methyl anthranilate 54%; alcohols as linalool, nerol, geraniol, benzyl alcohol, farnesol, terpineol, phytols 24%; phenols as eugenol 2.7%; ketones as *cis*-jasmone 2.7%; acids, aldehydes and other.

**Therapeutic actions** Nervine analgesic, sedative, antispasmodic, antidepressant, euphoric, aphrodisiac; antiseptic; balances hormones, hormone-like effects, probably via stimulation of the pituitary; galactagogue, parturient; cicatrising, anti-inflammatory, carminative, expectorant; uterine tonic; euphoric.

**Blends with** rose, lavender, sandalwood, citrus oils, clary sage, rosewood. Only a small amount is needed as the odour is intense.

**Other uses** Fragrance for perfumes (especially higher quality and oriental blends), soaps, toiletries, cosmetics; flavouring for food and beverages, e.g. jasmine tea.

 **Safety/precautions** Non-toxic, generally non-irritating, non-sensitising, though allergic reactions have occurred in some individuals. Avoid in pregnancy; may be used in labour.

# Lavender

**Name** Lavender

**Latin name** *Lavandula angustifolia* from the Latin *lavare* to wash, *angus* narrow, sharp, and *folius* leaf.

**Family** Lamiaceae/Labiatae

**Synonyms** *L. officinalis*, *L. vera*, garden lavender, common lavender, lavender 'Mailette'.

**Other species** There are at least 28 species in this genus and numerous subspecies and hybrids, e.g. *L. spica* or *spicata*, the English lavender; *L. latifolia*, *L. delphinensis* and *L. fragrans*.

**Description** An aromatic perennial subshrub, up to 1 m; stems woody; leaves grey-green, opposite, stalkless (sessile), entire (untoothed), very narrow, lanceolate/oblong-linear, finely hairy, smaller ones cluster in the axils; flowers in terminal spikes on peduncles, 10–20 cm, purplish-blue, in whorls, each flower has a tubular calyx and lipped corolla and contains oil glands. Most of the essential oil is yielded by the flowers.

**Habitat/distribution** Native to mountains bordering the western Mediterranean, near the snow line, 700–1,400 m; widely distributed in southern Europe and introduced to gardens world wide. Lavender prefers poor, well-drained soil. The higher the altitude the more it is exposed to the sun and to environmental stress, which tends to benefit the production of the volatile oil in the plant.

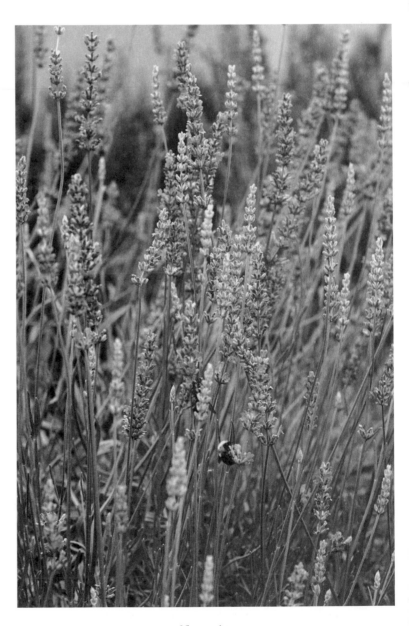

*Lavender*

**History** A lavender thought to be *L. stoechas* is mentioned by Dioscorides, who also lists its Egyptian name, indicating it was used by them. Theophrastus lists it among the 'coronary' plants. It was valued as an antidote to poison by the Romans. It is thought that lavender was first grown in England near Hitchin in Hertfordshire by Huguenot refugees in 1568 coming from the Cathar region of southern France. By the 1600s Culpeper declared it so well known as to not need description and classified the herb as hot in the 3rd degree, the flowers dry in the 2nd degree, and as good for 'all the griefs and pains of the head and brain that proceed of a cold cause, as apoplexy, falling sickness (epilepsy), dropsy, cramps, convulsions, palsies . . . it strengthens the stomach, frees the liver and spleen . . . provokes women's courses . . . expels afterbirth' (Culpeper, 1995). In the 19th and first third of the 20th century cultivation of English lavender – a varietiy or subspecies of *L. spica* – and production of essential oil was extensive around Mitchum in Surrey and Hitchin for toiletries (e.g. Yardley) and pharmaceuticals. English lavender was considered superior to French in the trade. Clones of this lavender were used to develop production in Norfolk. In the 1920s and 1930s Rene Gattefosse discovered and researched the healing properties of the essential oil and was midwife to the birth of modern aromatherapy.

**Cultivation** Wild. There are still populations of wild lavender varieties, which easily cross to produce 'natural hybrids' or subspecies. As with all plants, it is important that wild populations continue to exist in order to ensure the biodiversity of the species and its natural immunity. Wild populations display variations, e.g. in colour, size, form and scent. Wild varieties tend to be darker, bluer. It is cultivated extensively in gardens. Commercially grown varieties are usually hybrids and propagated by clones. These gradually weaken and have to be invigorated by crossing with wild stock. The majority of production is in southern France (Provence), and most of this is from clonal lavenders for the fragrance industry (perfumes, toiletries, cleansers, tourism) rather than from natural varieties for therapeutic purposes. It is also produced in Norfolk, the Crimea, Ukraine and areas bordering the Black Sea. In recent years lavender is being grown on Jersey and the Isle of Wight.

**Part used** Flower buds just before opening. About 130 kilo of flowers yields 1 kilo of essential oil. (Compare this with industrial clonal lavender yield of 1 kilo of essential oil from 40–60 kilo of flowers.)

**Extraction/adulterations** Steam distillation. Small quantities of concrete and absolute are produced. More than 30 different types are traded commercially (Price and Price, 1999). Check with suppliers to ensure authenticity of source and quality of distillation. Yields can be 'rectified' with addition of linalyl acetate to achieve industrial lavenders profile of 30% of the ester. A floral water is also produced and should smell 'like toffee'.

**Characteristics** A colourless or pale yellow liquid; a complex sweet-floral odour with a slighty fruity note. Middle note. (Old English lavender/*L. spica* or its subspecies have a slightly camphorous note. *L. stoechas* has a more spicy scent.)

**Energy** Warming, drying, amphoteric. Clears phlegm, calms and revives melancholy, cools choler, purifies blood. Reduces kapha, cools pitta, calms vata; satvik. Regulates qi, clears stagnation (liver–gall bladder, spleen), damp, and heat; tonifies yin.

**Chemical constituents** 300 known constituents featuring esters as linalyl acetate, geranyl acetate, lavandulyl acetate 45%; alcohols as terpinen-4-ol, α-terpineol, linalool, borneol, geraniol, lavandulol 36%; sesquiterpenes as β-caryophyllene 5%; ketones as octanone, camphor 4%; monoterpenes as ocimene, camphene, limonene 4%; oxides as 1.8-cineole, linalool oxide, caryophyllene 2%; aldehydes as citral 1%; aromatic alcehyldes as cuminaldehyde, benzaldehyde 1%; lactones and coumarins as coumarin, umbelliferone 0.3%; phenols, phenol ethers, trace. (Fine lavenders have ketones of the amyl group, while other sources have ketones of the camphor group (Price and Price, 1999, p. 330).)

**Therapeutic actions** Antibacterial, antifungal, antimicrobial; vulnerary, cicatrising, insect repellant; cytophylactic, anti-inflammatory; stomachic, carminative, choleretic, cholagogue; rubifacient, cardiotonic, hypotensive; diaphoretic; diuretic; emmenagogue; nervine analgesic, relaxant, antispasmodic, sedative, anxiolytic, tonic; stimulating, tonic to the whole system.

**Blends with** almost any other essential oil including geranium, marjoram, clove, cedarwood, clary sage, pine, vetiver, patchouli, rosemary, rose, jasmine. Blend with bergamot for acne. Lavender is a peacemaker and a drop will harmonise a blend and enhance its action.

**Other uses** Use floral water for children and frail, delicate patients. Encourage patients to use lavender in the bath. Compresses are very effective. Spraying essential oil into the air at regular intervals, e.g. via a nebuliser, will inhibit bacteria and prevent ear infections. Valnet (1982) records that a 4.5% strength kills staphylococcus, typhoid bacillus, diphtheria, gonococcus, pneumococcus, streptococcus. The vapour method is good for asthmatics who are prone to infections and for any infectious illness. Lavender is used as a fragrance in toiletries, soaps, perfumes; as flavouring agent in food products and beverages.

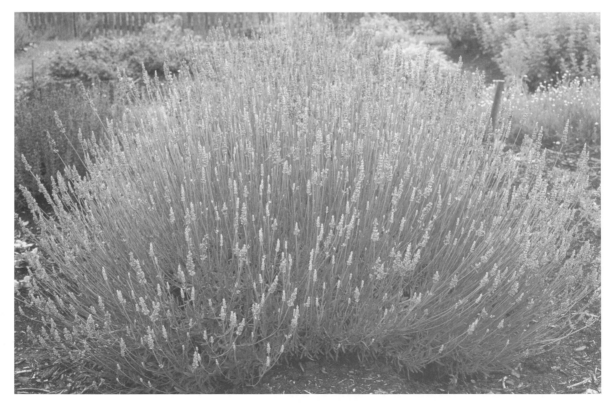

*Lavender*

- **Skin:** acne, dermatitis, eczema, psoriasis, herpes, allergies, inflammations, rashes; wounds, cuts, abrasions, burns including radiography burning, bruises, scars; ringworm, impetigo, athlete's foot; insect infestations, scabies, lice, bites, repellant; dandruff, alopecia; antivenom (Valnet).

- **Digestive:** liver problems, weak digestion, nausea, cramps, flatulence, congested bile, enteritis, parasites.

- **Respiratory:** asthma, bronchitis, cough, whooping cough, sinusitis, flu, tuberculosis.

- **Immune:** infections, inflammations, swelling, fever, tonsillitis, swollen glands; candida; chronic fatigue.

- **Circulatory:** strengthen the heart; palpitations, hypertension, varicose veins, phlebitis, Raynaud's.

- **Endocrine:** enhance production of endorphins; regulate menstrual cycle.

- **Muscular–skeletal:** osteo-arthritis, rheumatoid arthritis, muscle ache and fatigue, sciatica, sprain, strain.

- **Urinary:** cystitis.

- **Reproductive:** dysmenorrhoea, amenorrhoea, PMS, cramps, leucorrhoea, excellent for childbirth and post-partum, menopause; gonorrhoea.

- **Nervous:** depression, pain, cramps, anxiety, headache, insomnia, stress, tension, shock, vertigo, epilepsy.

- **Mental–emotional:** depression, mood swings, low self-esteem, worry, fear, anger, frustration (place a drop on the back of the neck).

- **Balancing:** uplifting, calming and stimulating according to need.

**Lavender**

*Lavandula angustifolia*

**Safety/precautions** Non-toxic, non-irritating, non-sensitising.

# Lemon

**Name** Lemon

**Latin name** *Citrus limonum*

**Family** Rutaceae

**Synonyms** *C. limon,* cedro oil, nimbu in India.

**Other species** Numerous varieties exist now. Closely related to lime – *C. aurantifolia/C. acida/C. medica,* cedrat (citron) and bergamot, *C. bergamina.*

**Description** A small tree 3–6 m with stiff thorns; leaves pale green, oblong to elliptic ovate; flowers 8–16 cm, white inside, pink outside, clustered in the axils; fruit yellow, oblong/ovoid ending in a nipple. The fruit is high in vitamin C.

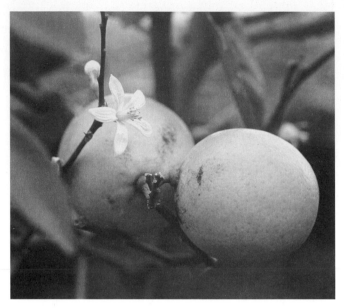

*Lemon*

**Habitat/distribution** Native of northern India, widely grown in southern Europe, Asia, Americas.

**History** Unknown in ancient Greece and Rome, it passed into European use via the Arabs, probably in the 13th century into Spain, Sicily. Used medicinally by Unani and Ayurvedic medicine and folk medicine of the Near East and India. Limes and lemons helped rid the British navy of scurvy in the 18th century. The French pioneers in aromatherapy, such as Gattefosse and Valnet (who used it for tuberculosis and serious infectious diseases), esteemed lemon highly.

**Cultivation** Wild in India; cultivated in domestic gardens and commercially in tropical countries around the world. Florida, California, South and Central America, West Indies, Mediterranean east to Asia.

**Part used** Fresh fruit peel.

**Extraction/adulterations** Expression from the peel. Today, the usual method is to mechanically abraise and pulp the fruit, and then the essential oil is separated from the juice and other constituents by a centrifugal separator. It takes about 3,000 lemons to produce a kilo of essential oil (Davis, 1995).

**Characteristics** A pale green-yellow liquid turning brown with age; a fresh lemon scent. Top note.

**Energy** Cooling, drying. Clears phlegm, cools choler and purifies blood. Reduces kapha and pitta, calms vata; satvic. Tonifies qi; clears heat, phlegm.

**Chemical constituents** Features terpenes as limonene, α-pinene, β-pinene, γ-terpinene, camphene, phellandrene, ρ-cymene, sabinene, myrcene 87%; small amounts of aldehydes as

## USES

- **Skin:** acne, oily skin; brittle nails, boils, chilblains, corns, warts, verrucas; herpes; cuts, bites, mouth ulcers, gingivitis.
- **Digestion:** dyspepsia, gastric acidity, infections.
- **Respiratory:** asthma, catarrh, bronchitis.
- **Immune/lymph:** colds, throat infections, fevers, flu, infections; stimulates production of leucocytes.
- **Circulation/lymph:** nosebleed, poor circulation, varicose veins, high blood pressure, cellulitis.
- **Muscular–skeletal:** arthritis, gout.
- **Mental–emotional:** cleansing, uplifting, refreshing/invigorating; depression, melancholy, attachment.

citral, citronellal, nonanal, octanal, decanal 3%; sesquiterpenes as β-bisobolene, α-bergamotene 2.5; alcohols as linalool, geraniol, octanol, nonanol, α-terpineol 2%; lactones, coumarins as bergaptene, bergamottin 2%, esters as neryl acetate, geranyl acetate, terpinyl acetate 1.5%.

(NB: According to Valnet (1982) lemon essence kills diphtheria bacilli in 20 minutes. Add juice of 1 lemon to a litre of water to kill or inhibit pathogens.)

**Therapeutic actions** Antiseptic, bactericidal, antiviral, increases leucocytes; carminative; diaphoretic, febrifuge; haemostatic, hypotensive, alterative, antisclerotic; astringent, rubifacient, cicatrising; immune stimulant; diuretic; tonic; vermifuge, insecticidal; antirheumatic. Antiscorbutic on ingestion of the juice.

**Blends with** other citrus oils, benzoin, ylang ylang, sandalwood, rose, lavender, geranium, juniper, eucalyptus, fennel.

**Other uses** Recommend patients to make use of the freshly squeezed juice to support aromatherapy treatments. The lemon is a versatile medicinal agent, useful for infections, fevers, digestive or respiratory complaints. Lemon juice is cleansing and tonic to the whole system. It helps restore alkalinity to an over-acid system because, on digestion, the citric acid is converted to carbonates and bicarbonates of potassium and calcium. Juice of baked lemon is good for cough, mixed with honey. Colonisers of India learned to enjoy a drink, nimbu pani, made with lemon or lime; a flavouring in foods, beverages, pharmaceuticals; a component in soaps, cleansers, perfumes, cosmetics, toiletries.

**Safety/precautions** It may cause dermal irritation or sensitisation in some individuals. Use in low dilution (1%); photo-toxic due to bergaptene, do not expose skin to sunlight after application.

**Name** Lemongrass

**Latin name** *Cymbopogan citratus*

**Family** Gramineae

**Synonyms** *Andropogan citratus*/West Indian lemongrass, Guatemala lemongrass, Madagascar lemongrass; *A. flexuosus*/East Indian lemongrass, Cochin lemongrass, 'vervaine indienne', French-Indian verbena; 'molissa oil' in India.

**Other species** There are several varieties in this species and chemotypes occur in each variety.

**Description** A perennial fragrant grass, up to 1.5 m; roots are a network of rootlets. The sliced stems are used in Thai cooking and can be easily sourced.

**Habitat/distribution** Native to tropical southern India/ Sri Lanka. Cultivated widely in West Indies, East India (Travancore), south-east Asia, Africa and Central America.

**History** Traditional and Ayurvedic remedy for indigestion, dyspepsia, vomiting, fevers, colic, flatulence, dysmenorrhoea, malarial dropsy.

**Cultivation** Widely cultivated for its essential oil and as a culinary herb.

**Part used** The grass leaf.

**Extraction/adulterations** Steam distillation of fresh and partly dried leaves. It has been used to adulterate lemon essential oil.

**Characteristics** A yellow or pale sherry-coloured liquid; intense, sweet lemony odour, reminiscent of lemon drops. Top note.

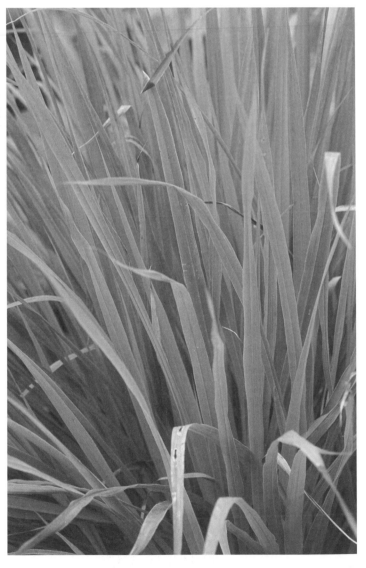

*Lemongrass*

- **Skin:** acne, candida, athlete's foot, ringworm, warts, deters pests; tonic to the skin and connective tissue.
- **Digestive:** flatulence, liver sluggishness, weak digestion, colic, nausea, vomiting, diarrhoea.
- **Immune:** infections, fevers.
- **Circulatory:** stimulate circulation, dilate the vessels.
- **Muscular–skeletal:** muscle strain/sprain, tired legs, neuralgia, arthritis/ rheumatic pain.
- **Urinary:** water retention, cellulite.
- **Reproductive:** stimulate milk flow, stimulate secretions, emmenagogue.
- **Nervous:** depression, low moods; exhaustion, stress, headaches.
- **Mental–emotional:** refreshing, cools and soothes hot emotions like anger and frustration.

**Lemongrass**
*Cymbopogon citratus*

**Energy** Cooling, drying, amphoteric. Cools choler, clears phlegm. Reduces kapha, cools pitta, strengthens agni. Drains damp, tonifies spleen and stomach, regulates qi in the middle burner.

**Chemical constituents** Features aldehydes as citral, which gives it the characteristic odour 80%; monoterpenes as mycrene, dipentene 14%; alcohols as linalool, geraniol, nerol, citronellol, farnesol 1.0%; sesquiterpenes 1.0%; ketones 0.3% as methyl heptenone; esters, acids and other.

**Therapeutic actions** Digestive tonic, sialagogue; antifungal, antiviral, antibacterial; anti-inflammatory; febrifuge; tonic; diuretic, galactagogue, emmenagogue; weak hypotensive and diuretic. Some research shows it has a sedative action on the central nervous system.

**Blends with** basil, citrus oils, lavender, geranium, niaouli, palmarosa, rosemary, tea tree.

**Other uses** Fragrance for toiletries, cosmetics, perfumes. Flavouring for foods. Citral, extracted from lemongrass essential oil, can be further converted to ionone, a substance with the fragrance of violets. Ionone has two isomers, each with a distinct odour.

**Comment** Lemongrass has been well studied by scientists and found effective against gram positive and gram negative bacteria, and also against candida albicans and aspergillus fumigatus fungi, even when airborne. Vaporisation is an effective disinfectant. The high aldehyde content makes the oil susceptible to oxidation. Correct storage is important.

 **Safety/precautions** Possible skin irritation in some persons. Citral on its own has caused dermal irritation, but this has not been confirmed by clinical experience using the essential oil, suggesting that components of the whole oil have a quenching effect.

# Lime

**Name** Lime

**Latin name** *Citrus aurantifolium* (Latin, gold-leaved)

**Family** Rutaceae

**Synonyms** *C. medica* var. *acida*, *C. latifolia*.

**Other species** *C. limetta*, Italian lime.

**Description** Evergreen tree up to 4.5 m; leaves ovate, smooth; flowers small, white, fragrant; fruit bright green, bitter-sour; half size of a lemon.

**Habitat/distribution** Native of southern India, though several of its common names (Mexican lime, West Indian lime) reflect its wide cultivation in the Americas.

**History** Lime is a traditional remedy in south Asia and in Ayurvedic medicine it is used similarly to lemon. When lemons, oranges and limes, with their vitamin C content, were found to cure scurvy among the crew of long sea voyages, they were planted in the colonised territories, including both East and West Indies, along the trading routes during the 17th and 18th centuries, to supply ships.

**Cultivation** Commercial cultivation in Florida, West Indies, Central America, Indian subcontinent and Italy.

**Part used** Peel, unripe and ripe.

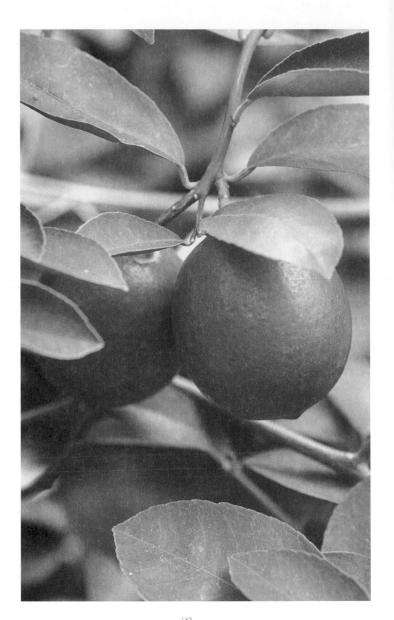

*Lime*

## USES

- **Skin:** acne, oily congested skin; brittle nails, boils, cuts, wounds, insect stings, mouth ulcers.
- **Digestion:** poor appetite, dyspepsia.
- **Immune:** respiratory fevers, colds, flu, infections, catarrh, congestion, cough, asthma.
- **Circulation/lymph:** high blood pressure, poor circulation, nosebleeds, cellulitis.
- **Muscular–skeletal:** arthritis.
- **Nervous:** stress, anxiety.
- **Mental–emotional:** uplifting, refreshing, mental fatigue, depression, anxiety, apathy.

**Extraction/adulterations** Expression of the unripe lime peel; also steam distillation of the ripe crushed fruit pulp, a by-product of the fruit industry.

**Characteristics** Expressed: a pale yellow to olive green liquid; fresh citrus odour. Distilled: a clear to pale yellow liquid; sharp lime odour. Top note.

**Energy** *See* lemon.

**Chemical constituents** Peel essential oil: features monoterpenes as limonene, camphene, myrcene, sabinene, ρ-cymene, pinenes, terpinolene 72%; aldehydes as citral 13%; esters as geranyl acetate, methyl anthranilate 7%; alcohols as α-terpineol, linalool, lactones and coumarins as bergaptene, limettin 2%; sesquiterpene bisabolene; and oxides, trace amounts.

**Therapeutic actions** Digestive, stomachic, aperitif, stimulates appetite while calming digestion; nervine antispasmodic, anxiolytic, sedative; refrigerant, febrifuge, anti-inflammatory; antiviral, antibacterial; circulatory tonic and hypotensive, styptic, anticoagulant, astringent; decongestant, mucolytic.

**Blends with** other citrus essential oils, lavender, geranium, nutmeg, rose, rosemary, vetiver, ylang ylang.

**Other uses** Fragrance and food industries; as a source for the production of citric acid.

 **Safety/precautions** *See* lemon. The oil contains bergaptene and is potentially photo-toxic; use with care.

# Mandarin

**Name** Mandarin

**Latin name** *Citrus nobilis* or *C. reticulata*

**Family** Rutatceae

**Synonyms** *C. deliciosa*, *C. madurensis*. Tangerine. The names tangerine and mandarin and satsuma tend to be used somewhat interchangeably. Lawless considers these to be distinct chemotypes. The fruit is called tangerine in the US, satsuma or mandarin in Europe, the Middle East and China. Satsuma is a Japanese term.

**Other species** Clementine.

**Description** An evergreen tree, up to 6 m; leaves glossy, fragrant; flowers white, fragrant. The peel of the tangerine is more yellow than mandarin and the fruit larger and rounder (Lawless, 1992).

**Habitat/distribution**
Native to China and the Far East. Mandarins are widely cultivated in the US (Texas, Florida, California), the Mediterranean basin (Italy, Spain, Algeria, Cyprus, Greece, Palestine and Israel), Brazil and Guinea. The original plant has been developed to have a looser, easy-peel skin, sweeter flavour and, in the case of tangerine, no pips.

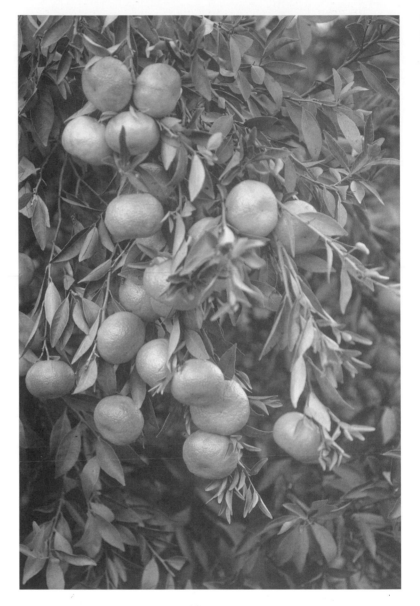

*Mandarin*

**History** The peel is an important minor tonic in traditional Chinese medicine for balancing and strengthening the digestion (middle burner, liver qi). These uses have followed its importation to the West. It was a fruit favoured by mandarins, the imperial officials in pre-revolutionary China.

## USES

- **Skin:** cell regenerator, stretch marks (use with wheatgerm oil as preventative during pregnancy), wound healing, acne, congestion, oiliness.
- **Digestive:** relieves bile congestion; dyspepsia, colic, flatulence and indigestion especially in children, pregnant women and elderly people.
- **Circulatory:** fluid retention, sluggish circulation/obesity.
- **Nervous:** insomnia, anxiety, low mood, tension, restlessness, stress; decreases hyper-sensitivity of the sympathetic nervous system.
- **Mental–emotional:** refreshing, dispels anxiety, uplifting.

**Cultivation** Widely cultivated in the US, Brazil, the Mediterranean and the Far East.

**Part used** Peel.

**Extraction/adulterations** Cold expression. A mandarin petitgrain is also produced from distillation of the leaves and twigs. Some suppliers offer green mandarin extracted from unripe fruit peel (Chinese medicine similarly also uses unripe peel); and red mandarin extracted from further ripened fruit. They have a different chemical profile.

**Characteristics** A yellow to orange, light liquid; a sweet, intense odour. Top note.

**Energy** Cooling, drying. Cools choler, revives melancholy, clears phlegm. Calms vata (increases vata in excess), reduces kapha and pitta; strengthens agni. Regulates stomach, lung and liver qi, removes stagnation, tonifies spleen.

**Chemical constituents** Features monoterpenes as γ-terpinene, limonene, pinenes, myrcene, ρ-cymene 90%; alcohols as linalool, citronellol, octanol 5%; esters as methyl anthranilate 1%; aldehydes as decanal, sinensal, citral, citronellal 1%; lactones and coumarins, trace; phenols and phenol ethers as thymol, trace; and other.

**Therapeutic actions** Digestive stimulant, tonic, stomachic, choleretic, cholegogue, lipolytic; nervine antispasmodic, sedative, tonic; antiviral; astringent, tonic to skin tissues.

**Blends with** citrus oils, geranium, lavender, Roman and German chamomile, jasmine, black pepper, palmarosa, rose, sandalwood, ylang ylang.

**Other uses** Fragrance for toiletries, cosmetics, perfume; flavouring for confections, soft drinks, liqueurs.

 **Safety/precautions** Non-toxic, non-irritant, non-sensitising.

# Marjoram

**Name** Marjoram

**Latin name** *Oreganum marjorana*

**Family** Lamiaceae/Labiateae

**Synonyms** *Marjoranum hortense*, pot marjoram, knotted marjoram, sweet marjoram, annual marjoram.

**Other species** Related to the pot or French marjoram (*O. onites* or *M. onites*), and the Spanish marjoram (*Thymus mastichina*) and *O. vulgare*.

**Description** A bushy, tender perennial in the Mediterranean, annual in colder climates; up to 60 cm; stem hairy; ovate dark green or light green leaves; flowers small, insignificant, white to pink in clustered spikes.

**Habitat/distribution** Native to the Mediterranean basin; widely cultivated in Europe, America, Asia, Australia.

**History** Marjoram has been used since ancient times in Egypt (e.g. in mummy garlands), Greece and the Middle East. It is mentioned in Hippocrates, Theophrastus, Dioscorides, Pliny. It was used in rituals, perfumes, incense, medicine, cooking and as a strewing herb. In European medicine of the Middle Ages, through the Renaissance and into the present, marjoram has been a medicinal and culinary herb. Culpeper esteemed it for warming and comforting the heart, which he understood to be an emotional as well as a physical organ, and for healing bruised or strained muscles.

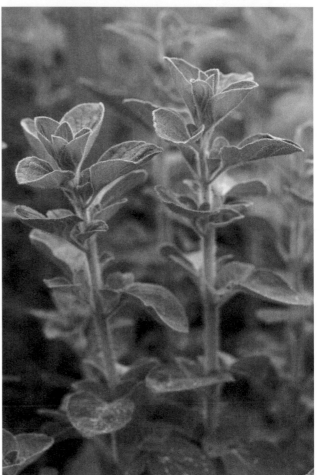

*Marjoram*

**Cultivation** Wild in the Mediterranean countries. It is grown as a perennial or annual depending on the climate.

**Part used** The flowering stems, dried.

**Extraction/adulterations** Steam distillation. An oleo resin is also produced in small amounts.

**Characteristics** A pale yellow liquid, darkening to amber as it ages; a woody-peppery, warm, slightly camphorous odour. Considered acceptable to men (Davis, 1995). Middle note.

## USES

- **Skin and connective tissue:** bruises, chilblains, ticks.
- **Digestive:** dyspepsia, colic, flatulence, constipation, nausea.
- **Respiratory:** coughs, sinus and respiratory congestion.
- **Immune:** infections, fevers (mild diaphoretic).
- **Circulatory:** hypertension, arteriosclerosis, balances heart function, fluid retention.
- **Muscular–skeletal:** arthritis, strains and sprains, overworked muscles, cramp, stiffness (multiple sclerosis, cerebral palsy).
- **Reproductive:** delayed or painful menses; cramps; sexual problems.
- **Nervous:** anxiety, insomnia, headache, tension, stress, depression, addictions, psychosis, obsessions, vertigo, confusion.
- **Mental–emotional:** comforts and revives the heart (cordial) or a lonely or grieving state; relieves mental fatigue, confusion, congestion (cephalic), obsessions and anxiety; uplifts.

**Energy** Warming, drying. Clears phlegm and choler (bile), comforts melancholy. Reduces kapha and vata, increases pitta, strengthens agni. Moves qi, calms heart, tonifies spleen, clears damp, warms the lower burner.

**Chemical constituents** Features alcohols as linlool, borneol, α-terpineol, terpinen-4-ol 50%; monoterpoenes as β-pinene, α-terpinene, γ-terpinene, ρ-cymene, myrcene, limonene, ocimene, sabinene 40%; sesquiterpenes as caryophyllene, cadinene 3%; esters as linalyl acetate, terpinyl acetate, geranyl acetate 2%; aldehydes as citral 1%; phenols and phenol ethers as carvacrol, eugenol, trace; other.

**Therapeutic actions** Digestive, stomachic, carminative, intestinal smooth muscle tonic, mild laxative, mild choloretic; nervine analgesic, sedative, antispasmodic, tonic; cordial, vasodilatory, hypotensive, cephalic but can be stupefying in large amounts (which anyway would not be used in therapy), diaphoretic; diuretic; emmenagogue; mild expectorant, antifungal, antiviral, antiseptic.

**Blends with** bergamot, cedarwood, chamomile, cypress, lavender, citrus oils, rosemary, ylang ylang.

**Other uses** Fragrance for toiletries, perfumes, cleansers, cosmetics. Flavouring for soft and alcoholic beverages. Marjoram is an important culinary herb; encourage patients to use it in cooking if you are prescribing the essential oil.

 **Safety/precautions** Avoid in pregnancy. Non-toxic, non-irritating, non-sensitising.

# May Chang

**Name** May chang

**Latin name** *Litsea cubeba*

**Family** Lauraceae

**Synonyms** *L. citrata,* exotic verbena, tropical verbena.

**Other species** *Litsea* is not related to verbena, despite some of its common names. It is related to cinnamon, bay laurel and rosewood, all in the Lauraceae family. There are several relatives on the Indian subcontinent, but these are not known for their essential oil.

**Description** A small tree; leaves narrow, fragrant; flowers small, white, clustered on a stalk, fragrant; fruits pepper-like and so named for the cubeb pepper of Java.

**Habitat/distribution** Native to tropical areas of east Asia, China.

**History** Traditional use in Chinese medicine for dysmenorrhoea, pain, chills, indigestion. Recent research points to a use in cardiac arrhythmia.

**Cultivation** Cultivated commercially in China, Taiwan, Japan. China is the main source of essential oil. May Chang is cultivated for the production of citral.

**Part used** Fruit.

**Extraction/adulterations** Steam distillation

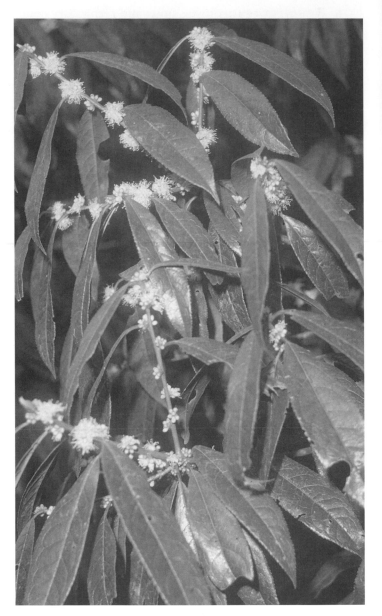

*May Chang*

## USES

- **Skin:** acne, dermatitis, oiliness, excessive perspiration.
- **Digestive:** indigestion, travel sickness.
- **Respiratory:** asthma, bronchitis.
- **Immune:** infectious diseases.
- **Circulatory:** hypertensive, cardiac arrhythmia.
- **Muscular–skeletal:** lower back ache, muscular aches.
- **Reproductive:** dysmennorhoea, promote breastfeeding.
- **Nervous:** pain.
- **Mental–emotional:** depression, low mood. Uplifting.

**Characteristics** A pale yellow liquid; intense, lemon-like odour, similar to lemongrass. Middle note.

**Energy** Warming, drying. Calms melancholy, purifies blood, clears phlegm. Calms vata, reduces kapha, increases pitta, strengthens agni. Moves blood, releases wind, regulates qi.

**Chemical constituents** Features aldehydes as citral, geranial, neral up to 85%; monoterpenes as limonene, myrcene, α-pinene, β-pinene 12.5%; alcohols as linalool, nerol 3.5%; esters as linalyl acetate 1.65%; sesquiterpenes as caryophyllene 0.51%.

**Therapeutic actions** Digestive, stomachic; emmenagogue, galactagogue; antiseptic, disinfectant, insecticidal; nervine analgesic, sedative; cordial, regulates cardiac rhythm, hypotensive; bronchial dilator; astringent tonic to skin tissues.

**Blends with** basil, bergamot, geranium, ginger, jasmine, lavender, citrus oils, ylang ylang, rosemary, rosewood.

**Other uses** Fragrance for toiletries, perfumes, soaps, fresheners; flavouring for fruit products; industrally used to obtain citral.

**Safety/precautions** Non-toxic, non-irritant, possible sensitisation in some individuals.

# Melissa

**Name** Melissa, lemon balm

**Latin name** *Melissa officinalis* from the Greek *meli* honey and bee.

**Family** Lamiaceae/Labiatae

**Synonyms** Balm, bee balm, heart's delight, honey plant. Balm is an abbreviation of balsam.

**Other species** A variegated variety exists. Related to all the mints.

**Description** A fragrant perennial herb, up to 60 cm. Root short; stem square, branching; leaves opposite, ovate, toothed, fragrant; flowers in loose clusters from axils of leaves, whitish, sometimes pink or yellow.

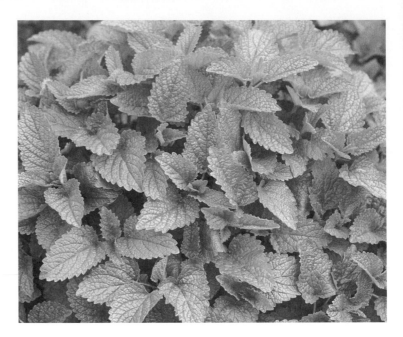

*Melissa, lemon balm*

**Habitat/distribution** Native to southern Europe: the Mediterranean, southern central Europe. Introduced in temperate zones of Europe, Americas, Australia. Melissa enjoys a sunny position with some shade, damp soil. The essential oil in the leaves does not survive into the dried, stored material.

**History** Known since ancient times and prized by Greeks and Romans for being attractive to bees, melissa was indicated by Dioscorides for use for healing wounds. Probably introduced to Britain by the Romans. Medicinal use was developed by Arab physicians specifically for anxiety and depression and they introduced melissa to European medicine. It was esteemed by Paracelsus as the 'elixir of life' for its reviving properties. It is 'sovereign for the brain, strengthening the memory, powerfully chasing away melancholy' (John Evelyn, quoted in Grieve, 1984). It was an ingredient in Carmelite water. Melissa is so popular in France that it became known as 'thé de France'.

**Cultivation** Wild. Cultivated in Hungary, Egypt and Italy, more recently Wales and Ireland.

**Part used** Fresh leaves, flowering stem.

**Extraction/adulterations** Steam distillation. Though strongly aromatic, there is relatively little essential oil present, the yield is low and consequently the price of melissa is higher. It is frequently adulterated with lemongrass or citronella, so insist on the real thing from suppliers; a 'nature identical' is not authentic.

## USES

- **Skin:** allergies, insect bites, eczema. Use in low concentrations.
- **Digestive:** indigestion, dyspepsia, colic, flatulence, nausea. Especially good for children (low dilution).
- **Respiratory:** asthma, bronchitis, cough, catarrh, hyperventilation.
- **Immune:** fevers, infections, colds, flu, bronchitis, herpes simplex and zoster (shingles), chickenpox, mumps.
- **Circulatory:** hypertension.
- **Reproductive:** delayed menses, irregular periods/ovulation (apply prepared cotton wool directly over ovaries), difficulties of conception, dysmenorrhoea.
- **Nervous:** nervine tonic, depression, anxiety, migraine, tension, stress, shock, vertigo, insomnia, paranoia.
- **Mental–emotional:** depression, anxiety, paranoia, shock, bereavement. Both soothing, calming and invigorating, uplifting to the mind and spirit.

**Characteristics** A pale yellow liquid; fresh, light lemon odour. Middle note.

**Energy** Cooling, stimulating. Revives and calms melancholy, cools choler, purifies blood, clears phlegm. Balances and calms vata, reduces kapha and pitta; balances agni. Moves qi (e.g. stagnant qi in the heart, stomach, lower burner, lung), moves blood, clears heat, wind, phlegm.

**Chemical constituents** Features aldehydes as citronellal, citral 50%; sesquiterpenes as β-carylphyllene, germacrene, α-copaene 20%; ketones as methyl heptenone 7%; oxides as 1.8 cineole, caryophyllene oxide 4%; esters as geranyl acetate, neryl acetate, citronellyl acetate 1.2%; monoterpenes as limonene, *trans*-ocimene 1%; traces of lactones and coumarines; other components 11%.

**Therapeutic actions** Digestive, carminative, stomachic; nervine sedative; diaphoretic; febrifuge; hypotensive, cordial; anti-allergic, antihistaminic; bactericidal, antifungal, antiviral; uterine tonic; vermifuge, insect repellant.

**Blends with** basil, geranium, jasmine, lavender, citrus and lemon-scented oils, marjoram, cedarwood.

**Other uses** Herb pillows, pot-pourris, summer teas. Fragrance for toiletries, cosmetics, perfumes; flavouring for foods, alcoholic and soft beverages.

**Safety/precautions** Non-toxic. Possible skin sensitisation and dermal irritation in some individuals. Avoid in pregnancy. Use in low concentrations for skin applications and for children.

# Myrrh

**Name** Myrrh

**Latin name** *Comiphora myrrha* var. *molmol*

**Family** Burseraceae

**Synonyms** *Balsamodendrom myrrha*, gum myrrh, common myrrh, hirabol myrrh.

**Other species** *C. molmol,* the Somalian myrrh; *C. mukul,* the guggul of India; *C. abyssinica,* Arabian or Yemen myrrh.

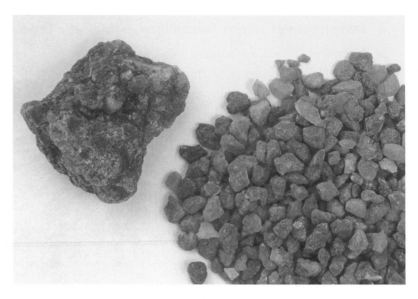

*Myrrh*

**Description** A bush of up to 3 m or small tree up to 10 m; trunk thick with numerous irregular knotted branches with stout, clustered branchlets spreading at right angles and terminating in a sharp spine; leaves few and very small, trifoliate, borne at the ends of branchlets; flowers white. A gum discharges naturally from the bark when the tree is wounded.

**Habitat/distribution** Native to the Horn of Africa: Ethiopia, Somalia; and to the Arabian peninsula. Other species grow in India. Myrrh grows on basaltic soil in hot, dry areas.

**History** A most precious medicine and incense, myrrh has been used from ancient times in Egypt, Palestine, Greece, Persia, Rome and Indian subcontinent for religious rituals/communion with deities, fumigations, sanitation, mummification, perfumes, ointments and unguents, medicines. One of the 3 gifts to the newborn Jesus. It was discussed by Theophrastus in his treatise on odours, by Disocorides in his herbal. Myrrh has always been traded extensively and valued for its wound healing (antiseptic) properties, used continuously into the present day in herbal and traditional medicine and in pharmacy. The *British Pharmacopoiea* lists it as an astringent; myrrh tincture is still available from chemists.

**Cultivation** Wild. Cultivated in its native areas.

**Part used** 'Tears' or oleo-gum-resin, the pale yellow exudative discharge of the trunk after wounding is collected. It hardens to a reddish brown substance which is brittle, often marked with white, and a little oily; traded in various sizes. The gum is mucilaginous.

**Extraction/adulterations** Resinoid and resin absolute by solvent extraction. Essential oil by steam distillation. Crude drug can be adulterated with stones, nuts, false myrrhs.

- **Skin:** mature, weak or damaged, chapped or cracked skin, wounds, eczema, ringworm, fungal infections, athlete's foot, haemorrhoids. Use on wounds slow to heal, ulcers.

- **Oral:** mouth ulcers, oral hygiene, gingivitis – an extremely effective specific; use the tincture diluted for a mouthwash.

- **Digestive:** diarrhoea, dyspepsia, flatulence, loss of appetite, candida.

- **Respiratory-immune:** catarrh, colds, flu, bronchitis, sore throat, coughs, mucous membrane, irritation.

- **Muscular–skeletal:** arthritis.

- **Reproductive:** delayed menses, pelvic inflammatory disease, thrush, leucorrhoea (vaginal douches).

- **Mental–emotional:** calms the mind, clears confusion, revealing the way forward.

**Myrrh**
*Commiphora myrrha*

**Characteristics** Resinoid is a dark reddish brown, very viscous substance; warm spicy, balsamic odour. The essential oil is pale yellow to amber, viscous; warm, sweet-spicy, balsamic odour. Base note.

**Energy** Warming, drying. Clears phlegm, reduces choler, purifies blood, calms and revives melancholy. Calms and rejuvenates vata, reduces and rejuvenates kapha, increases pitta (in excess). Blood moving; tonifies yang, lungs and spleen; clears damp and phlegm, disperses wind-cold.

**Chemical constituents** Features alcohols as myrrh alcohols 40%; sesquiterpenes as elemene, heerabolene, cadinene, copaene, curzerene, lindestrene 39%; ketones as methyl isobutyl ketone, curzerenone 6%; phenols/pheonol ethers as eugenol 3%; aldehydes as 2-butanal 2%; traces of esters as myrrholic ester, acids as myrrholic acid, aromatic aldehydes as cinnamaldehyde, cuminaldehyde; monoterpenenes as limonene, dipentene, pinene.

**Therapeutic actions** Vulnerary, cicatrising, astringent, balsamic, rejuvenating; antimicrobial, fungicidal; anti-inflammatory, blood purifying; carminative, stomachic; tonic to mucous membranes, uterine muscle and whole system; emmenagogue; expectorant.

**Blends with** frankincense, sandalwood, benzoin, cypress, jasmine, thyme, juniper, geranium, patchouli, pine, lavender, mints, tea tree, rosewood.

**Other uses** An ingredient in oral pharmaceuticals, such as toothpaste, mouthwash, gargles. A fixative and fragrance in toiletries, soaps, cosmetics, perfumes (oriental and floral notes). A flavour ingredient in foods and beverages.

**Safety/precautions** Avoid in pregnancy. Non-irritating, non-sensitising but possibly toxic in high concentrations.

# Myrtle

**Name** Myrtle

**Latin name** *Myrtus communis* from the Greek *myrtos* the myrtle tree and the Latin *communis* common.

**Family** Myrtaceae

**Synonyms** Common myrtle, Corsican pepper

**Other species** *Myrica cerifera*, the wax or bay myrtle of southern United States. *M. gale*, the British bog myrtle.

**Description** A small evergreen tree or shrub, 1–3 m; much branched; leaves glossy, dark green, opposite, ovate to lancelote, entire, 3–5 cm, with transparent oil glands visible, fragrant; flowers pure white or rosy, fragrant, numerous stamens, 5-petalled, 2 cm; fruit a bluish berry.

**Habitat/distribution** Native to the Mediterranean and western Asia; grows up to 800 m altitude, myrtle was introduced elsewhere, e.g. Europe. It prefers full sun, and the protection of a south-facing wall in northern climates.

**History** Known and used in ancient Egypt, the Near East, Greece and Rome, myrtle was sacred to Aphrodite-Venus. It was the symbol of beauty and youth and decorated temples and sanctuaries. It has been used in bridal crowns in these lands down to the present day. Theophrastus and Dioscorides discuss it,

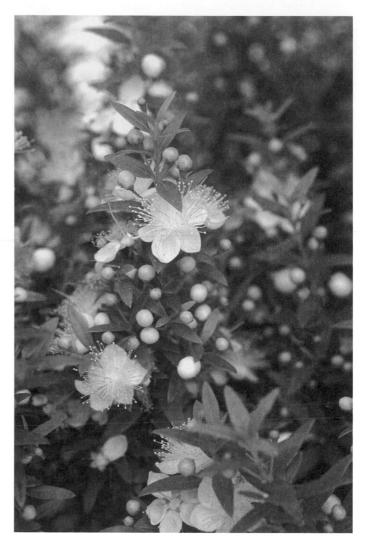

*Myrtle*

- **Skin:** acne, open pores, oiliness; haemorrhoids.
- **Repiratory:** asthma, bronchitis, chronic cough, tuberculosis, chest congestion. Myrtle's mild but effective nature makes it an ideal chest rub for children's ailments, or elderly patients.
- **Immune:** colds, flu, infectious diseases.
- **Nervous:** restlessness, poor sleep, anxiety, irritability. It is useful for treating addictions.
- **Mental–emotional:** uplifting, refreshing, enhances self-esteem and tolerance.

the latter citing it for respiratory ailments, bites of poisonous beasts and insects, intestinal inflammations. In the 16th century it was an ingredient of 'Eau d'ange' (angel water) skin lotion.

**Cultivation** Mediterranean countries of Europe, North Africa, former Yugoslavia. Propagated from cuttings.

**Part used** Leaves, twigs, sometimes the flowers.

**Extraction/adulterations** Steam distillation.

**Characteristics** Pale yellow to orange liquid; fresh, sweet odour, slightly reminiscent of eucalyptus. Middle note.

**Energy** Warming, drying. Clears phlegm, purifies blood. Reduces kapha and pitta, calms vata. Clears cold, wind, damp from lungs and skin.

**Chemical constituents** Features esters as linalyl acetate, myrtenyl acetate 37%; oxides as 1.8-cineole 30%; monoterpenes as α-pinene, β-pinene, limonene 16%; alcohols as α-terpinen-4-ol, myrtenol, geraniol 0.8%; phenols as carvacrol 0.6%.

**Therapeutic actions** Astringent, balsamic; bactericidal, antiseptic; anticatarrhal, expectorant; nervine calmative.

**Blends with** bergamot, lavender, rosemary, clary sage, lime, ginger, clove.

**Other uses** Included in eau de colognes, toilet waters; a culinary herb.

 **Safety/precautions** Non-toxic, non-irritating, non-sensitising.

# Niaouli

**Name** Niaouli

**Latin name** *Melaleuca viridiflora* from the Greek *melan* and *leuco*, black and white, because the bark of some species is dark and light; from the Latin *viridiflora* green-flowered.

**Family** Myrtaceae

**Synonyms** *M. quinquenervia* var. *cineol*. Broadleaved paperbark tree, gomenol (the French name, after Gomen, a town in French East Indies, now New Caledonia, from which it was first exported). A variety known as *M. viridiflora* 'Type A' has been developed to provide a source for nerolidol; this is also rich in linalool. It is less available now since perfume industry has developed a synthetic source of nerolidol. Aromatherapists use the cineole rich variety. The genera is complex and botanists are not in agreement on identification and classification (Gibbs).

**Other species** Niaouli is related to other *melaleucas*: cajeput, tea tree and to eucalyptus.

**Description** An evergreen tree 8–12 m, sometimes as high as 24 m; bark spongy or papery, greyish white; leaves lanceolate-elliptical, stiff, leathery, 5-veined, very fragrant; flowers in sessile (stalkless) spikes, yellowish/greenish to white; fruit in small, woody capsules with flattened tops.

**Habitat/distribution** Native to Australia, New Caledonia, Indonesia, Tasmania, New Guinea, niaouli thrives in swampy or rocky soil, low and higher altitudes (1,000 ft). Quickly colonises disused land.

**History** Traditionally niaouli has been used by Aboriginal peoples for aches and pains, respiratory conditions, cuts, infections. They shared their knowledge with European colonisers, one of whom introduced it to France in the 18th century from specimens in New Caledonia, a French colony. It was first 'discovered' by botanists on Captain Cook's voyage to Australia in 1770. Since its introduction to Europe it has been popular, especially in France, for treating respiratory infections (Gibbs, 1997).

**Cultivation** Wild. Cultivated in its native areas. More recently in plantations in Madagascar.

**Part used** Leaves and young twigs.

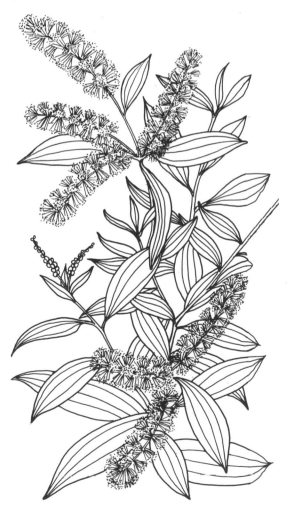

*Niaouli*

- **Skin:** acne, boils, cuts, wounds, insect bites, oiliness, ulcers, burns. Gentle yet powerful. Applied to skin before radiation therapy it helps protect against burning and reduces severity of burns (Davis, 1995).

- **Digestive:** enteritis, gastric and duodenal ulcers, intestinal parasites.

- **Respiratory-immune:** asthma, bronchial infections, colds, fever, flu, coughs, sinusitis, sore throat, whooping cough, pneumonia. Gentle yet powerful.

- **Circulatory:** poor, sluggish.

- **Muscular–skeletal:** arthritis, aches and pains.

- **Urinary:** cystitis, urinary tract infections.

- **Reproductive:** vaginal douche.

- **Mental–emotional:** clears the head, aids concentration, stimulating and uplifting.

**Niaouli**

*Melaleuca viridiflora*

**Extraction/adulterations** Water or steam distillation over 6 hours. It is sometimes subject to adulteration with kerosene, or even eucalyptus. Do not confuse with *M. leucodendron*, cajeput, when sourcing.

**Characteristics** Watery white or pale yellow or greenish yellow in colour, liquid; strong, hot, fresh sweet-camphorous odour reminiscent of eucalyptus and cardamom; sweeter than cajeput or eucalyptus; a hint of bitter almond. Top note.

**Energy** Warming, stimulating. Clears phlegm, invigorates melancholy, purifies blood, cools choler. Reduces kapha, lowers pitta, may aggravate vata in excess; stimulates agni. Disperses wind, clears phlegm and liver qi stagnation, tonifies wei qi.

**Chemical constituents** Features oxides as 1.8-cineole (eucalyptol) 60%; alcohols as α-terpeneol, viridiflorol, nerolidol, globulol 15%; esters as terpinyl valerate, terpinyl acetate, terpinyl butyrate 15.%; monoterpens limonene, α-pinene, β-pinene 2%; traces of sesquiterpenes, aldehydes and other constitutents.

**Therapeutic actions** Strongly disinfectant, antiseptic, antiviral, antibacterial; anticatarrhal, expectorant–decongestant, balsamic; diaphoretic; cicatrising; gastric tonic; nervine; immune stimulant; antirheumatic; regulating, vermifuge, oestrogen-like.

**Blends with** basil, cajeput and other *melaleucas*, rosemary, marjoram, fennel, juniper, thyme, citrus oils, mints, melissa.

**Other uses** Pharmaceutical preparations: gargles, cough drops, toothpaste.

 **Safety/precautions** Non-toxic, non-irritating, non-sensitising (contrast with *M. leucodendron*).

# Orange bitter

## Neroli Petitgrain Bigarade

The extractions from the different parts of the bitter orange tree are grouped together as they originate from one tree.

**Name** The flower: Orange blossom/neroli
The leaf: Petitgrain bigarade, the bitter orange, Seville orange
The peel: Orange bigarade/Seville
The common name 'orange' comes from the Sanskrit *nagaranga* through the Arabic *naranj*.

**Latin name** *Citrus aurantium* var. *amara*

**Family** Rutaceae

**Synonyms** *C. vulgaris*, *C. bigaradia*.
The flower: orange blossom, orange flower, neroli, neroli bigarade
The leaf: petigrain, petitgrain bigarade, Paraguay bigarade
The peel: Seville orange, oil of bigarade

**Other species** *C. aurantium* var. *dolcis*, sweet orange, is also extracted as an absolute and an essential oil. It is less fragrant and fine and is also known as Portugal neroli.

**Description** A glabrous evergreen tree to 8 m; branches spiny; leaves alternate, ovate-oblong, very fragrant; flowers fragrant, white or pink at axils, single or few; fruit globe-shaped, of darker orange than the sweet

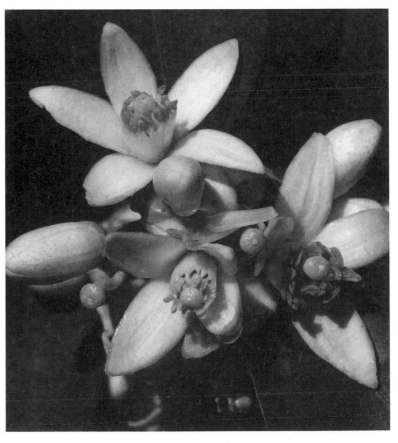

*Neroli orange bitter*

orange, fragrant. The leaf stalk of the bitter orange tree distinguishes it from the sweet, being broadened out in the shape of a heart.

**Habitat/distribution** Native to Asia. It has been introduced and naturalised in southern Europe/the Mediterranean basin, in the United States, Central and South America, and elsewhere. It prefers dry soil, sun. In Provence, where it has been traditionally cultivated and distilled, the flowering season is in May.

**History** Orange trees have been used from India to China for food and medicine since ancient times. In Chinese medicine the peel is used to treat prolapsed uterus and is an important remedy for digestive conditions. The orange was known to the Greeks and Romans and has been used in Unani medicine. The flowers were called neroli after an Italian princess who made it famous as her preferred perfume. Essential oil of neroli is an important ingredient in eau de cologne. In Grasse, Provence, the flowers traditionally are candied.

**Cultivation** Wild and cultivated commercially widely: traditionally in Provence, Calabria, Sicily, Spain, Madeira; California, Florida; the West Indies; Central and South America; Asia. The flowers begin three years after grafting, reaching their maximum number at about 20 years. It flowers in May but may flower again in autumn if conditions are right, though the oil is inferior. The yield is very dependent on conditions; settled warm, dry weather is best (Grieves, 1984).

**Part used** Flower for neroli.
Leaves and twigs for petitgrain.
Peel of fruit for bitter orange/bigarade.

**Extraction/adulterations** Neroli: solvent; an absolute is produced by solvent extraction; enfleurage was traditionally used. Steam distillation of freshly picked flowers; a hydrolat is yielded. The yield in distillation is greatly influenced by the temperature and atmospheric conditions prevailing, decreasing in cool, damp, changeable weather. A tree can produce up to 30 kg of blossoms. One tonne of flowers can yield up to 1 kg of essential oil. Neroli may be adulterated with petitgrain.
Petitgrain: steam distillation of leaves and twigs. A hydrolat is also yielded.
Bigarade/bitter orange: cold expression (hand or machine) of the peel of almost ripe fruit.

**Characteristics** Neroli: The essential oil is a deep brown, viscous liquid; a bitter-sweet intense odour. The absolute is a dark brown or orange, viscous liquid; fresh, delicate, intense sweet-floral odour. Base note.
Petitgrain: a pale yellow or amber liquid; fresh floral-sweet-slightly woody odour. Top note.
Bigarade: a dark yellow or brown-yellow liquid; fresh, dry, slightly sweet-floral odour. Top note.

**Energy** Neroli: cooling, balancing moist and dry. Cools choler, enhances sanguine, calms and revives melancholy. Reduces excess pitta, calms vata. Calms heart, clears heat, regulates qi.
Petitgrain: cooling, balancing moist and dry. Cools choler, enhances sanguine, calms and revives melancholy. Reduces excess pitta, calms vata. Tonifies spleen qi, calms heart, clears heat, releases qi stagnation.
Bigarade: cooling, balancing moist and dry. Cools choler, enhances sanguine, calms and revives melancholy, promotes digestive fire. Reduces excess pitta, calms vata, strengthens agni. Tonifies spleen qi, releases qi stagnation.

## Therapeutic actions

| **Neroli** | **Petitgrain** | **Bigarade** |
|---|---|---|
| nervine stimulant | nervine antispasmodic, | nervine sedative |
| antidepressant | stimulant | carminative, stomachic |
| antispasmodic | digestive, stomachic | choleretic |
| cordial | antiseptic | antiseptic, fungicidal |
| digestive, carminative | | anti-inflammatory |
| bactericidal, antiseptic | | astringent |
| fungicidal | | tonic |
| tonic – cardiac, circulatory | | blood thinning |
| aphrodisiac | | |

**Chemical constituents** Neroli: features alcohols as linalool, α-terpeneol, geraniol, nerol, nerolidol, farnesol, benzyl aocohol, phenylether alcohol 40%; terpenes as limonene, β-pinene 35%; esters as methyl antranilate, linalyl acetate, geranyl acetate, neryl acetate 14%; aldehydes as citral 2%; ketones as jasmone 0.5%.

Petitgrain: features esters as linalyl acetate, geranyl acetate, neryl acetate 55%; alcohols as linalool, geraniol, nerolidol, α-terpenol 30%; terpenes as α-pinene, limonene, ρ-cymene, ocimene, myrcene 10%; lactones as limettin, bergaptene trace; phenols as thymol trace.

Bigarade: features terpenes as limonene, α-pinene, myrcene, terpinolene, camphene, ρ-cymene, ocimene 90%; esters as linalyl acetate, geranyl acetate, citronellyl acetate 2%; aldehydes as citral, undecanal 2%; sesquiterpenes as farnesens, copaene, humulene 0.5%; alcohols as linalool, nerol, α-terpeneol, citronellol 0.3%; oxides as 1.8 cineole; ketones trace.

### Blends with

Orange blossom/neroli: other citrus oils, all oils, sandalwood, geranium, clary sage.

Petitgrain: lavender, rosemary, geranium, bergamot, jasmine, palmarosa.

Bigarade: lavender, rosemary, geranium, bergamot, jasmine, palmarosa.

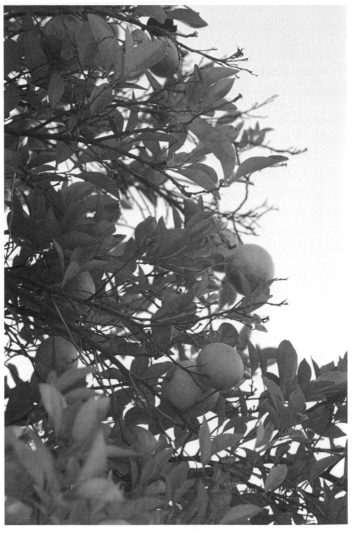

*Neroli orange bitter*

# USES

| Neroli | Petitgrain | Bigarade |
|---|---|---|
| 🔹 **Skin:** | | |
| scars, stretch marks, broken veins, mature/ sensitive skin, wrinkles | acne, excess perspiration, oily skin and hair | dull, oily complexions, mouth ulcers |
| 🔹 **Digestive:** | | |
| diarrhoea, colic, wind, nervous dyspepsia | dyspepsia, flatulence | constipation, dyspepsia, spasm |
| 🔹 **Respiratory:** | | |
| (no particular indications) | bronchitis | bronchitis, asthma |
| 🔹 **Immune:** | | |
| (no particular indications) | (no particular indications) | colds, flu, chill |
| 🔹 **Circulation:** | | |
| palpitations, poor circulation | (no particular indications) | fluid retention, obesity, blood clots |
| 🔹 **Nervous:** | | |
| anxiety, depression, tension, stress, shock, PMS | insomnia, nervous fatigue, depression, convalescence, stress, tension | tension, stress, vertigo |
| 🔹 **Mental–emotional:** | | |
| low self-esteem, depression, hysteria | cheering, uplifting, detaching | cheering, uplifting, stimulating |

**Other uses** Hydrolats of neroli and petitgrain can be used as facial toners and for children, weak or delicate patients. Fragrance for perfumes, cosmetic and toiletries; flavouring for foods and beverages, liqueurs, e.g. the immature fruits – 'orange berries' – flavour curacao; flavouring for pharmaceuticals.

 **Safety/precautions**
Neroli: non-toxic, non-irritating, non-sensitising, non-phototoxic.
Petitgrain: as neroli.
Bigarade: phototoxic, avoid exposure of skin to sun after application; otherwise safe. Limonene may cause contact dermatitis in some individuals.

# Palmarosa

**Name** Palmarosa

**Latin name** *Cymbopogon martini* var. *martinii*

**Family** Graminaceae

**Synonyms** *Andropogon martini, A. martini* var. *motia*; (east) Indian geranium, Turkish geranium, Indian rosha, motia.

**Other species** Related to lemongrass and citronella and to another species, *C. martinii* var. *sofia* or gingergrass, a different chemotype. The two are sometimes distilled together in India.

**Description** A grass; long slender, fragrant leaves; flowers in terminal spikes.

**Habitat/distribution** Native to Indian subcontinent, from north-west (including Pakistan) to south. Cultivated in Africa, Indonesia, Brazil and Comoro Islands.

**History** Traditional use in native habitat. Traded to the west through Bombay (hence 'Indian'), Constantinople (hence 'Turkish') and Bulgaria.

**Cultivation** Wild. Cultivated.

**Part used** Leaves, fresh or dried.

**Extraction/adulterations** Steam or water distillation. Palmarosa itself has been used to adulterate rose oil.

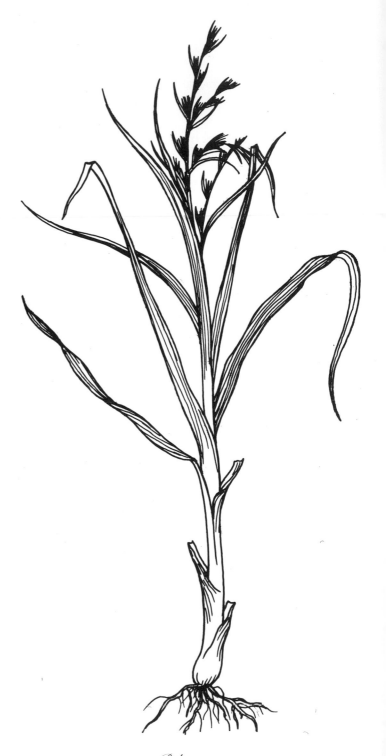

*Palmarosa*

- **Skin:** acne, dermatitis, infections, wounds, scars, sores, wrinkles; chapped, dry skin (hydrating).
- **Digestive:** anorexia, atonia, enteritis, dysentery.
- **Immune:** rich in alcohols, which are anti-infectious. Colds, flu, fevers.
- **Nervous:** tension, stress, exhaustion.
- **Mental–emotional:** calms and uplifts.

**Palmarosa**

*Cymbopogon martini*

**Characteristics** Pale yellow or olive, liquid; geranium or rose-like odour. Top note.

**Energy** Cooling, moistening (hydrating). Reduces choler, purifies blood, calms melancholy. Calms vata, cools pitta, enhances rasa dhatu. Moves stomach qi; disperses wind.

**Chemical constituents** Features alcohols as geraniol, citronellol, farnesol, linalool, nerol, elemol 85%; aldehydes as citral, citronellal 7%; esters as gernayl acetate, genranyl formate, geranyl isobutyrate, geranyl hexanoate, neryl formate 5%; sesquiterpenes as β-caryophyllene; monoterpenes as dipentene, limonene; ketones as methyl heptenone; and others.

**Therapeutic actions** Antiseptic, bactericidal (particularly intestinal pathogens); digestive tonic, enhances appetite, stomachic; astringent, hydrating, regulates sebum production; stimulating, tonic, cicatrising, febrifuge.

**Blends with** ylang ylang, geranium, rose, rosewood, sandalwood, cedarwood, lavender, citrus oils.

**Other uses** Fragrance for toiletries, soaps, perfumes, cosmetics. Some limited use as flavouring (tobacco). It is used as a source for isolated geraniol.

**Safety/precautions** Non-toxic, non-irritating, non-sensitising.

# Patchouli

**Name** Patchouli

**Latin name** *Pogostemon cablin*

**Family name** Lamiaceae/Labiatae

**Synonyms** *Pogostemon patchouli*, Puchput; Tamil 'paccali'; Philippine 'cablin'. Other species related to Java patchouli, *P. heyneanus*, false patchouli. There are about 40 species, 20 in India alone.

**Description** A perennial bushy herb, up to 1 m; roots extensive, branching, going deep, slightly fragrant; stem erect, hairy; leaves large, opposite, fur-like hairs, soft toothed, fragrant; flowers white, tinged with purple on axillary and terminal spikes.

**Habitat/distribution** Native to tropical south and south-east Asia (southern India, Sri Lanka, Malaysia, Indonesia, Philippines).

**History** Patchouli has been traditionally used in the East to ward off infectious diseases, to treat fever, cold, nausea, vomiting diarrhoea, abdominal pain, bad breath, headaches, snake and insect bite; as an insecticide. Traditionally valued as an aphrodisiac, it is also used in perfumes and to perfume textiles in India, and by Arabs to scent and possibly protect carpets. The Chinese produce a perfume.

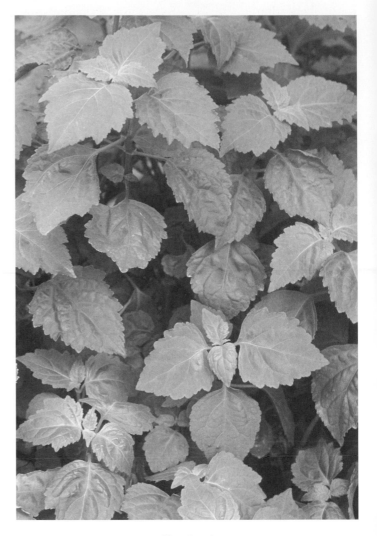

*Patchouli*

**Cultivation** Wild. Cultivated in its native areas, in China, South America (West Indies, Paraguay), Mauritius, Vietnam. The crop is harvested 2 or 3 times a year. It is packed in bales for export to distilleries abroad, if not extracted locally.

**Part used** Dried leaves, usually dried and fermented.

**Extraction/adulterations** Steam distillation. Locally distilled oil is superior. A resinoid is also produced for use as a fixative. India, Taiwan, Brazil and Seychelles produce the essential oil locally. A solvent extraction is also done to double the yield.

## USES

- **Skin:** acne, cracked, chapped skin, wounds, sores, inflammations, allergies, eczema (seborrhoeic); athlete's foot, fungal infections/impetigo, ringworm.
- **Digestive:** nervous digestion, nausea, flatulence, enteritis; possibly habits of over-eating.
- **Immune-respiratory:** fevers, lowered immunity.
- **Circulatory:** varicose veins, haemorrhoids, fluid retention, cellulite.
- **Genito-urinary:** fluid retention, cellulite; frigidity.
- **Nervous:** tension, stress, anxiety, depression, exhaustion, low libido.
- **Mental–emotional:** calming, grounding, clearing and uplifting.

**Characteristics** An amber or brownish-yellow tinged with green, viscous liquid; sweet-earthy-herbaceous tenacious odour, improving with age. Base note.

**Energy** Warming, grounding, uplifting. Clears phlegm, cools choler, revives and calms melancholy. Reduces kapha, cools pitta, calms, rejuvenates vata; balances agni. Clears cold and damp-heat, tonifies wei and spleen qi.

**Chemical constituents** Features alcohols as guaiol, bulnesol, pogostol, patchouli alcohol 25–50%; sesquiterpenes as α-guaiene, patchoulenes, α-bulnesene, seyschellenes, cadinene, caryophyllene, aromadendrene 50%; oxides as guaiene oxide, bulnesene oxide, caryophyllene oxide 6%; ketones patchoulenone, isopatchoulenone 2%; monterpenes as α-pinene, β-pinene, limonene 1%; remainder 8%.

**Therapeutic actions** Antimicrobial, antiviral, bactericidal, fungicidal; febrifuge, diaphoretic; vulnerary, astringent, cicatrising, cell rejuvenating; digestive, stomachic, carminative, anti-emetic; diuretic; antidepressant, immuno-stimulant.

**Blends with** vetiver, sandalwood, cedarwood, geranium, clove, lavender, rose, neroli, bergamot, myrrh, clary sage. Use with discretion: only a small amount in a blend as it may overpower other components.

**Other uses** Fragrance and fixative for cosmetics, soaps and oriental type perfumes, incense. Flavouring in food products and beverages.

 **Safety/precautions** Non-toxic, non-irritating, non-sensitising.

# Peppermint

**Name** Peppermint

**Latin name** *Mentha* x *piperita*, botanically a hybrid of *M. aquatica* and *M. spicata*, spearmint.

**Family** Lamiaceae/Labiatae

**Synonyms** Brandy mint, balm mint.

**Other species** Other varieties exist such as black peppermint. Related to other mints such as spearmint, garden mint.

**Description** An aromatic perennial to 1 m; stems square, erect, branched above; leaves opposite, ovate or lanceolate, toothed, green or purplish (e.g. black peppermint); flowers on terminal spikes from axils of upper leaves, 3–7.5 cm, irregularly arranged in whorled clusters, mauve, sometimes white; root produces numerous runners by which plant may be propagated as flowers are infertile.

**Habitat/distribution** Native to Europe, peppermint likes damp soil; distributed wild along hedgerows, ditches and near dwellings.

**History** The use of mints goes back millennia. A sample was found in an Egyptian tomb of 1000–3000 BC. The Greeks and Romans used them at festive or ritual occasions. It is mentioned in an Icelandic herbal of the 13th century. Although some mints were recommended in Dioscorides, it is difficult to identify the species. It is known that peppermint was first identified in the 17th century in Hertfordshire and introduced by Ray into his *Historia plantarum* (1704), after which it began to be used medicinally and cultivated from the mid 18th to mid 20th centuries. English peppermint has been considered the finest in pungency and flavour. In France a 'red mint' variety has been cultivated. English plants are cultivated in France and Italy, and most recently the United States. True peppermint cannot be cultivated on the same field for more than 2 years. The soil has a strong influence on the fragrance and flavour. The distilled oil has remained in the *British Pharmacopoeia* for intestinal complaints and has recently been redeveloped for treatment of irritable bowel syndrome (IBS).

**Cultivation** Wild. Cultivated widely now, particularly in the US. Peppermint does not breed true from seed, but is propagated from divisions of the stolen (roots) in autumn.

**Part used** Flowering stems.

**Extraction/adulterations** Steam distillation. Yield is approximately 3–4%. Adulterated with cornmint, *M. arvense*.

**Characteristics** A pale yellow or greenish liquid; pungent-peppery, minty, refreshing and invigorating odour. Top note.

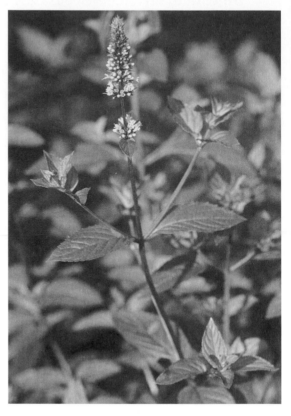

*Peppermint*

## USES

- **Skin:** congestion, acne, eczema, dermatitis, ringworm, scabies, toothache; skin tonic.

- **Digestive:** IBS, candida, intestinal dysbiosis, colic, cramp, dyspepsia, ulcers, flatulence, nausea, travel sickness, cirrhosis, enteritis, gallstones, hepatitis, jaundice, worms.

- **Respiratory-immune:** colds, flu, infections, fevers, bronchitis, rhinitis, sinusitis, otitis, laryngitis, cough, asthma.

- **Circulatory:** palpitations, low blood pressure.

- **Muscular–skeletal:** cramp, aches and pains (effective local analgesic–anasthetic), arthritis, tendonitis, repetitive strain injury.

- **Urinary:** cystitis, nephritis, prostate (benign hyperplasia).

- **Reproductive:** dysmenorrhoeal, delayed menses, cramp, assist childbirth; impotence.

- **Nervous:** pain, neuralgia, headaches, migraine, mental fatigue, sciatica, tension, stress, vertigo, exhaustion.

- **Mental–emotional:** uplifts, invigorates, opens the mind, clears doubt and confusion; improves concentration.

**Energy** Warming/cooling, drying. Amphoteric. Clears phlegm, cools choler, uplifts, invigorates melancholy, purifies blood. Calms vata (may aggravate on excessive use), reduces kapha and pitta. Tonifies, moves and clears qi/qi stagnation especially in the stomach-intestines. Peppermint is unique in its combination of warming stimulating/cooling calming and balancing effects.

**Chemical constituents** Features alcohols as menthol, neomenthol, isomenthol, linalool 42%; ketones as menthone, isomenthone, pulegone 30%; oxides as 1.8 cineole, caryophylllene oxide 7%; esters as menthyl acetate 6%; sesquiterpenes as germacrene, β-caryophyllene 6%; monoterpenes as phillandrene, α-pinene, β-pinene, menthene, limonene 6%; lactones and coumarins as aesculetene, menthofuran, trace; and others 3%.

**Therapeutic actions** Digestive stimulant and tonic, stomachic, carminative, hepatic, cholagogue; nervine antispasmodic, analgesic, tonic; mucolytic, expectorant, febrifuge; anti-inflammatory; diaphoretic; antiseptic, antimicrobial, antiviral; cordial, vasoconstrictor; cephalic; astringent (e.g. stems milk flow); emmenagogue, uterine tonic; vermifuge.

**Blends with** mints, citrus oils, benzoin, rosemary, cajeput, niaouli, tea tree, eucalyptus, lavender, basil, marjoram, cypress, juniper, thyme.

**Other uses** A good quality peppermint tea helpful for digestive problems, fatigue, colds, flu, fever, respiratory–mucous congestion. The essential oil is used as a flavouring in pharmaceuticals, foods (confection, chewing gum), beverages, tobacco; a fragrance in toiletries, toothpastes and mouthwashes, cosmetics, perfumes, cleansing products.

**Safety/precautions** Avoid in pregnancy, lactation and for children under 3 years. Non-toxic, non-irritating. Possible sensitisation in some due to menthol. Use in higher dilutions. Avoid alongside homoeopathic remedy.

# Pine

**Name** Pine

**Latin name** *Pinus sylvestris* from the Latin *sylvestris*, of woods and forests.

**Family** Pinaceae

**Synonyms** Forest pine, Scots pine, Norway pine.

**Other species** Many species of pine yield essential oil from heartwood, needles, twigs, e.g. the eastern white pine, *P. strobus* of the US.

**Description** A tall tree, up to 40 m with a flat crown; bark reddish and deeply fissured; needles long, growing in pairs, fragrant; cones pointed.

**Habitat/distribution** Native to Eurasia, introduced and naturalised elsewhere.

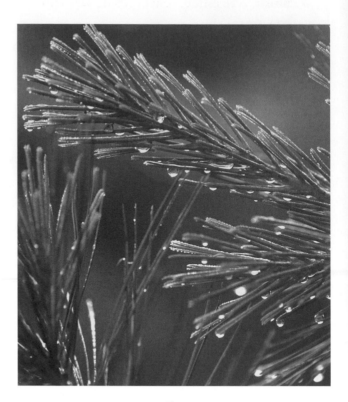

*Pine*

**History** Pines have been used throughout history to produce terebinth/turpentine from the oleoresin, which exudes from the bark: until the discovery of America, Europeans used native species, e.g. *P. palustris,* to produce terebinth; after 1492 *P. strobes* from the south-eastern US became the main source. Turpentine, as well as being used as a solvent, has been traditional as a rubifacient, for sprains and strained muscles, to relieve rheumatic swellings and to kill parasites. The roots of *P. sylvestris* have been used to produce tar. Pine was used in ancient Greek medicine and is still current in Unani medicine. It was recommended by Avicenna for pneumonia.

**Cultivation** Wild. Cultivated in the eastern US, Europe, Russia, Baltic states and Scandinavia.

**Part used** Needles.

**Extraction/adulterations** Steam distillation. An inferior essential oil is produced from wood chippings so check for authenticity. A gum turpentine is also produced by steam distillation from the oleoresin. Assuming harvesting and distillation are optimum, the best quality comes from trees cultivated in northern, colder temperatures.

**Characteristics** A colourless or pale yellow liquid; a strong, balsamic or resinous odour, conjuring the freshness of the outdoors. Enjoyed by men. Middle note.

**Energy** Warming, stimulating, drying. Softens, clears phlegm, purifies blood, cools choler. Reduces kapha and pitta. Tonifies lung qi, kidney yang and wei qi, clears phlegm; moves stomach and liver qi.

## USES

- **Skin:** allergies, eczema, psoriasis (cortisone-like); scabies, lice; sores; cuts excessive perspiration.

- **Digestive:** congested liver/low bile production, hepatitis; weak digestion, indigestion.

- **Respiratory-immune:** asthma, bronchitis, catarrhal congestion, sinusitis, colds, flu, tuberculosis.

- **Endocrine system:** adrenal exhaustion, auto-immune inflammatory conditions.

- **Muscular–skeletal:** aches and pains, sprains, strains; arthritis and rheumatic swellings; fatigue (multiple sclerosis).

- **Urinary system:** cystitis, urinary tract infection, gout.

- **Reproductive:** impotence, frigidity; low fertility (male and female).

- **Nervous:** stress, exhaustion, fatigue; neuralgia, pain.

**Chemical constituents** Features montoterpenes as α-pinene, β-pinene, limonene, $\Delta^3$-carene, camphene, phellandrene, dipentene, terpinene, myrcene, sabinene 70%; alcohols as borneol, terpinen-4-ol, cadinol 5%; esters as bornyl acetate, terpinyl acetate 5%; sesquiterpenes as caryophyllene, cadinene, copaene, guaiene, farnesene 5%; oxides, acids, ketones and aldehydes in trace amounts and other undetermined components 15%.

**Therapeutic actions** Antimicrobial, parasitical, antiviral, bactericidal, antiseptic (powerful for lungs), insecticidal; vermifuge; deodorant, balsamic, antiscorbutic; expectorant, mucolytic; antirheumatic; diuretic; cholagogue, choleretic; adrenal cortex stimulant, circulatory and nervous system stimulant; hypertensive; nervine analgesic, tonic; reproductive tonic; digestive tonic (stimulates gastric secretions).

**Blends with** rosemary, tea tree, sage, thyme, eucalyptus, cedarwood, juniper, lemon, niaouli.

**Other uses** Fragrance in soaps, cleansing products, toiletries (e.g. bath products), some perfumes; flavouring in food products and beverages.

 **Safety/precautions** Non-toxic, non-irritating, except in high concentration, possibly skin sensitising. Avoid in presence of allergies, use higher dilution for massage. (NB: Dwarf pine e.o. is hazardous; obtain authentic *P. sylvestris* oil.)

# Rose

**Name** Rose species, cabbage rose

**Latin name** *Rosa* x *centifolia*

**Family** Rosaceae (many medicinal and food plants are in the Rosaceae family: apples, meadowsweet, lady's mantle, hawthorn).

**Synonyms** Rose maroc, French rose, Provins rose (Provence rose).

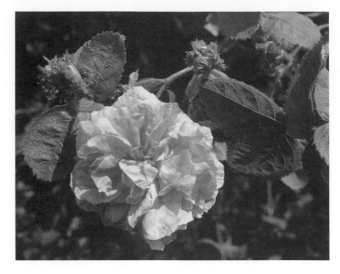

*Cabbage rose*

**Other species** There are many species native to temperate climates world-wide; many hybrids have been developed, over 10,000 varieties are cultivated. Species native to Britain include the dog rose, *R. canina*, and the eglantine rose, *R. eglanteria*, Rose de Mai, a hybrid of *R. gallica* (a wild rose of southern France) and *R. x centifolia*. Main source of essential oil of *R. x centifolia*. (See *R. x damascena*.) *R. indica*, the tea rose, is found in India and *R. rugosa* in China and Japan.

**Description** An herbaceous shrub up to 8 m; leaves alternate, usually pinnate, with stipules at the base of stalks; flowers a mass of conspicuous, pink or rosy petals; stems thorny.

**Habitat/distribution** The rose is believed to have originated either in northern Perisa on the Caspian sea or in Faristan on the Persian Gulf. From Persia cultivation spread across Mesopotamia to Greece, the Mediterranean and southern European countries and eastward into India in ancient times.

**History** Our relationships and associations with the rose are ancient, rich and complex. Remains of roses have been found in Egyptian tombs; they are depicted in Minoan frescos (1900 BC); they appear on Assyrian and Greek tablets and coins. Rose is prescribed in ancient Chinese medical texts. A macerated oil was traded among Mediterranean peoples for perfume and healing. King Midas of Phrygia sent a 60-petaled, strongly-scented rose to the Greeks, according to Herodotus. In Greece and Rome it was used for celebrations, banquets, nuptual rites and religious festivals and funerals. It was sacred to Dionysius and Aphrodite-Venus, symbolising both worldly and spiritual love, life and renewal. Paestum, in southern Italy, was a centre of cultivation during Emperor Nero's reign, probably of *R. gallica*. The ancient associations of the rose were transferred to Christianity: the white rose symbolised Christ's spiritual aspects and the red rose his human form. It was also associated with the Virgin Mary, representing her unselfish love and devotion. The rose's sweet flowers borne on a thorny stem symbolise the triumph of good over evil, or of love over hatred. The apothecary rose, *R. gallica* officinalis, has been traditional in herbal medicine for its cooling, anti-inflammatory and astringent properties. It is said that the idea for distillation came when the fragrance of thousands of petals strewn on the waters on a warm day filled the air.

**Cultivation** Cultivated commercially in plantations in France, Morocco, Tunisia, Italy, former Yugoslavia, China. Cultivated in gardens in temperate zones world wide.

**Part used** Flowers, rose buds, with the calyces cut off.

- **Skin:** conjunctivits (use rose water); dry, chapped, cracked or sensitive skin, eczema; ageing skin; herpes; gingivitis.
- **Digestive:** liver and bile congestion, nausea.
- **Respiratory-immune:** asthma, couchs, bronchitis, tuberculosis.
- **Circulation:** palpitations, poor circulation, Raynaud's.
- **Reproductive:** PMS; irregular periods, painful periods, leucorrhoea, uterine disorders, menopausal symptoms; low libido, impotence; of use pre-partum to help ligaments soften enabling pelvic bones to expand.
- **Nervous:** insomnia, anxiety, stress, tension, headaches; low self-esteem.
- **Mental–emotional:** depression, anxiety. Uplifts and strengthens, gives confidence. Harmonises the different aspects of ourselves and inspires our highest nature.

**Rose, cabbage**
*Rosa x centifolia*

**Extraction/adulterations** Steam distillation. An absolute and a concrete are also produced. *See* damask rose (page 284). Distillation requires very low temperatures and careful handling. The distillation water is itself distilled to recover the essential oil. Sometimes the essence is produced by enfleurage. The presence of hydrocarbon stearopten makes the essence congeal at cool temperatures and this can be used to verify authenticity. Adulterated with palmarosa.

**Characteristics** Essential oil: a pale yellow; fluid liquid, congealing at cooler temperatures; a rich, sweet, floral, tenacious odour. Absolute: a red-orange viscous liquid; rich, sweet-spicy, rosy odour. Base note.

**Energy** Cooling, drying/moistening. Cools choler, nourishes and purifies blood, revives and soothes melancholy. Tridosic; regulates and strengthens agni; satvic. Nourishes and regulates blood, tonifies yin, clears stagnant qi; clears heat (stomach, lower warmer).

**Chemical constituents** Over 300 constituents have been identified, including: alcohols phenyl ethanol 63%, citronellol 18–20%, geraniol and nerol 63%, farnesol 0.2–2%, stearopten 8%.

**Therapeutic actions** Antiseptic, antiviral, antitubercular; anti-inflammatory; astringent, cicatrising, vulnerary; digestive stomachic, appetite regulator, hepatic; alterative, circulatory haemostatic, blood nourishing, cardiac tonic; nervine sedative, antidepressant; emmenagogue, uterine tonic.

**Blends with** neroli, lavender, jasmine, geranium, sandalwood, clary sage, patchouli.

**Other uses** *See* damask rose.

**Safety/precautions** Non-toxic, non-sensitising, non-irritating.

# Rose

**Name** Rose species, damask rose

**Latin name** *Rosa x damascene*

**Family** Rosaceae

**Synonyms** Damask rose, Bulgarian rose, Turkish rose.

**Other species** There are many subspecies and cultivars: *R. x damascene* var. *alba*, *R. x damascena* 'Kaznalik rose'. It is closely related to *R. x centifolia*. Rose de Hai, a cross of *R. damascene* and a *R. rugosa* ('General Jacqueminot'), is also now distilled.

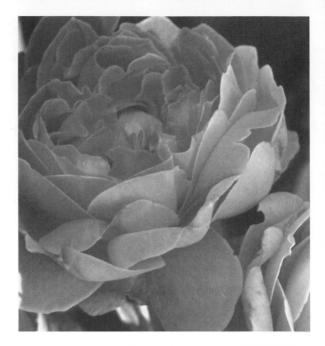

*Damask rose*

**Description** A herbaceous shrub up to 1–2 m; stems thorny; leaves alternate, usually pinnate, with stipules at the base of stalks, grey-green, hairy beneath; flower in multiple petals, pink to white, fragrant; hips long and thin.

**Habitat/distribution** The damask rose prefers a sandy or well drained soil, well exposed to sun but protected from cold and wind. The cultivation of the rose is so ancient that it is difficult to identify native habitats unless for wild roses.

**History** *See* also *R. centifolia*. Damask is a cross between *R. gallica* and *R. phoenica,* a rose from the Middle East. Tablets found at the palace of Nestor in Pylos, Greece, show that rose essence preserved in olive oil was a significant commodity of trade in the 13th century BC. The ancient Greek poet Sappho called the rose the Queen of Flowers. It is also central to Unani medicine and Sufism. It is thought Avicenna developed the distillation of rose essence. For Sufis the rose (gulkand) is 'the Mother of Scents' and 'Queen of the Garden'. Sufism holds it to have been created from the soul burning with such light that it perspired and Allah formed the rose from the drops of perspiration. The rose and its symbolism were also important in alchemy.

**Cultivation** The damask is now mainly cultivated in Bulgaria, France and Turkey. Recently cultivation and distillation has begun in England of *R. x damascena* 'Kaznalik', and others. The flowers are picked before sunrise.

**Part used** Rose buds, petals.

**Extraction/adulterations** Steam distillation, with rose water a by-product; a concrete and absolute are produced by solvent extraction. It takes about 4,000 kg of flowers to yield 1 kg of otto. It can be adulterated with geraniol, its alcohol component that has a rose-like scent, and historically with spermacetti to give it correct consistency at cool temperatures. The essential oil is called an otto, rose otto or attar (not to be confused with aytar, the Indian distillation of an essence in sandalwood e.o.).

**Characteristics** The otto: a pale yellow liquid, tinged with green; a rich, deep, floral, sweet rose odour. The absolute: a reddish-orange or olive viscous liquid; a rich, sweet, spicy-floral

## USES

- **Skin:** conjunctivits (use rose water); dry, chapped, cracked or sensitive skin, eczema; ageing skin; herpes; gingivitis.
- **Digestive:** liver and bile congestion, nausea.
- **Respiratory-immune:** asthma, couchs, bronchitis, tuberculosis.
- **Circulation:** palpitations, poor circulation, Raynaud's.
- **Reproductive:** pms; irregular periods, painful periods, leucorrhoea, uterine disorders, menopausal symptoms; low libido, impotence.
- **Nervous:** insomnia, anxiety, stress, tension, headaches; low self-esteem.
- **Mental-emotional:** depression, anxiety. Uplifts and strengthens, gives confidence; enhances feminine principle in men and women. Helps harmonise the different aspects of ourselves and inspires our highest nature.

odour. Base note. The distilled otto is preferred for aromatherapy, at least for physical applications. The genuine essence will congeal in cool temperatures.

**Energy** Cooling, drying/ moistening. Cools choler, nourishes blood, revives and soothes melancholy. Tridosic, rejuvenating; regulates and strengthens agni; satvic. Nourishes and regulates blood, tonifies yin, clears stagnant qi, clears heat (stomach, lower warmer).

**Chemical constituents** Features alcohols as citronellol, geraniol, farnesol, nerol, linalool, phenylethyl alcohol 60%; montoterpenes as stearoptene, camphene, myrcene, cymene, pinenes, ocimene 20%; esters as citronellyl acetate, geranyl acetate, neryl acetate 5%; phenols, phenol ethers as methyl eugenol 1.5.%; sesquiterpenes as caryophyllene 1%; aldehydes as neral 0.5%; oxides as rose oxide 0.3%.

**Therapeutic actions** antiseptic, antiviral, anti-tubercular; anti-inflammatory; astringent, cicatrizing, vulnerary; digestive stomachic, appetite regulator, hepatic; alterative, circulatory haemostatic, blood nourishing, cardiac tonic; nervine sedative, anti-depressant; emmenagogue, uterine tonic.

**Blends with** many essential oils. It may be used to harmonise or 'round off' a blend, using only a very small amount.

**Other uses** Rose water was the original ingredient in cold cream. Fragrance in toilet waters, cosmetic, soaps and the finest perfumes. Flavouring in foods. Rose fragrance is a component in about 46% of men's and 98% of women's fragrances.

 **Safety/precautions** Non-toxic, non-irritating, non-sensitising.

# Rosemary

**Name** Rosemary

**Latin name** *Rosemarinus officinalis* from the Latin *ros* dew and *marinus* sea: dew of the sea.

**Family** Lamiaceae/Labiateae

**Synonyms** *R. coronarium*, compass-weed, polar plant, incensier (old French).

**Other species** There are many different cultivars.

**Description** An evergreen perennial shrub, up to 180 cm; branches become woody on maturing; leaves simple, opposite, leathery, densely woody beneath; flowers pale blue, small on short axillary racemes, blooming in late spring, early summer. The essential oil is concentrated in the calyces.

**Habitat/distribution** Native to Mediterranean, introduced elsewhere.

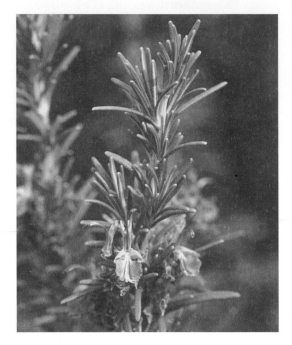

*Rosemary*

**History** Rosemary has been used continuously since ancient times in Egypt, Greece, Rome for sacred, ritual and medicinal purposes. It was recommended by Hippocrates and Dioscorides. In Greece it was considered a gift of Aphrodite to humankind. Statues of gods were garlanded with it and it was used as incense. Because it strengthens the memory it became a sign of fidelity between lovers and used at marriages. The Spanish associate it with the Virgin Mary, saying that its flowers changed from white to blue when she took shelter under it during the Flight to Egypt. It was burned against evil spirits, and used to fumigate hospitals. In Marseille, it was an ingredient of the medieval Four Thieves' Vinegar, the protection used by workers who plundered the corpses of Black Plague victims. 'It helps a weak memory and quickens the senses' (Culpeper, 1995). It is an ingredient of eau de cologne and of Queen of Hungary Water.

**Cultivation** Wild. Propogated by seed, by cuttings, and by layering. Cultivated commercially in California, Russia, Middle East, Britain, France, Spain, former Yugoslavia, China, Morocco.

**Part used** Flowering tops. Sometimes the whole plant but this produces an inferior oil.

**Extraction/adulterations** Steam distillation. A chemotype *R. officinalis* ct. *verbenone* is also distilled.

**Characteristics** A colourless or pale yellow liquid; a strong, fresh, penetrating green/herbal odour. Middle note.

**Energy** Warming, stimulating, drying. Clears phlegm, cools choler, purifies blood, invigorates melancholy; comforting (Culpeper). Reduces kapha, warms, unblocks obstructed vata; strengthens agni. Tonifies yang; moves blood and qi (clears stagnations).

## USES

- **Skin:** infestations, lice, scabies; acne, dermatitis, eczema, regulates sebum; hair care: stimulates growth, reduces oiliness, reputed to inhibit greying.

- **Digestion:** weak digestion; intestinal infections, diarrhoea, constipation, dyspepsia, colitis, flatulence; fatty liver/hyper-cholesterolaemia, jaundice, cirrhosis, gallstones.

- **Respiratory-immune:** asthma, bronchitis, whooping cough, flu.

- **Circulatory:** palpitations, cardiac failure of nervous origin, hypotension; varicose veins, arteriosclerosis; fluid retention, gout, poor or sluggish circulation, cellulite.

- **Endocrine:** glandular disorders, chorosis, weak adrenal glands.

- **Muscular–skeletal:** contusions, cuts, wounds, sores, arthritis, rheumatic pains, gout; massage before athletic or dance performance to strengthen and prepare muscles.

- **Reproductive:** dysmenorrhoea, vaginal douche for leucorrhoea; impotence.

- **Nervous:** fatigue, weakness in children, vertigo, fainting; migraine; temporary paralysis; loss of senses, e.g. poor sight, loss of smell, speech impairment; as adjunctive treatment for multiple sclerosis.

- **Mental–emotional:** uplifts, refreshes; improves concentration and memory. Strengthens; purifies.

**Chemical constituents** Features oxides as 1.8-cineole, caryophyllene oxide 30%; monoterpenes as α-pinene, β-pinene, camphene, myrcene, limonene, ρ-cymene 30%; ketones as camphor, carvone, thujone, octanone 25%; sesquiterpenes as caryophyllene, humulene 3%; alcohols as terpineol, linalool, borneol, terpinen-4-ol 3%; esters as bornyl acetate, fenchyl acetate 1%; others 8%.

**Therapeutic actions** Antiseptic, antifungal, antiviral, bactericidal; cicatrising, astringent; cytophylactic; stomachic, digestive stimulant, carminative, hepatic, cholagogue, choloretic; nervine analgesic, tonic, antispasmodic; diaphoretic, diuretic, cephalic; adrenal, circulatory and general tonic; parasiticide, vermifuge; cardiotonic.

**Blends with** lavender, citronella, thyme, pine, basil, peppermint, cedarwood, petitgrain, eucalyptus, tea tree, niaouli, cajeput.

**Other uses** Fragrance for soaps, cleansers, cosmetics, perfumes; flavouring for food products and beverages.

**Safety/precautions** Avoid use in presence of epilepsy, although in high dilution it may help treat the condition (Davis, 1995, Valnet, 1982). Non-toxic, non-irritating (in dilution), non-sensitising. Contra-indicated in conditions of high blood pressure.

# Sage

**Name** Sage

**Latin name** *Salvia officinalis* from Latin *salvere* to save or be in good health and *officium* of the pharmacy, medicinal.

**Family** Lamiaceae/Labiatae

**Synonyms** Garden sage, narrow-leaved sage (northern Europe), broad-leaved (warmer countries) white sage, true sage. Red or purple sage is a natural variety of this species. The genus is very large, with native species found in many temperate climes. There are many ornamental members.

**Other species** Several different species exist. *S. triloba,* which is antifungal, antibacterial, helpful for menopause but low in ketones, is also distilled.

**Description** A subshrub, up to 30–70 cm. Stems woody at base, branched, white and woolly when young; leaves oblong, usually entire, grey-green, petiolate, fragrant; flowers blue-violet, irregular, lipped, 5 to 10 arranged on terminal spikes, fragrant.

**Habitat/distribution** Native to the northern Mediterranean, especially the eastern Adriatic coasts.

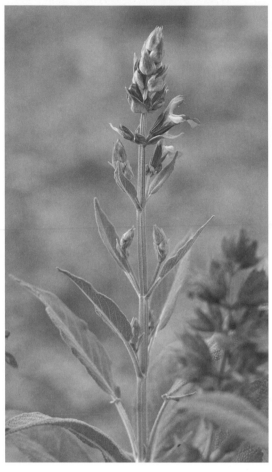

*Sage*

**History** An ancient herb, used by Egyptians, Greeks and Romans and many ancient peoples of the Mediterranean, Near and Middle East for both cooking and healing. Continuous use down to the present, particularly valued for sore throats, oral infections or inflammations. When introduced to the Chinese, they came to prefer it to their own teas.

**Cultivation** Wild, collected on the Croatian and Dalmation coasts; cultivated world wide including the Mediterranean, e.g. France, Italy, Greece, Turkey, and Britain, USA, China. Propagated from cuttings. Enjoys a thin, limestone soil in full sun conditions which produce a more penetrating, spicy-dry odour.

**Part used** Dried leaves.

**Extraction/adulterations** Steam distillation. An 'oleoresin' is further produced from exhausted material.

**Characteristics** Pale yellow; fluid liquid; herbaceous, warm, penetrating, slightly camphorous odour. Top note.

## USES

- **Skin:** wounds (especially slow to heal), ulcers, insect bites, toothache, alopecia.
- **Digestive:** congestion of bile, poor appetite, dyspepsia.
- **Respiratory–immune:** asthma, bronchitis, coughs.
- **Circulatory:** low blood pressure, poor circulation.
- **Endocrine:** adrenal weakness, abnormal sweating.
- **Muscular–skeletal:** arthritis, rheumatic aches and pains.
- **Reproductive:** candida (thrush), leucorrhoea, genital herpes; menopause: hot flushes.
- **Nervous:** trembling, debility.
- **Mental–emotional:** memory weakness, loss of concentration, confusion, fatigue.

**Energy** Warming, drying. Clears phlegm, purifies blood, strengthens vital heat, revives melancholy. Reduces kapha and vata, increases pitta (in excess), strengthens agni, promotes satva. Tonifies qi (lungs, spleen, stomach), removes damp.

**Chemical constituents** Features ketones as α-thujone, β-thujone, camphor, fenchone 35%; monterpenes as α-pinene, β-pinene, phellandrene, camphene, myrcene, limonene, ρ-cymene 20%; sesquiterpenes as caryophyllene, humulene, cadinene 12%; aromatic aldehydes 10%; oxides as 1.8-cineole, caryophyllene oxide 8%; alcohols as borneol, viridiflorol, linalool, terpinen-4-ol 8%; phenol ethers as mythyl chavicol and phenols as thymols 3.5%; esters as bornyl acetate, linalyl acetate 2.5%; aldehydes as hexanal.

**Therapeutic actions** Antimicrobial, antiseptic, antifungal, antiviral, bacterial; anti-inflammatory, alterative (lymphatic and blood cleansing), febrifuge; cicatrising, astringent, antigalactagogue, inhibits sweating; digestive, stomachic tonic, laxative; diaphoretic, diuretic; circulatory stimulant but amphoteric; nervine antispasmodic; emmenagogue, abortifacient, possibly oestrogenic; expectorant, mucolytic.

**Blends with** rosemary, lavender, lemon and citrus oils, eucalyptus and melaleucas.

**Other uses** Encourage patients to use sage leaf infusion in conditions indicated and to use liberally in cooking. An ingredient in proprietary oral products (toothpastes, gargles, mouthwashes). Fragrance in soaps, cosmetics, shampoos, antiperspirants, colognes, perfumes. Flavouring for food products, beverages.

 **Safety/precautions** Avoid in pregnancy (abortifacient) and while lactating; avoid in patients with epilepsy and high blood pressure (neurotoxic in large or prolonged doses). Use in higher dilutions, short term only.

# Sandalwood

**Name** Sandalwood

**Latin name** *Santalum album*

**Family** Santalaceae

**Synonyms** White sandalwood, Mysore sandalwood, santal, saunders oil.

**Other species** A species native to Australia, *S. spicatum* has a similar fragrance but a dry-bitter top note. Islands of the south Pacific have *S. austroclaedonicum* and Hawaii has a native species. Other members of the genus are grown in Japanese islands and in Chile. Do not confuse with 'West Indian sandalwood' (*Amrys balsamifera*, Rutatceae), or with *S. rubrum*, red sandalwood.

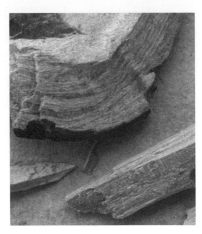

*Sandalwood*

**Description** A modest sized tree of around 9 m; branches slender, drooping; bark smooth, grey-brown; leaves opposite, leathery, showing variation in size and shape (elliptical, ovate, lanceolate), evergreen; flowers in terminal clusters, pale yellow to pink-purple, unscented. The tree is parasitic when young, the roots needing to attach to roots of other plants. This habit disappears as tree matures.

**Habitat/distribution** Native to south India in dry forests of the Deccan plateau, particularly in Mysore state; also grown near Coimbiatore in Tamil Nadu where it prefers hard, rock, ferruginous soil – the conditions that produce a richer scent in the tree. Indian sandalwood is in very short supply due to several factors. Sandalwood trees are difficult to raise, being susceptible to spike disease, which destroys young saplings. They take 30–40 years to reach maturity, the optimal time for harvesting. The wood is so valued that the trees are preyed on by poachers, and much sandalwood is sold illegally. All cultivation, harvesting and sale of products is regulated by the Indian state governments, but this has not been able to stop the diminishing of availability. More planting has been undertaken but it will be many years before the maturity is reached. In recent years cultivation of the species native to New Caledonia (Fiji), a group of islands in the South Pacific, has begun and this sandalwood essential oil is now available for aromatherapists.

**History** Sandalwood is one of the most important plants in Indian culture. It has been used for spiritual, ritual and medicinal puposes, and in perfumes and incense for millennia. Interiors of temples are carved extensively in sandalwood; furniture and decorative objects also. In Ayurvedic medicine it is considered the best substance for cooling pitta fire (specifically in genito-urinary conditions), and used both as an essence and in remedies made from the powder. It is the most *satvic* herb, one that promotes emotional, mental and particularly spiritual peace, clarity and harmony. It is important to the Jain religion, Hinduism, Buddhism, Islam and helpful for preparing the mind for meditation. Buddhist monks brought its use to China and it became valued there, so much so that in the 19th century Chinese tea merchants only accepted sandalwood, gold or spices for their tea. It also traditionally has erotic associations. In perfumery it is made into an *aytar* (attar) and acts as a fixative for distillation of fragile scents such as rose: distilled sandalwood is placed in the receiver of the distillation unit and the charge, e.g. rose, is very gently distilled and its essence received into the sandalwood essence.

## USES

- **Skin:** inflammations, dermatitis, eczema, psoriasis, acne, chapped, damaged, or cracked skin, dry and oily skin; aftershave.
- **Digestive:** nervous digestion, diarrhoea, nausea.
- **Respiratory:** asthma, bronchitis, whooping cough, sore throat.
- **Urinary:** cystitis, urinary tract infections, burning on passing urine.
- **Nervous system:** spasms, over-excitability, insomnia, anxiety, stress, tension.
- **Mental–emotional:** depression, irritability, anger, paranoia, obsessions, jealousy, low self-esteem, confusion.

**Cultivation** Wild. In plantations in southern India, Indonesian islands of Timor and Sunda and New Caledonia. The trees are not cut down but uprooted. The larger parts are used for furniture, panelling, carving, the sawdust and smaller parts used for distillation.

**Parts used** Heartwood and roots of mature trees; powdered, dried. The roots a contain higher percentage of essential oil by weight. .

**Extraction/adulterations** Water or steam distillation. Traditional distillation is done in a *deg* still at very low temperatures over a long period, from 10 days to several weeks. Traditionally the powder is first soaked in water for 48 hours to enhance extraction of the essential oil.

**Characteristics** A pale yellow, greenish or brownish viscous liquid; deep, very subtle, woody-sweet odour. Base note.

**Energy** Cooling, drying and moistening. Calms and cools choler, purifies blood, calms and revives melancholy. Reduces pitta (specifically in the urinary system), calms vata; rejuvenative; satvic. Yin tonic; clears damp-heat, phlegm-fire.

**Chemical constituents** Features alcohols as sanatalols, tricycloekasantalol, borneol 80%; sesquiterpenes as santalene, curcumene, farnesene 10%; traces of monterpene limonene; phenols, ketones as santalone; and other components as yet undetected 7.5%.

**Therapeutic actions** Nervine sedative, antispasmodic, antidepressant, aphrodisiac; antiseptic, antibacterial; astringent, cicatrising; diuretic, expectorant; carminative; anti-inflammatory, febrifuge; tonic.

**Blends with** rose, jasmine, lavender, geranium, patchouli, vetiver, myrrh, bergamot, petitgrain, neroli.

**Other uses** Fragrance and fixative in perfumes, toiletries, cosmetics, soaps; incense; flavouring for food products, beverages.

**Safety/precautions** Non-toxic, non-irritating, non-sensitising.

# Spanish sage

**Name** Spanish sage

**Latin name** *Salvia lavandulaefolia* from the Latin *salvere* to save or be in good health and *lavendulae-folia* lavender-like leaves.

**Family** Lamiaceae/Labatiae

**Synonyms** Lavender-leaved sage

**Other species** Several different varieties exist. *S. triloba,* which is antifungal, antibacterial, helpful for menopause but low in ketones, is also distilled. *S. fruticosa*.

**Description** Evergreen subshrub, up to 30–70 cm. Stems, square, woody at base, branched; leaves oblong, narrow, usually entire, grey-green, petiolate, fragrant; flowers blue-violet, smaller than garden sage, irregular, lipped, terminal spikes, fragrant. The fragrance is like that of spike lavender.

**Habitat/distribution** Native to mountains of Spain; distributed to mountains of south-west France, the former Yugoslavia.

**History** Used in traditional and folk medicine in Spain as a 'cure all', e.g. digestive problems, infections, fevers (plague), menstrual, nervous and rheumatic problems, infertility.

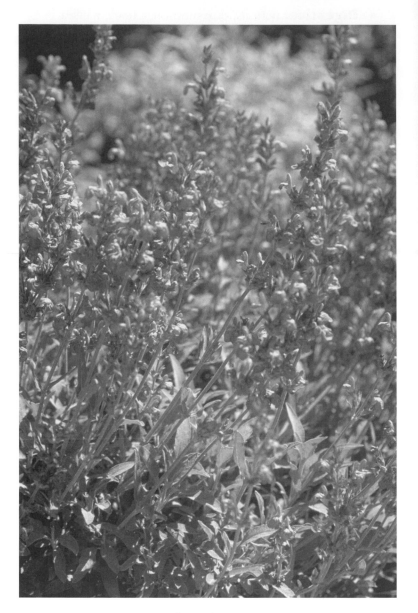

*Spanish sage*

## USES

- **Skin:** acne, eczema, dermatitis, allergies; cuts, wounds; alopecia, dandruff; oral – gingivitis.
- **Digestive:** liver, bile congestion, jaundice.
- **Respiratory:** asthma, coughs, laryngitis, colds, fever, flu.
- **Immune-circulatory:** excess sweating.
- **Reproductive:** amenorrhoea, dysmenorrhoeal, PMS; infertility.
- **Nervous:** headache, migraine, stress, tension; debility, fatigue.
- **Mental–emotional:** depression, fatigue; uplifts and invigorates.

**Cultivation** Wild.

**Part used** Leaves.

**Extraction/adulterations** Steam distillation.

**Characteristics** Pale yellow fluid liquid; herbaceous, camphorous, pine-like odour.

**Energy** Warming, drying. Clears phlegm, cools choler, purifies blood, revives melancholy. Reduces kapha and pitta, calms vata; rejuvenative. Clears heat, phlegm; regulates qi in the middle and lower warmer.

**Chemical constituents** Features alcohols as linalool, α-terpineol, borneol, sabinol, geraniol 35%; monoterpenes as α-pinene, β-pinene, sabinene, myrcene, camphene, limonene, ρ-cymene 25%; oxides as 1.8-cineole 18%; ketones as camphor 15–34%; sesquiterpenes as caryophyllene, humulene, bergaptene 2%; esters as linalyl acetate, bornyl acetate, sabinyl acetate, terpinyl acetate 2%; traces of acids and other components.

**Therapeutic actions** Antimicrobial, antiseptic, anti-inflammatory; astringent, vulnerary; carminative; alterative; emmenagogue; nervine analgesic, antispasmodic, antidepressant.

**Blends with** rosemary, lavender, citronella, eucalyptus, juniper, clary sage, pine, cedarwood.

**Other uses** Fragrance in soaps, toiletries, perfumes, cosmetics; flavouring in food products, especially meat and in beverages.

 **Safety/precautions** Relatively non-toxic, non-irritating, non-sensitising. Use in moderation. Avoid in pregnancy.

# Spearmint

**Name** Spearmint

**Latin name** *Mentha spicata* from the Latin *spicata* spear.

**Family** Lamiaceae/Labiatae

**Synonyms** Formerly *M. viridis*, garden mint, Our Lady's mint, Sage of Bethlehem, pea mint.

**Other species** Closely related to peppermint, cornmint, lemon balm.

**Description** Erect, hairless perennial; stems square, branched, 30–60 cm. Leaves smooth, opposite, lance-like and curled, deeply serrated, fragrant; flowers pale lilac on terminal spikes at ends of leaf stalks.

**Habitat/distribution** Native to southern Europe, Mediterranean, and probably Eurasia; naturalised in Europe, Americas, Australia, the Middle East. Varieties are also native to the Himalayas, Persia. Cultivated widely, including the US and Japan.

**History** Introduced to northern and western Europe by the Romans. Spearmint has been used in folk medicine and cooking for centuries. It is mentioned in Pliny, and by Dioscorides as having a healing, binding and drying quality and used to stay bleeding. It was known to stop milk curdling and this was transferred to the stopping of milk curdling in the stomach, i.e. the improvement of digestion. Culpeper recommended it for 'cold liver', vomiting, poor digestion, dog and insect bites, childbirth and many ailments.

**Cultivation** Wild and in gardens since ancient times. Propagation by division of the stolens (roots). Replace after four years. Seed cultivars do not breed true.

**Part used** Leaves and flowering tops.

**Extraction/adulterations** Steam distillation. The distilled water or hydrolat is excellent for hiccough, colic, nausea, indigestion and flatulence.

**Characteristics** A pale yellow or olive light liquid; warm, green-minty, penetrating odour. Top note.

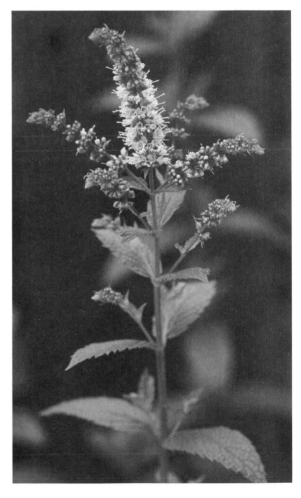

*Spearmint*

## USES

- **Skin:** inflammations, acne, dermatitis, congestion. Oral hygiene.
- **Digestive:** dyspepsia, colic, flatulence, dysbiosis, bile congestion, nausea, vomiting, irritable bowel syndrome.
- **Respiratory-immune:** colds, flu, coughs, bronchitis, asthma, sinus congestion, sinusitis.
- **Nervous:** headache, pain, spasm, stress, fatigue, exhaustion.
- **Mental–emotional:** uplifting and stimulating, refreshing and invigorating.

**Energy** Warming, drying. Clears phlegm, cools choler, purifies and cools blood; balances melancholy. Reduces kapha; calms vata and clears obstruction; balances pitta; strengthens agni. Tonifies spleen yang; clears heat; moves and regulates qi.

**Chemical constituents** Features ketones as carvone, dihydrocarvone, menthone 55%; alcohols as linalool, menthol 22%; monoterpenes as limonene, α-pinene, β-pinene, phellandrene, camphene 12%; esters as *cis*-carvyl acetate, *trans*-carbyl acetate, dihydrocarbyl acetate 3.5%; sesquiterpenes as caryophyllene, elemene, farnesene, bourbonene 3.5%; oxides as 1.8-cineole 2.2%; acids and others.

**Therapeutic actions** Similar to peppermint, but milder. Antiseptic; digestive tonic and stomachic, carminative, cholagogue, hepatic; mucolytic, expectorant; nervine antispasmodic, local anaesthetic; febrifuge; astringent; stimulant; cephalic.

**Blends with** citrus oils, lavender, thyme, basil, marjoram, eucalyptus, tea tree, cajeput, niaouli, rosemary, jasmine, ylang ylang.

**Other uses** Fragrance for toiletries, soaps; flavouring for toothpaste, chewing gum, foods, beverages, confections.

**Safety/precautions** Avoid in pregnancy and with children under 3. Non-toxic, non-irritating, non-sensitising.

# Tea tree

**Name** Tea tree

**Latin name** *Melaleuca alternifolia* from the Greek *melan* black and *leuco* white, for its varied bark. Latin *alter* alternating and *folia* leaves.

**Family** Myrtaceae

**Synonyms** Ti tree, narrow-leaved paperbark tree, melasol.

**Other species** There are many members of the *melaleuca* genus and tea tree is related closely to cajeput and niaouli.

**Description** A tree similar in form to its relative cajeput, but smaller and with more narrow leaves: a spongy, shiny, peeling bark; pendulous branches bearing oblong tapering, strongly-veined and narrow leaves (cypress-like); flowers borne on terminal spikes, yellow or purplish, without stalks, small with numerous stamens; fruit a brown capsule.

**Habitat/distribution** Native to Australia, particularly New South Wales.

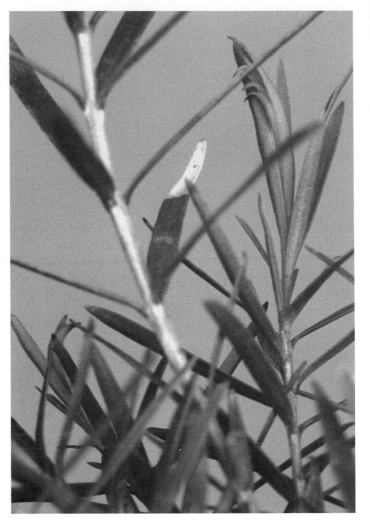

*Tea tree*

**History** Used by the Aboriginal peoples for millennia for treating cuts, wounds, skin infections. They would crush the leaves and make a poultice for the affected part, covering it with warm mud. Botanists with Captain Cook 'discovered' tea tree for the rest of the world in the 18th century, but it lost prominence until the 1920s when research discoveries made it known again as a medicine in a bottle. The essential oil was found to very effectively dissolve pus and make the surfaces of wounds and cuts clean. This was in the days before antibiotics when wounds could often lead to septicaemia. As an ingredient in soap it was tested on typoid bacilli and found 60 times as rapid in killing the bacteria as any other disinfectant. In the 1930s it was used by dentists for pyorrhoea, gingivitis, nerve-capping and haemorrhages and by doctors for sore throats, skin infections and gynaecological conditions. It was given to soldiers in the Second World War as part of their first aid kits. In 1985 a basic level of oil quality was established by the Australian Standard government agency. In the 1990s cultivation of the trees and production of the oil was increased markedly. Tea tree has been one of the most scientifically studied of the essential oils.

## USES

- **Skin:** acne, dermatitis, eczema, burns – including radiography burns; gingivitis, mouth ulcers, cold sores, herpes; boils, wounds, insect bites, insect infestations (lice), haemorrhoids; athlete's foot, verrucas, warts, ringworm; sweaty feet.

- **Digestive:** flatulence, congested bile, candida.

- **Respiratory-immune:** cold, flu, asthma, bronchitis, catarrhal congestions, sinusitis, whooping cough, tuberculosis; viral diseases such as chickenpox, mumps, herpes.

- **Circulatory:** varicose veins, heart weakness.

- **Genito-urinary:** leucorrhoea, thrush, pruritis, candida, vaginitis; cystitis.

- **Nervous:** shock, trauma, hysteria, stress.

- **Mental–emotional:** invigorating, stimulating, depression, lethargy, general fatigue.

**Cultivation** Wild and cultivated in plantations in Australia.

**Part used** Leaves and twigs.

**Extraction/adulterations** Steam and water distillation. May be adulterated with other *melaleuca* species.

**Characteristics** A pale, yellow-green or a watery-white liquid; stimulating, penetrating, warm camphorous odour. Top note. Tea tree is an assertive essential oil.

**Energy** Warming, stimulating, drying. Clears phlegm, cools choler, purifies blood, strengthens melancholy but may aggravate it in excess. Tridosic: reduces kapha and pitta, unblocks vata. Tonifies yang and wei qi, clears external wind, cold, and damp (especially in lung).

**Chemical constituents** Features alcohols as terpinen-4-ol, α-terpineol, globulol, viridiflorol 45%; monoterpenes as α-pinene, α-terpinene, γ-terpinene, ρ-cymene, limonene, terpinolene, myrcene 41%; oxides as 1.8-cineole, 1.4-cineole 7%; sesquiterpenes as aromadendrene, viridiflorene, cadinene, caryophyllene 6%; traces of acids.

**Therapeutic actions** Antimicrobial, antifungal, antibacterial, antiviral, antiseptic, parasiticidal, vermifuge; astringent, cicatrising, vulnerary; anti-inflammatory, febrifuge, mucolytic, diaphoretic; stimulates leucocytosis; digestive stomachic, carminative, hepatic, cholagogue; nervine analgesic, antispasmodic; circulatory stimulant and tonic.

**Blends with** rosemary, cajeput, clary sage, cypress, marjoram, lavender, niaouli.

**Other uses** An ingredient in toiletries, soaps, shampoos, deodorants, oral products, and in aftershaves or colognes for men.

**Safety/precautions** Non-toxic, non-irritating, possibly sensitising in some people.

# Thyme

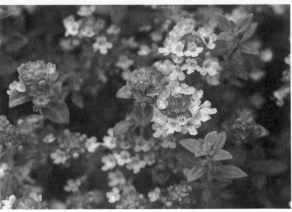

*Thyme*

**Name** Thyme

**Latin name** *Thymus vulgaris* from the Greek *thymbra* or *thumon* through Latin *thymum*, its ancient names plus *vulgaris* common.

**Family** Lamiaceae/Labiatae

**Synonyms** Garden thyme, common thyme, red thyme, white thyme.

**Other species** *T. serpyllym*, 'Mother-of-thyme', a creeping thyme of the Mediterranean and gardens; *T. zigis*, a thyme of Spain. Lemon thyme is a lemon scented variety of *T. vulgaris* and there is also a *T.* x *citriodorus*, a hybrid. There are at least nine chemotypes of *T. vulgaris*, which seems to enjoy diversifying itself and producing different chemotypes at different altitudes. These include: thymol and carvacrol (rich in phenols), linalool, geraniol and thusanol-4-ol (rich in alcohols), α-terpenyl acetate (rich in esters). Taxonomic identification of thyme species is not straightforward. There may be 400 species or 100 species with 400 names (Price and Price, 1999).

**Description** Perennial aromatic subshrub; stems square, woody 10–30 cm, branched; leaves small opposite, grey-green, with or without stalks, linear-elliptical, entire; flowers small in dense terminals, lilac to white.

**Habitat/distribution** Native to western Mediterranean and southern Italy; introduced elsewhere. Prefers dry or well drained, rocky soils in full sun, to 2,500 m altitude.

**History** An ancient herb of Mediterranean peoples, though possibly not the exact same species as was known to Greek and Roman authors (Hippocrates, Dioscorides, Pliny). This was more likely *T. capitatus*. Thyme was introduced to northern Europe perhaps by the Romans, but perhaps by others only in the 9th or 10th centuries. It was in general cultivation in the north by the 16th century. In 1785 a German apothecary, Neumann, first isolated the essential oil and introduced it as a powerful antiseptic substance thymol. This was used as a disinfectant in hospitals at least until the First World War.

**Cultivation** Wild, collected from the wild in native areas. Cultivated throughout the Mediterranean basin and more northern European countries, especially Hungary, Germany, and in the USA, Russia, China.

**Part used** Flowering parts, fresh or partially dried.

**Extraction/adulterations** Steam or water distillation. 'Red thyme' is the crude distillate while 'white thyme' is produced by re-distillation and rectification. It is not a complete oil and is often subjected to adulteration. An absolute is also produced for use in perfumery.

**Characteristics** A red, brown or orange liquid; a warm, penetrating, green or herbaceous, fresh odour. Top note. White thyme is a paler colour, and has a milder scent.

- **Skin:** acne, boils, wounds, dermatitis, eczema, insect bites and infestations, oily skin; oral infections; alopecia.
- **Digestive:** dyspepsia, weak digestion, poor appetite, flatulence, intestinal dysbiosis, spasms, diarrhoea.
- **Respiratory-immune:** coughs, whooping cough, asthma, bronchitis, colds, flu, congestion of catarrh, sinusitis, sore throat, laryngitis; fevers, viral infections.
- **Circulatory:** poor or weak circulation, oedema, cellulite; low blood pressure.
- **Muscular–skeletal:** muscle strain, sprain, fatigue, spasm; arthritis, rheumatic pains, gout; obesity.
- **Urinary:** cystitis, urinary tract infections.
- **Reproductive:** delayed or painful periods.
- **Nervous:** weakness, fatigue, stress, especially mental, headache, insomnia.
- **Mental–emotional:** depression, low mood, weak concentration, mental fatigue, day-dreaming. Uplifts and invigorates, revives.

**Energy** Warming, stimulating, drying. Clears phlegm and congested choler, purifies blood; revives melancholy. Reduces kapha and pitta, calms vata; strengthens agni. Tonifies yang and wei qi, disperses cold, damp; moves blood.

**Chemical constituents** Features phenols as thymol, carvacrol 40%; monoterpenes as ρ-cymene, γ-terpinene, α-pinene, camphene, myrcene, limonene, terpinolene 25%; alcohols as borneol, linalool, terpinen-4-ol 17%; ketones as camphor, thujone 9%; oxides as 1.8-cineole 4%; esters as linalyl acetate, terpinyl acetate 2%; sesquiterpenes as β-caryophyllene 1.5%; traces of acids.

**Therapeutic actions** Antimicrobial, bactericidal, antifungal, antiviral, antiseptic, disinfectant, parasiticide, anthelmintic; astringent, balsamic, rubifacient, cicatrising; digestive, stomachic, aperitif and carminative; nervine antispasmodic and tonic, antitussive; mucolytic, expectorant; stimulates production of leucocytes; immuno-stimulant, emmenagogue.

**Blends with** bergamot, citrus oils, rosemary, lavender, marjoram, pine, cypress, clary sage.

**Other uses** Encourage patients to drink thyme tea whenever thyme is indicated. A concentrated thyme tea decocted with raw molasses sugar is a specific for whooping cough. Thyme is an ingredient in oral hygiene products, cough lozenges. Thymol is still used in surgical dressings and industrial disinfectants. Thyme is used as a fragrance in toiletries, soaps, aftershaves, a flavouring in food products and beverages.

**Safety/precautions** Avoid in pregnancy and in patients with hypertension. May cause sensitisation in some persons. Use in high dilution and moderation/short term. Alcohol-rich chemotypes are generally less toxic and sensitising, safer for children, sensitive and elderly patients.

# Valerian

**Name** Valerian

**Latin name** *Valeriana officinalis* – the origin of the name is uncertain. Suggestions include its being named for Valerius, a notable person, or from *valere* to be in health. The name is not that of the ancients; Hippocrates and Dioscorides refer to it as *phu*. 'Valerian' was first used in the 9th–10th centuries. *Officinalis* from the Latin for 'of the pharmacy'.

**Family** Valerianaceae

**Synonyms** All-heal, great wild valerian, garden heliotrope, amantilla, setwall.

**Other species** Up to 150 known species, some native to Japan, India and Pakistan. It is related to the Indian *V. wallachii* and to the Himalyan *Nardosatchys jatamansi* (probably the spikenard of the Bible). There are several nards known and used in the East.

**Description** A perennial herb 20–150 cm; root stock aromatic; stems slightly grooved; leaves pinnate, incised, leaflets toothed or entire, lanceolate; flowers a terminal inflorescence, white to pinkish. Not to be confused with another British wildflower, also commonly called valerian, which is not aromatic.

**Habitat/distribution** Native to Europe (including the British Isles) and west Asia; naturalised in North America. Valerian grows wild in marshy thickets, on damp grassland and along hedgerows, where its height makes it prominent at flowering time.

**History** A herb of ancient usage. Several valerians are mentioned by Dioscorides: a celtic nard of the Alps, three types of 'nardos' (Syrian and Indian); 'phu' or nard of the woods; the latter seems closest to our valerian. Galen praised it. Arab physicians use/used it in Unani medicine. It was used in the Middle Ages and Renaissance. It was promoted for epilepsy in 1592 by Fabius Calumna, who cured himself of

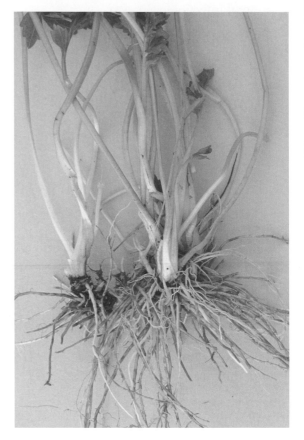

*Valerian*

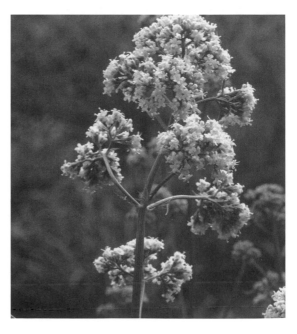

*Valerian*

## USES

- **Digestive:** intestinal colic.
- **Circulatory:** raised blood pressure, oedema.
- **Muscular–skeletal–nervous:** cramp, spasm.
- **Nervous system:** insomnia, nervous indigestion, migraine, restlessness (restless legs), tension.
- **Mental–emotional:** anxiety, nervousness. Stabilising, grounding.

the disease with it. Culpeper esteems it highly as 'of special value against the plague being drunk and the root smelled' (Culpeper, 1995). Tincture of valerian was used in the First World War for shellshock. In medieval times its scent was very popular and roots were placed among linens. To us today it is less attractive. The aroma becomes stronger on drying of the root. Cats are strongly attracted to it and will seek it out to eat if they are injured. Culpeper also says it heals inner and outer wounds.

**Cultivation** Wild. Cultivated by botanical growers in Belgium, France, The Netherlands, Hungary, Germany, Scandinavia, former Yugoslavia, Russia and China.

**Part used** Root.

**Extraction/adulterations** Steam distillation.

**Characteristics** Dark green to dark brown, it darkens with age; liquid; warm, balsamic musky-wood odour. Base note.

**Energy** Warming, drying. Calms and comforts melancholy. Reduces kapha, calms vata. Clears cold, wind (liver). Take caution in using it for hot individuals, use for short time only. It may be stupefying for some individuals.

**Chemical constituents** Features esters as bornyl acetate, isovalerate, eugenyl isovalerate; monoterpenes as pinenes; sesquiterpenes as caryophyllene; ketones as valeranone, ionone; alcohols as patchouli alcohol and borneol; aldehydes as valerianal.

**Therapeutic actions** Nervine sedative, antispasmodic, anodyne; hypotensive; stomachic carminative, diuretic.

**Blends with** patchouli, lavender, pine, citrus oils, rosemary, cedarwood.

**Other uses** An ingredient in nervine pharmaceuticals and herb teas. A fragrance in soaps, perfumes (mossy and woody fragrances). A flavouring in tobaccos, root beer, liquors, apple flavourings.

 **Safety/precautions** Non-toxic, non-irritant, possibly sensitising. Use with moderation and short term only.

# Vetiver

**Name** Vetiver

**Latin name** *Vetiveria zinzanioides*

**Family** Gramineae

**Synonyms** *Andropogon muricatus*, Khus-khus grass.

**Other species** It is related to the Sudanese *Vetiveria nigritana*.

**Description** An aromatic perennial grass; leaves narrow, parallel veined; root a network of white rootlets, aromatic; flowers in terminal racemes.

**Habitat/distribution** Native to south India (Coromandel coast, Mysore), Sri Lanka, Indonesia. Introduced to other tropical areas.

**History** Used in folk, Ayurvedic, Siddha and Unani medicine of Indian subcontinent for millennia.

The rootlets are woven into mats and blinds and hung from lintels and porches to give relief from the heat. Water is sprayed on them to cool and scent the air. Used as a cooling drink for fevers, inflammations and irritability of the stomach. A paste is made of the root and applied as a poultice to burns and hot skin conditions. The grass is smoked with benzoin to relieve headache. The distilled essence is given to check vomiting in cholera and is used in perfumery. It is sown to prevent erosion of soils.

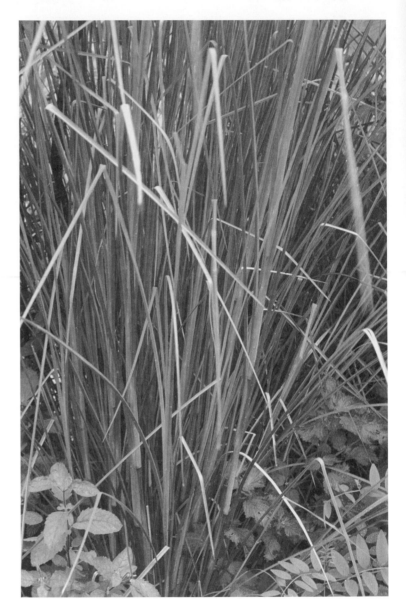

*Vetiver*

## USES

- **Skin:** acne, cuts, wounds, inflammations, dermatitis, eczema, ageing skin, insect bites.
- **Digestive:** loss of appetite, anorexia.
- **Immune:** fevers, inflammations, heat stroke.
- **Reproductive:** menopause, post-partum depression, hormone balancing and tonic, aphrodisiac.
- **Nervous:** insomnia, anxiety, stress, tension.
- **Mental–emotional:** depression, disconnection, confusion, irritation, hot emotions such as anger, jealousy, hatred. Calms and grounds.

**Cultivation** Wild. Cultivated in Indian subcontinent, Sri Lanka, East and West Indies, Java, Réunion. Some distillation is undertaken in Europe and the US.

**Part used** Roots and rootlets, chopped, dried and soaked.

**Extraction/adulterations** Steam distillation. A resinoid is produced by solvent extraction for perfumery.

**Characteristics** A dark brown, olive or amber viscous liquid; cooling, deep, earthy-sweet odour. Base note.

**Energy** Cooling, moisturising. Cools choler and blood, calms melancholy. Calms vata, increases kapha, cools pitta; rejuvenating. Tonifies yin, clears heat, nourishes blood.

**Chemical constituents** Features alcohols as vetiverol, ketones as vetivone, monoterpenes as vetivenes and other compounds.

**Therapeutic actions** Antiseptic, bactericidal, anti-inflammatory, febrifuge, alterative; nervine sedative, antispasmodic; aperitif; circulatory stimulant, rubifacient and promotes production of red blood cells; hormone balancing.

**Blends with** rose, neroli, jasmine, lavender, ylang ylang, patchouli, clary sage, geranium.

**Other uses** Fragrance and fixative in perfumes, toiletries, soaps; preservative in food products.

**Safety/precautions** Non-toxic, non-irritating, non-sensitising.

# Yarrow

**Name** Yarrow

**Latin name** *Achillea millefolium* from the Greek hero of the Trojan war, Achilles, whose only weak point was his heel; and from the Latin *mille* thousand and *folium* leaves.

**Family** Asteraceae/Compositae

**Synonyms** Thousand heal, milfoil, soldier's woundwort, herbe militaris, staunchweed, devil's plaything.

**Other species** Many varieties of yarrow exist, some are garden ornamentals; *A. ligustica*, Ligurian yarrow. *A. moschata*, musk yarrow is also distilled, producing an oil rich in cineole.

**Description** An aromatic perennial herb; roots creeping, spreading; stem erect, furrowed 8–60 cm; flowers minute, in round, flat clusters on terminal cymes, white, sometimes pinkish, each like a tiny, flattened daisy, blooming summer into autumn; leaves alternate, bi-pinnate and finely cut giving them a feathery appearance. They form many leaflets hence the appellation 'millefolium'. The whole aerial parts arc slightly hairy. The flowers and leaves are pungent with a bitter taste.

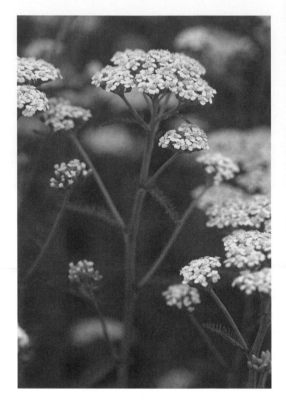

*Yarrow*

**Habitat/distribution** Native to Europe, widespread in temperate zone, naturalised in the US.

**History** A herb of ancient use among the early Greeks, and European peoples from the Mediterranean to the Orkneys. Achilles is said to have learned its uses from the healer Chiron and commended its virtues to posterity (Culpeper, 1995). It has always been valued as a styptic and healer of wounds and also with folk traditions of warding off evil sprits and with divination. In China the stems have been used for divination using the *I Ching*. Dioscorides mentions it to stop bleeding, fluxes of the womb and dysentery. Culpeper adds that it can be used for wounds, ulcers, fistulas, gonorrhoea, loss of hair; it has a binding quality. Currant in herbal medicine for coronary thrombosis, hypertension, fevers and wounds. The fresh leaf is used for toothache.

**Cultivation** Wild, self-sowing. Cultivated. Yarrow is adaptable to many soils; prefers sunny position. Propagate by division of roots in spring or autumn.

**Part used** Dried herb/aerial parts in flower.

**Extraction/adulterations** Steam distillation.

**Characteristics** A dark blue or olive green liquid; herbaceous, sweet, slightly camphorous odour. Middle note.

## USES

- **Skin:** wounds, bleeding, burns, ulcers; acne, eczema, rashes, scarring; hair loss.
- **Digestive:** diarrhoea, dysentery, sialagogue, cramp, poor digestion, bile congestion, flatulence, indigestion.
- **Immune:** fevers, flu, colds; inflammatory conditions (rheumatoid arthritis).
- **Circulatory:** hypertension; varicose veins, haemorrhoids.
- **Muscular–skeletal:** osteo-arthritis, rheumatoid arthritis.
- **Urinary:** cystitis.
- **Reproductive:** dysmenorrhoea, amenorrhoea, leucorrhoea, fibroids.
- **Nervous:** insomnia, stress, tension, neuralgia.
- **Mental–emotional:** promotes clarity and perception, helpful for making decisions.

**Energy** Cooling, drying. Clears phlegm, cools choler, purifies blood; calms melancholy. Reduces kapha and pitta, calms vata (mildly) – but may aggravate it if used to excess; strengthens agni. Tonifies kidney, spleen qi, moves qi and blood; clears damp, heat, wind (especially liver) and stagnation.

**Chemical constituents** Features sesquiterpenes as chamazulene, caryophyllene, germacrene, dihydroazulene 45%; monterpenes as limonene, α-pinene, β-pinene, sabinene, camphene, myrcene 28%; ketones as isoartemesia, camphor, thujone 9%; oxides as 1.8-cineole, caryophyllene oxide 7%; alcohols as borneol, terpinen-4-ol, cadinol 7%; esters as bornyl acetate 2%; lactones and coumarines as achilline; phenols as eugenol.

**Therapeutic actions** Styptic, vulnerary, astringent, cicatrising; antiseptic (urinary); diaphoretic; diuretic, anti-inflammatory, febrifuge; stomachic, digestive carminative, choloretic; circulatory tonic, hypotensive, peripheral vasodilator; nervine antispasmodic; antirheumatic; regulates menstrual cycle.

**Blends with** cedarwood, pine, chamomile, valerian, vetiver, juniper, clary sage, rosemary, citrus oils.

**Other uses** Fresh, young leaves may be eaten in salads. Use an infusion of the dried herb as a rinse for hair loss and skin problems. Drink it for colds, flu and fevers. Use tea infusions or essential oil drops in water for footbaths, sitz baths, compresses, douches for conditions listed. Yarrow can be used as a substitute for hops in brewing and as a snuff or substitute for tobacco, helping to break addictions. It is used to some extent in pharmaceutical preparations for the skin and in perfumes and aftershaves. Yarrow is an ingredient in vermouths and bitter aperitifs.

 **Safety/precautions** Avoid in pregnancy and with young children; non-toxic, non-irritating, possibly sensitising in some individuals.

**Name** Ylang ylang

**Latin name** *Cananga odorata* var. *genuina*

**Family** Annonaceae (Custard apple family)

**Synonyms** *Unona odorantissimum*, flower of flowers.

**Other species** Ylang ylang is related closely to *C. odorata* syn. *C. odorata* var. *macophylla* (large-leaved). Taxonomic distinction between the two is not firmly established (Davis).

**Description** A tree, up to 20 m; flowers pink, mauve or yellow depending on the variety, yellow is considered to produce the finest oil.

**Habitat/distribution** Native to tropical Asia, Indonesia and the East Indies islands, Philippines. Cultivated in the Philippines, Madagascar.

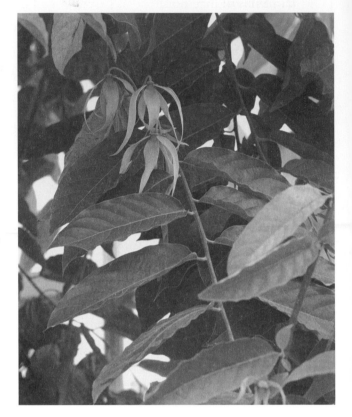

*Ylang ylang*

**History** It has been traditionally used by indigenous peoples and the general population: e.g. as an aphrodisiac (the flowers are spread on the nuptial bed), and for asthma, rheumatic aches, malaria, headaches, stomach problems, opthalmia. It is used as an ointment in the Mulucca islands for skin care, skin diseases and insect bites, and to prevent infections, fight fevers and for hair care. The Victorians introduced its use as a hair tonic called macassar oil; they used white linen on the backs of chairs, called antimacassars, to prevent oil damage.

**Cultivation** Wild. Cultivated for production of essential oil is greatest in Madagascar, Réunion, Comoro islands.

**Part used** Flowers. The best oil comes from flowers picked in the early mornings and in early summer.

**Extraction/adulterations** Steam distillation in stages: first 'ylang ylang extra' (40%), then grades 1, 2, 3 ( the 'tail', often sold as 'Cananga oil', for scenting soap). A 'complete' oil is also produced of the whole oil, but sometimes this is a reconstructed blend of grades 1 and 2. An absolute and concrete are also produced. Adulterated with cananga oil, the tail of the distillation.

**Characteristics** Ylang ylang extra: a pale, yellow, fluid liquid; intense, sweet and heavy floral, balsamic with a 'creamy' top note (Lawless). Base note. Sometimes called 'poor man's jasmine' because it is intensely sweet and floral, like jasmine but less expensive.

## USES

- **Skin:** infections, bites; both dry and oily skin, allergies, irritation; stimulates hair growth.

- **Digestive:** may be of use in psychological disorders affecting eating habits, nervous digestion.

- **Circulatory:** hypertension (slows heartbeat), tachycardia, palpitations with associated over-rapid breathing (hyperpnoea) and with high blood pressure, shock, fright, anxiety, or anger-frustration.

- **Endocrine:** female and male tonic, stimulating ovaries and testicles (Cady); adrenalin secretion.

- **Reproductive:** impotence, frigidity, infertility, menopause.

- **Nervous:** insomnia, restless sleep or legs; anxiety-fear-panic, depression, shock, trauma; stress, severe tension.

- **Mental–emotional:** shock, trauma, depression, especially in women; cools hot emotions; helps enhance self-esteem.

**Energy** Cooling, moistening. Cools choler and blood; revives and clams melancholy. Calms and balances vata, cools pitta, increases kapha. Tonifies both yin and yang; strengthens kidney yang deficiency; clears heat, damp, and heart-fire; regulates qi.

**Chemical constituents** Ylang ylang extra features: sesquiterpenes as β-caryophyllene, cadinene, farnesene, germacrene, humulene 40%; alcohols as farnesol, geraniol, linalool benzyl alcohol 20%; esters as methyl benzoate, benzyl acetate, benzyl benzoate, geranyl acetate 15%; phenols and phenol ethers as methyl eugenol, eugenol, safrole, ρ-cresyl methyl ether 10%; monoterpenes as pinenes 0.4%; aldehydes 0.1%; ketones 0.1%; acids trace; remainder 14.4%.

**Therapeutic actions** Antiseptic, anti-infectious; hormone tonic, regulates secretion of adrenalin; euphoric antidepressant; nervine sedative, circulatory stimulant, hypotensive; febrifuge; balances sebum production. Ylang ylang is possibly antimalarial (Price and Price).

**Blends with** geranium, jasmine, lavender, citrus oils, benzoin, rose, vetiver; blend with bergamot or sandalwood when indicated for men who may otherwise dislike its sweetness.

**Other uses** Fragrance for toiletries, soaps, cosmetics, perfumes (extra used for finest perfumes); flavouring for beverages, fruit flavours and desserts.

**Safety/precautions** Non-toxic, non-irritant, non-sensitising in most people though a few cases of sensitisation have been reported. Scent may cause headaches or nausea in some people.

# 12 AROMATHERAPY IN THE COMMUNITY

After reading this chapter you will:
- appreciate the potential aromatherapy has within healthcare and education services
- recognise special considerations necessary when giving aromatherapy in these settings
- understand some basic procedures for initiating a contact with the relevant authority
- be familiar with relevant protocols for working within these areas.

There has been a growing acceptance of the therapeutic benefits of aromatherapy within the medical and health care professions, and to a lesser extent within the education service. This is in large part due to the effort of aromatherapists to reach out to the community and share their healing touch. Another reason is that many nurses have become interested in massage and aromatherapy and introduced it into their work.

In 1988 the International Federation of Aromatherapists created a special group within its membership to introduce aromatherapy into medical establishments. This was carried out also by Shirley Price Aromatherapy members. Aromatherapists on their own initative have also volunteered themselves. Therapists of the Aromatherapy – in – Care project introduced themselves first to hospices, then to hospitals and other settings and volunteered their skills to patients, beginning with cancer sufferers, and extending to other groups who might benefit. Aromatherapists have also lectured in hospitals and presented papers at nursing conferences to expand awareness. Trials have been conducted in healthcare settings. Among medical professions, the Royal College of Nursing has taken a lead by setting up a special interest group to investigate complementary therapies. It is now called the Complementary Therapy Forum. Some GP's now make aromatherapy available to patients in the surgery; others are willing to refer to an aromatherapist.

As a result, most hospitals and hospices are at least familiar with aromatherapy and there is tremendous scope for individual therapists to extend their practice into this area. Some examples of areas where aromatherapists have been working include: care of the elderly; patients suffering from stress, anxiety, depression or psychiatric disorders; stroke patients; people with learning difficulties; the disabled; cardiac rehabilitation patients; patients in intensive care; pre- and post-operative patients; burns patients; mothers and babies and those who are deaf and deafblind.

Unless you are already a qualified nurse or other health care professional, you will be unlikely at this stage to receive payment for your treatments; it would still be only on a voluntary basis at least initially. Until the benefits are proven by scientific trials, many health managers would not be willing to employ an aromatherapist. Still, once a practitioner has been giving treatments for a length of time, the benefits will begin to be felt not only by individuals, but by the staff and the accountants as well! For example, patients often recover more quickly, have a greater sense of well being, in spite of their medical conditions, and these translate into less stress for staff and often less medication so that the presence of aromatherapy can actually reduce costs.

## Benefits observed by aromatherapists

Price and Price in *Aromatherapy for Health Professionals* (1999) have compiled the experience of aromatherapists working in health care and report that patients have benefited in the following ways: improved sleep; easing of tension in muscle spasms (e.g. cerebral palsy); improved co-operation; improved interest in activities; more acceptance of touch by carers; reduction in anxiety in coronary patients; lowering of blood pressure; improved regularity of bowel movements with abdominal massage and essential oils and reduction in the need for tamazepam (a sedative and tranquiliser).

Fauve Armstrong, a nurse-aromatherapist, and Vera Heidingsfeld, an educator, have worked with deaf and deafblind residents at a centre in Bath. They report that one patient, who had for years refused physical contact (violently), thrown tantrums and self-mutilated, gradually became more accepting of tactile contact and progressively more sociable and cooperative with staff. They also report that residents benefited from the chance to practice making personal choices and communicating these to others. (Armstrong and Heidingsfeld, 2000.)

## Working in a health care setting

These are some steps you can take to arrange to give aromatherapy in a health care setting – hospice, hospital, care home or GP surgery.

1   Decide which area you wish to work in. For example, do you want to work with psychiatric patients, with terminal cancer patients, with the elderly, or with those recovering for an operation?
2   Research the condition and the relevant oils you may wish to use for it; and any contra-indications or special precautions.
3   Find out the name and position of the appropriate person to contact. This may be the nurse or physician in charge of the ward or section of the service.
4   Write a proposal introducing aromatherapy and specifying what you are willing to offer. Include:
    ♦   an introduction of yourself and your qualifications and why you are offering the service
    ♦   a brief explanation of aromatherapy and how it could benefit patients
    ♦   notes of any contraindications or precautions possible
    ♦   an explanation of the likelihood of side effects and how they would be avoided

♦ the type of sessions you could offer: e.g. length, number of times a week, number of patients, type of application (if, massage, then which part of the body) etc.

♦ include a copy of any research you can find to support the validity of treatments

♦ what materials, equipment, type of space you will need. If essential oils are to be stored on the premises, provision should be made for them to be locked up as with medicines.

4   Write to the person in charge outlining your proposal and asking for an appointment to discuss it. Be prepared to discuss with this person:

♦ your training, experience and why you wish to offer the service

♦ the safety of the treatments

♦ what you would expect in terms of benefits, the issues of contraindications and of side effects and how these would be avoided

♦ the need to obtain consent of the patient

♦ the need to obtain the consent of staff

♦ issues of privacy and how these could be managed

♦ the possibility of giving an introductory talk to members of the staff and a group of interest patients to make them aware of the benefits.

♦ the protocols under which you would be working.

## Protocols

Protocols are the rules and standards of behaviour and activity under which the therapist will work. They are agreed in advance by all those involved or responsible for the patient's care.

They could include the following:

♦ The practitioner will be qualified to a professional standard.

♦ The practitioner will practice the therapy in consultation with the relevant medical staff. Written permission for the treatments is to be given by the physician in charge.

♦ The practitioner should have full knowledge of the patient's medical history.

♦ The patient/client/responsible relative or carer must give informed consent to the treatment by the practitioner.

♦ The practitioner will draw up a treatment plan, outline the objectives of the treatment and the parameters of the treatment: how often, for how long, method of application, area of application and essential oils chosen.

♦ The practitioner will document within the patient or client's care plan the relevance of the treatment and observations made during and after treatment.

♦ The practitioner will evaluate and record the effectiveness of the treatment given.

♦ The practitioner will consult and liase with the relevant medical staff during care for the benefit of the patient.

Discuss and agree protocols under which you will work in the care area before beginning to give treatments. Arrange for these to be in written form.

**Progress Check**

1    What are some advantages of volunteering to do aromatherapy in the community?
2    What are protocols?
3    Why is it a good idea to give sample treatments to relevant staff and a responsible family member?
4    What is the purpose of giving an introductory talk on aromatherapy to those concerned?

**ACTIVITY**

1    With a small group of students brainstorm a list of settings in which you would like to volunteer.
2    Draw up a list of possible oils you would use for the condition and discuss the merits of each.
3    Discuss and draw up a list of possible problems you may have to overcome to obtain permission to treat.
4    Role-play a situation in which each of you has a chance to make a presentation to a healthcare manager discussing your proposal.
5    Expand the suggested protocol by thinking of other details that could be included.

## Aromatherapy in education

There is scope for aromatherapy to be applied in an educational setting as well. There are several situations in which aromatherapy can be used. For example, essential oils such as rosemary, peppermint, juniper are known to help with concentration and memory. Others, like lavender, ylang ylang, petitgrain can help with anxiety and stress, such as before exams.

Most pupils and students can pass through such times without the need for extra support but some may benefit significantly from the help aromatherapy can give. Even students who are coping well could still benefit form the support of aromatherapy.

Those with learning difficulties, whether these come from a difficult situation in the home, a physical disability, a condition such as autism, attention deficit disorder (ADD) or hyperactivity (or their combination, ADHD), can definitely benefit. It is generally recognised that feelings of inadequacy, frustration, and lack of self-esteem can lead to tension, anxiety, or resentment and these in their turn to either withdrawal or aggressive, unsocial, or challenging behaviours in a classroom. A vicious cycle of negative feelings and behaviour leading to unrewarding outcomes can become established. As part of a holistic programme of care, aromatherapy can help to break this cycle.

In addition to the benefits of caring, therapeutic touch, the fragrance dimension of aromatherapy can act as a catalyst for better communication between the pupil and teacher and as a basis for building rapport rather than antagonism. When chosen with the active participation of the pupil, the essential oils provide a positive feedback mechanism. With repeated, consistent use they help to gradually change the inner mood of the pupil and the climate of the classroom or setting (Dodd,1988; Pitman, 2000).

## GOOD PRACTICE

When aiming to help at the psychological level, a lower amount of essential oils is needed in a blend, 1–1.5%.

## Preparation

Here again, preparation in terms of research by the aromatherapist is essential. Formulate your objectives and a preliminary plan of execution. A prerequisite is consultation with parents and teachers, obtaining informed consent, and the establishing of the protocols. An introductory session of experiential learning with the pupil(s), teacher(s) and ideally parent(s) is also advised.

## Selection of essential oils

As with any patient or client, the selection should be made on an individual basis if at all possible. With the aim of healing the mind and emotions, an important aim is to bring the whole organism as close to a state of equilibrium as possible, as from this state the optimum functioning of all aspects is more likely. This can mean stimulation or relaxation or their combination, depending on the circumstances. The following assumes you have already assessed the pupil and is a suggested procedure only and may need to be adapted to particular cases.

1   Decide on only one or two areas of focus in the therapeutic strategy and select three essential oils that will positively affect each. If possible choose a variety of notes and types of fragrance, e.g. fruity, floral, spicy.
2   In consultation with the teacher, decide on the appropriate methods of application, including home use if possible.
3   Arrange to present this range to the pupil and allow them to choose the ones they like best. Be prepared to revise your selection and re-present some essential oils if necessary.
4   Prepare the application(s) and again present the now blended essential oils to check that the synergistic blend is still desired. Repeat steps 3 and 4 if necessary.

5   Commence the treatments. If possible have the pupil as well as the teacher and parent keep a record of any responses. Record your own observations as well.

6   At regular intervals, evaluate the results and make appropriate adjustments to the programme and record these.

**Comments by students at King Arthur's School aromatherapy project:**

One said it helped in her history lesson: "I get stuck and if I take my oils it helps me do more work."

"In school when using them I felt a little happier. I think they helped a little bit with school work, but don't know how. My concentration has improved." (Pupil couldn't be more specific.)

"Helps me concentrate on work"

"Helped me to work out the spellings a lot."

"[I] seem to be reading better and don't get angry as much . . . I'm calmer and joining in more activities."

"Helps me concentrate on work sometimes and makes me work harder as well."

"Haven't noticed any effect on my school work."

"Feel joyful, more relaxed . . . My brother teases me and I get angry at him and I use the inhalation and it helps me."

**GOOD PRACTICE**

When offering the essential oils, blend each with the carrier and rub it on your own and the pupil's hand. This can provide an opportunity for positive physical contact with pupils or patients who are uncomfortable with caring touch.

**ACTIVITY**

1   Research and compile a list of essential oils that could benefit a child with ADHD. Give reasons for each choice.

2   Prepare a brief talk to a group of pupils preparing for their GCSE exams on the benefits of essential oils for study.

3   Compose a letter to the Coordinator of a care home proposing an aromatherapy-in-care project and outlining the benefits it could bring to residents and staff. Quote at least one piece of published research to support your proposal

*Aromatherapy for Health Professionals*, Shirley and Len Price, Churchill and Livingstone (1999).

"Aromatherapy for deaf and deafblind people living in residential accommodation", Favre Armstrong and Vera Heidinsfeld, *Complemetary Therapies in Nursery and Midwifery,* 6, 2000.

"Aromatherapy and children with learning difficulties", Vicki Pitman, *Aromatherapy Today.*

*Perfumery: the psychology and biology of fragrance*, G. Dodd and S. Van Toller, Chapman and Hall, 1988.

# PROFESSIONAL DIMENSIONS AND RESEARCH

**13**

After working through this chapter you will be able to:

- understand the nature and scope of the legal responsibilities of a practitioner
- understand the need to conform to local requirements for businesses
- appreciate the advantages and privileges of belonging to a professional association
- know the requirements for reporting serious cases of disease or possibly dangerous symptoms
- appreciate the need for continuing professional development
- adopt the high standards of ethics and conduct of a professional aromatherapist
- understand the role of research in professional aromatherapy.

Aromatherapy can be practised in a variety of situations, ranging from the private clinic offering individual consultations and therapy to beauty therapy salons, residential holiday or recreation centres and hospitals, care homes, GP surgeries and hospices. No matter what the context, awareness of legal and ethical responsibilities is very important.

## Health and safety guidelines

An aromatherapy practice needs to conform to certain health and safety guidelines:

- Fire-fighting equipment is on site and kept in good working order. Equipment is readily accessible and suitable for fires that are likely to occur and someone on site is trained in their use.
- Clear evacuation exits are present, room contents do not obstruct exits and members of staff are trained in evacuation procedures.
- First aid equipment is on site and kept up to date. The aromatherapist needs to have trained in first aid and to keep the training up to date.
- The practice is accessible to disabled people.
- If practitioners are employed, the employer and employee must conform to the Health and Safety at Work Act 1974. The Act's main provisions are set out in the table below.
- Gas safety regulations must be followed.
- Electricity at work regulations must be followed.
- Correct hygiene procedures must be followed.

If you work as a beauty therapist privately or in a beauty salon, or work in a health spa, you may need to be familiar with other regulations as well.

As a practitioner, you will also need to be aware of health and safety regulations in regard to:

- the handling and correct storage of dangerous substances
- the recognising, rectifying, recording and reporting of any hazards on the premises
- the correct action to deal with spillages and breakages
- the required procedures for dealing with clinical waste
- the reporting of accidents.

## Insurance

Public liability insurance and professional indemnity insurance is not statutory at the time of writing, but is required of members by responsible professional organisations. It provides important cover for aromatherapists. It covers the aromatherapist for claims made by members of the public as a result of injury or damage to people or personal property resulting directly from the site of treatment or from the treatment itself. Such damage is said to be due to 'professional negligence'. A good insurance plan can also include provision of free legal advice.

**GOOD PRACTICE**

Ensure that your practice is fully covered by public liability and malpractice insurance – and keep the cover up to date.

## Legal responsibilities

### Local authority licence

Some, though not all, local authorities do require a licence for aromatherapy practices. The by-laws of your authority must be learned and observed. Licences are usually for a year, are charged for and allow an inspection by Environmental Services officers who have authority to fine or cancel registration of the business if it does not conform to the standards laid down by the authority. The aim is to protect the public by requiring practitioners to conform to the regulations as set forth in the licence. When setting up a business giving aromatherapy treatments, check with the Environmental Services department of your local authority to see if you need a licence to operate or a special treatment licence.

### Trade Descriptions Act 1968

Aromatherapists are also bound by the provisions of the Trade Descriptions Act 1968. An important provision of the Act is the one against making any false statements as to services offered, or claims about the effectiveness of a treatment, and claims to cure or diagnose specific ailments. This Act, together with Cosmetic Products Regulations 1996 and the General Product Safety Regulation 1994 (No. 2328), is also important for any own label products sold by the aromatherapist, e.g. products that you may create for retail sale such as massage blends, or creams and lotions, and even if they don't include essential oil. Any such product must be properly labelled.

The Trade Descriptions Act also lists Prohibited Functions within the field of medicine that unqualified persons are forbidden to perform. These include the treatment of venereal disease, and dentistry, midwifery and veterinary surgery. It is also an offence under the law to publicise or advertise any article or description so as to lead to the use of the article to treat certain diseases. These include: Bright's disease, glaucoma, diabetes, cancer, cataract, epilepsy or fits, tuberculosis, locomotor ataxia, paralysis.

## Medicines Act 1968

There is a distinction in law between a product, such as a blend of essential oils for massage, individually prescribed for a single client after a consultation, and the sale of a retail product. Individually prescribed products, such as the blend you create for a patient's massage or home blend, currently come under the Medicines Act 1968, section 12, which allows herbal prescriptions to be prepared after an individual consultation with the therapist. This legal situation is currently under review and it is likely, though not certain as we go to press, that aromatherapists who wish to practise in this way will in future be regulated, like herbal practitioners, under a statutory self-regulation arrangement. This means that the title 'aromatherapist' will have a legal definition and only those who conform to certain training standards are eligible to practise.

## Data Protection Act 1984

If a practitioner uses a computer to store personal data about clients, they must register with the Data Protection Registrar or be liable to prosecution. The Act only applies to information relating to living persons stored on computer. Information and forms are available from post offices. Registration is for three years and involves a fee. Clients who feel they are affected by lost or incorrect information or wrongful disclosure without consent may make a claim to the Registrar and are entitled to see the data relating to them.

## Performing rights

If recorded music or a radio is played in a place of business, a fee may be payable. For information contact the Performing Rights Society, 29–33 Berners Street, London W1T 3AB (tel: 0207 5805544) and/or Phonographic Performance Ltd, Ganton House, 14–22 Ganton Street, London W1F 7QU (tel. 0207 4370311). If radio or television broadcasts are used, similarly the premises must hold a licence.

## Children under 16

When treating a child under 16, the practitioner must also be careful. It is an offence under the law for a parent or guardian to fail to provide adequate medical aid for a child, and by treating a child who is not also under medical care, the aromatherapist may be said to be 'aiding and abetting' an offence. Precautions you can take include the following:

- Make it clear to the parent or guardian that you are not qualified to treat a disease or diagnose a medical condition.
- Ensure that the parent or guardian has informed the GP that he or she is seeking complementary treatment.
- Before treating a child who is or appears to be near age 16 but in fact is not, obtain a parent's permission in writing; for example, if the child is seeking to be treated without a parent's consent.

**Progress Check**

1    If you treat a child, it is advisable to compose a brief statement for the parent or guardian to sign. What should this document include? Why is this procedure advisable?

2    What are some of the provisions of the Trade Descriptions Act that relate to the aromatherapist?

3    Describe what is meant by 'professional negligence'.

4    Other than the local council, where else might you be able to find out if a local authority has licence requirements or procedures?

## Professional life

### Professional organisations

It is highly recommended that aromatherapists belong to a good professional organisation. Some addresses are listed in *Resources* at the end of this book. Your teacher should also be able to advise you. Membership has numerous advantages, which should at least include the following:

♦    A register of professionally qualified members whose names can be given to members of the public enquiring for an aromatherapist in their area.

♦    Aromatherapy is promoted, with accurate information being given to the media and the medical profession to educate them to the value of aromatherapy.

♦    A subscription to a periodical journal, which communicates information about various aspects of aromatherapy and provides a forum for discussion of issues and subjects of professional interest or relevance to members.

♦    Provision of insurance at competitive rates.

♦    Sale of books and other items of use to practitioners.

♦    Organising of regional support groups for members.

♦    Support for professional development by organising an ongoing educational programme of seminars and workshops.

♦    Promotion and development of high educational and training standards for practitioners.

♦    Keeping members informed of developments in the field of aromatherapy, and complementary medicine in general, at both national and international levels as monitored by the organisation.

♦    Supporting, monitoring and engaging in research projects into the benefits of aromatherapy.

♦    Working with other organisations in the field of complementary medicine for the benefit of professionals and the public.

◆ Assessment and accreditation of training courses to high professional standards and providing a list of such courses for information to prospective students.*

(*Note: If statutory self-regulation does become law, this aspect of the professional organisation may in future come under the remit of a general council for aromatherapy.)

Through membership of a professional organisation the practitioner can be in contact with aromatherapists from Europe and throughout the world. Attending international conferences of aromatherapy is also a way to link with practitioners from other countries.

## Professional discipline

A good professional organisation also will have in place a clear statement of investigative and disciplinary procedures as part of its **Code of Practice** or **Code of Ethics**. Such a code includes a description of the professional conduct expected of members. Its provisions will cover: confidentiality, the responsibility to work within the limits of training, the avoidance of prescribing or diagnosing medically, the duty to report infectious diseases and to advise clients to seek medical help for symptoms, record keeping, prohibitions about claims seeking to attract business unfairly, and bringing discredit on aromatherapy.

Failure to abide by the code will incur discipline and disciplinary procedures are also set out in the code. These will be followed in the event of a complaint being received by someone against a member practitioner. The aim of such codes is to ensure that high standards of practice and ethics are adhered to by members in order to protect the public. As regards the practitioner, the procedures help protect him or her from false allegations and aim less to punish than to help by providing means by which the member may be enabled to raise his or her standard of treatment. This role may also in future become part of the function of a general aromatherapy council.

**GOOD PRACTICE**

Be discreet in conversations and in any promotional talking that you do, as well as in any literature or advertisements that you produce. Do not make unwarranted claims about aromatherapy and do not denigrate a fellow professional in public.

## Referrals to medical and other professionals

A qualified aromatherapist always works within the limits of his or her own training and expertise. When faced with a patient whose needs are assessed as being outside the range of the practitioner's expertise, in the patient's best interest the aromatherapist has no hesitation in making a **referral** to another practitioner – whether this be a medical physician, a practitioner of another complementary discipline, counsellor or other professional. New patients should be asked if they have consulted a doctor about their symptoms and, if they have not, they should be advised to do so. This advice should be recorded in the case record.

In addition, the aromatherapist is obliged to report certain types of disease conditions to a doctor or medical authority. These include:

- sexually transmitted diseases (STDs)
- any bleeding reported in the stools, urine, sputum or vomit; vomit with dried blood (like coffee grounds); non-menstrual bleeding, vaginal bleeding with pregnancy or after a missed period
- pain in the eye or temples of elderly or rheumatic people, with local tenderness – sign of a possible stroke
- stiff neck and/or high fever, photophobia – possible sign of meningitis
- any sudden difficulty breathing, breathing is cut-off, rapid or laboured – sign of possible heart condition or severe respiratory condition
- drowsiness or loss of consciousness, dizziness, vomiting following an injury.

## Other relevant responsibilities

Practitioners are also advised to be aware of government legislation regarding the following:

- the prevention of discrimination on the basis of gender, race or religious affiliation
- protection from physical and mental abuse.

These are found in such Acts as Children Act 1989, Social Services Act 1970, Protection of Children Act 1999, Youth and Justice and Criminal Evidence Act 1999, Crime and Disorder Act 1998, Sex Offenders Act 1997, Care Standards Act 2000, Children Leaving Care Act 2000, Data Protection Act 1984 and Human Rights Act 1998.

## Continuing professional development

As discussed at the beginning of this textbook, basic training in aromatherapy is only the beginning. A good aromatherapist is under an obligation to continue to develop professional skills in all areas by engaging in further training on a regular basis, at least bi-annually. **Continuing professional development** may be specifically in aromatherapy skills or in areas that have a direct bearing on the understanding of health and disease. Professional development can include participation in research, teaching and publishing articles, and time given voluntarily for the running of a professional association. Professional aromatherapy involves lifelong learning.

Attendance at further training seminars and workshops has added advantages for the aromatherapist. It is an opportunity to share experiences with fellow practitioners and to glean new insight and information from others' experiences. Such events usually stimulate the practitioner to try new approaches and think in new ways to the benefit of the practitioner and patient alike.

Developing aromatherapy skills and expertise also involves continuing self-education, developing further our self-understanding and awareness. We can never know all there is to know, but we can continually extend our range of understanding.

**REMEMBER**

The aromatherapist accepts the responsibility to refer a client to the GP or other suitable practitioner if circumstances indicate this is necessary.

## Complementary and alternative medicine (CAM) and government regulation

Within the last few years in the UK, complementary medicine therapies such as aromatherapy have become recognised as valid forms of treatment by other health care professionals and the government. They are very popular with the public. The Prince of Wales, long a supporter of CAM, was instrumental in setting up the Foundation for Integrative Medicine, now renamed the Foundation for Integrative Health; the new title highlights the fact that complementary medicine can and should be integrated into our National Health Service. In addition, the government has been facilitating the work of the various professional bodies towards consolidation, with a view to agreeing training standards and course curricula, and the form of a council accountable to the public. The House of Lords established a select committee to investigate complementary therapies and its report has been published (web address in *Resources*). Most of its recommendations are already in hand among professional aromatherapists who have been cooperating to establish common standards of training and competency via the Aromatherapy Consortium and Healthwork UK.

## Research and the professional aromatherapist

The House of Lords Select Committee strongly recommended that an understanding of basic scientific research methods and outcomes should be included in training and that more research should be done in CAM so the public can use it with knowledge and security.

Historically, as regards scientific research aromatherapy has greatly relied on research conducted by essential oil chemists, perfumers or psychologists to support the efficacy experienced by clinical practitioners.

There is in fact a lot of research available, but from the perspective of aromatherapy practitioners, the problem has been one of knowing how to access it, as well as how to understand and evaluate its findings. Some experience in the language and style and especially in research **methodology** is needed. (Methodology is the way the research is designed and conducted.) It is also true to say that little research has been done into aromatherapy by clinical aromatherapists themselves or about the clinical, therapeutic use of essential oils. This is partly due to lack of funding. Obtaining funds for research is itself something that requires skill and training and is usually outside the remit of an individual practitioner. It is also to do with the problem that a holistic approach, which focuses on individualised treatments, is difficult to match with a **quantitative** and statistical approach. However, much has been done to overcome these issues and the situation is now changing. Professional bodies are putting into place protocols and guidance, and encouraging and supporting their members to engage in research.

## Research methodology

The fundamental aim of all scientific research is to learn more about the world of nature, what is true about it and what is not. The first step is to formulate a viable **hypothesis**, or question that the research is then designed to test. A hypothesis is a suggested explanation for something that has been observed. For example, lavender oil is observed by practitioners to be calming for patients. A hypothesis might be – patients exposed to lavender essential oil experience calming sensations. Traditionally scientific research has favoured the quantitative approach to collecting the data (the raw facts, something that can be measured). For example, it asks what can we detect and in what quantities? It then conducts a trial to collect data.

How could we test the hypothesis about lavender? How can we measure what looks like a feeling or sensation? A simple research project might be as follows: first choose the subjects to be studied, trying to get them to be as similar as possible. Then measure the subjects' saliva for levels of stress hormones when they are calm and record this. This becomes a base line against which future changes are measured. Then subjects could receive a challenge of some kind (perhaps watching a clip from a horror movie), after which half of them could receive 5 minutes' exposure to essential oil of lavender in a particular controlled environment and half would not. Then their saliva will be measured again and the two records compared to see if any change in levels occurred and how the two groups differed. The data will be evaluated and a conclusion will be drawn as to whether the hypothesis has been proven. In this example, the effort is to reduce everything to measurable units and care is taken to control for unwanted variables.

Quantitative research goes to great lengths to control for variables that might confuse the results. For example, subjects will all be of a certain age, sex and health status, and all will receive the exposure in the same environment at the same time of day, etc. A double blind trial is thought to provide the highest degree of accuracy because it tries to eliminate the possibilities of the scientist interfering with the data collection in some way and also to correct for the placebo effect. In our example, another group of subjects could be exposed to an inert substance – perhaps a mist is sprayed but it is only water.

Science likes to measure things and if something cannot be measured, as far as science is concerned it doesn't exist. What it can investigate is thus dependent on and limited to the technological development of its instruments. However, such a reductionist approach has its drawbacks.

Growing out of social sciences, such as sociology and psychology, and professions such as nursing, a different methodology has been developed called **qualitative** research. It is particularly relevant to health issues because it acknowledges and accounts for the subjective experience of the persons studied. Data is collected on these aspects in a way that allows for subjective experience to be evaluated. For example, subjects may be asked to rate their symptoms on a scale before, during and after the trial. As with quantitative research, steps are taken to minimise bias and collect accurate data. More recently still a third approach, using several hypotheses and several research methods in the same study, has been developed to try to address the complexity of human health dynamics; it is called triangulation.

## Basic stages in research

Research attempts to test or answer a question or hypothesis formed about the nature of the world. Broadly speaking, the process of conducting research trials involves the following steps:

- conceiving and focusing of the hypothesis to be tested; it cannot be vague or too broad
- identifying and developing the appropriate methodology: how the hypothesis will be tested
- writing a grant proposal, applying for and obtaining funding from the appropriate external funding body
- conducting the research, collecting the data, evaluating the results, drawing conclusions
- writing up the results and submitting the research for peer review
- publishing the results so others can benefit.

## Evaluating research

It is important that when learning about the results of research, for example reading a summary of it or a report about it in the media, the aromatherapist has the skills to evaluate the research. Do not take the report of the research at face value. Much scientific research is in fact flawed. Just because it is published does not mean research results stand up to scrutiny. The practitioner must evaluate the research to see if it is valid. Questions should be asked, such as:

- What type of methodology was used? Was it appropriate to the topic?
- Was the design of the trial sound? Were there any variables unaccounted for or not corrected for? Was the procedure correct? Was it appropriate to the condition/situation/subjects?
- Was the sample investigated representative?
- Do the results prove a causal connection or only suggest an association that must be further investigated?

## Medical audit

One type of research that can be within the means of the clinical aromatherapist is called the audit, or medical audit. Basically it involves monitoring one's own practice in order to assess and evaluate some aspect. Topics for monitoring are very varied, for example it can include such hypotheses as: What is the level of patient satisfaction with the care they are receiving? How many patients presenting with PMS/headache/pain is this clinic seeing in the course of a year? Auditing involves setting up an information-gathering procedure, such as: for a set period, having each patient complete a survey form before, during and after a series of treatments. The data collected is then evaluated and conclusions are drawn. This type of research can be useful to both the therapist – as it helps evaluate the effectiveness of his or her treatments – and to the profession, as it can supply a reservoir of clinical experience, which can be used to formulate research trial questions or provide raw data for other types of research.

Conducting research is a difficult but very rewarding task. It can be a means of methodical self-evaluation of our skills and professionalism as well as identifying new areas for aromatherapy development or areas needing improvement. It can identify particular conditions that benefit consistently from aromatherapy. For example, UK hospital trials have shown that essential oil of lavender massage, as distinct from relaxing massage alone, helps reduce high blood pressure.

Research can explore new methods in a coherent, organised way. Research can highlight areas where application of research findings could inform conventional medicine, for example, by showing cost-effectiveness of aromatherapy treatment relative to conventional care. In summary, research can be of benefit to both practitioners and the public.

## ACTIVITY

1 Find out more about the Foundation for Integrative Health and its activities or about the House of Lords Select Committee Report. Make a report to your fellow students.

2 In a group, discuss the ethics of scientific research relative to a holistic therapy.

3 Using the internet or by writing to professional associations, try to find some research into aromatherapy or essential oils for health that has been published and accepted. Review and evaluate it and make a report to your fellow students.

4 Find out more about the difference between quantitative and qualitative research. How could you use each in an aromatherapy trial? Give some examples.

5 Brainstorm an idea for an aromatherapy research trial. Phrase it in the form of a hypothesis and sketch out a methodology that might be employed. Report on this to your fellow students.

 **Progress Check**

1 What are the benefits of conducting research?

2 What are some drawbacks of the quantitative approach in research?

3 How does qualitative research differ from quantitative research?

4 How might research be flawed?

## Key Terms

You need to know what these words mean. Go back through the chapter or check in the glossary to find out.

- Code of Ethics
- Code of Practice
- continuing professional development
- hypothesis
- methodology
- qualitative research
- quantitative research
- referral

| | *Health and Safety at Work Act 1974* |
|---|---|
| Employer | Safeguards as far as possible the health, safety and welfare of themselves, their employees, contractors' employees and members of the public. |
| | Ensures all equipment is kept up to standard. |
| | Ensures the environment is kept free of toxic fumes. |
| | Ensures safety equipment is regularly checked. |
| | Ensures all staff know safety procedures and provides safety information and training. |
| | Ensures safe systems of work. |
| Employee | Takes reasonable care to avoid injury to themselves and others. |
| | Co-operates with others. |
| | Does not interfere with or misuse anything provided to protect their health and safety. |

**Fig. 13.1** *The main provisions of the Health and Safety at Work Act 1974*

## Further information

House of Lords Report on Complementary and Alternative Medicine
www.publications.parliament.uk/pa/ld/ldsctech.htm

NORA Natural Oils Research Association
www.acemake.com/NORA

Aromatherapy Consortium
PO Box 6522, Desborough, Kettering, Northants NN14 2YX.
info@aromatherapy-regulation.org.uk
Tel: 0870 7743477

After working through this chapter you will be able to:

- understand the importance of drafting a business plan and where to get help in its preparation
- understand your responsibilities for maintaining accounts, filing tax returns and paying National Insurance contributions
- know how to contact advisory services or help lines that can be of help to you in managing the business side of your aromatherapy practice
- begin to formulate ways of promoting your practice in the local community
- understand the important elements involved in public speaking, which can be of help in giving talks to promote your practice.

This chapter is adapted from *Good Practice in Salon Management* (1997) by Dawn Mernagh-Ward and Jennifer Cartwright, Nelson Thornes, Cheltenham.

Gaining a qualification in aromatherapy is the necessary first step to a successful practice. But it is only the first step. Working with clients is our goal but to do this we have to put in place a structure and administration that enables us to do so. To achieve this takes a lot of hard work.

As complementary medicine is becoming more accepted by the public, opportunities for giving aromatherapy increase. At the same time, there is increased competition as more practitioners are trained.

## Foundations of a professional practice

### Identify your preferred place and style of practice

Perhaps the first thing you need to do is to decide in what kind of setting you want to practise aromatherapy. For example, would you like to work independently in your own private clinic, with other complementary practitioners in a group practice, within a general medical practice (this is increasingly a possibility), in a hospital, hospice or care home? Or would you prefer the setting of a beauty or health salon, a gym or health club, or a health retreat, spa or holiday centre? Would you like to work on a self-employed or on an employee basis? It is possible in some areas to combine some of these. You may decide that you prefer to give some, or even all, of your treatments voluntarily; some aromatherapists are in a position to donate their skills, for example, to a local hospice.

### Employed and self-employed work

Bear in mind that there are differences between being self-employed and employed. If you are employed, your employer is responsible for

National Insurance contributions, and for working out your tax as part of pay as you earn (PAYE). Safety and health regulations are also the employer's responsibility. However, while your money is not put at risk and you are not directly responsible for profits or losses, you may have little or no say in the running of the business. If you are self-employed, you are responsible for taxes, contributions, health and safety, as well as capital risks, but you can also enjoy creating your own enterprise.

If you are self-employed you also need to decide if you want to work full-time or only part-time. This will determine to what extent you promote yourself.

## ACTIVITY

Start a file or folder to store all your business information in an orderly fashion.

If you decide to work from home, bear in mind that a room used exclusively for business may become liable for a business rate of tax and liable for capital gains tax when the property is sold. On the other hand, you can claim the full cost of expenses associated with the room on your **tax return**.

## ACTIVITY

With fellow students discuss and draw up a list of the advantages and disadvantages of :

(a)  running a clinic from home
(b)  working from a group practice of complementary therapists
(c)  making home visits to clients.

## Drafting a business plan

Before setting yourself up in business it is a good idea to create a **business plan**. Even if you don't need to show it to a bank manager, this encourages you to think realistically about what you need and do not need for your practice. Any bank will be able to advise you on drawing up a business plan. They usually require this as part of the application for a loan.

## ACTIVITY

The Department of Trade and Industry produces booklets that can help small businesses. Call 0870 150 2500 and ask for copies of these relevant to your profession.

The information asked for on a business plan includes such things as: your training, qualifications and experience, a customer profile or idea of your target market, proposed charges or a comparison with competitor's charges, setting up and running costs, projections about profits and income from the business, cash flow statements and forecasts. A **cash flow forecast** is a way of working out how much cash a business is likely to generate in a future period. After you have been in business, it can be calculated on the basis of past receipts and payments made on a regular basis. The cash flow itself is found in the difference between outgoings and receipts over a given period.

### Business help and advice

Many other agencies, besides banks, exist to help new businesses. Among the places offering free help are: the Training and Enterprise Council, Chamber of Commerce, Local Enterprise Agency, business enterprise trusts and small business advisory centres.

Business Link is a network of offices that provide a single point of access for all key local business support agencies, including the Training and Enterprise Council, Local Enterprise Agency, Chamber of Commerce and local authority. The address of local Business Link offices is in the telephone directory.

## ACTIVITY

1 Write to three banks and ask them for some information on preparing a business plan. Compare the information from the banks with the sample provided here and draw up a plan, which seems best suited to your practice.
2 Find out exactly which business start-up support agencies are active in your area. Contact each one and discover what help they can give you. Keep the information in your business file or folder.

 **Progress Check**

1 What is Business Link?
2 How would you formulate a cash flow forecast once you have been in business for one year?
3 What are some differences between self-employment and employee status?

## Planning and starting up

When you are planning the start of your practice, remember that in a business sense, practising aromatherapy involves more than giving the treatment. In order to give the treatment you need to have secured such things as the worksite, transportation to work, the equipment and supplies. There are overheads involved in running a clinic, even if yours is only a proportional contribution. In addition, keeping client records, ordering supplies and paying bills, and promoting your business through talks and advertisements takes a certain amount of administration time, which must be allowed for in your overall concept. From the beginning, set up a regular routine for your business administration. Do your paperwork, whether client records or your **accounts**, on a regular basis.

Some practitioners enjoy running the business aspects of their practice and enjoy creating or making available retail products to offer their patients. Others find such aspects more of a challenge as they might prefer to concentrate on the healing treatments, but it is a challenge that can be met. Attending to the business aspects enables us to give the treatments in the best circumstances and environment.

Once in business, you must notify:

1  your local tax office
2  your local Social Security office
3  Customs and Excise, if your annual turnover is above a certain amount, currently £54000
4  your local Job Centre, if you are registered with one.

## Maintaining accounts, tax and insurance

If you are self-employed you need to keep full and accurate records of all your business transactions. These include:

- all income received
- all business expenses incurred
- drawings for yourself
- any loans put into the business
- capital expenditure items.

This information is filed as an annual return with the Inland Revenue every year. These may be examined at any time, so must be carefully and accurately kept. Bear in mind that accounts may also be required for reasons unconnected with tax, for example, by your bank when considering an application for a business loan.

### Income tax

Each year in April you will receive a tax return to fill in, giving information on the year's earnings, any capital gains and your net profit – the amount left over after expenses and eligible deductions for the year. If your earnings exceed your tax allowances, the money you are allowed to earn each year before paying tax, you will be assessed and required to pay tax. Your allowance is calculated by the Inland Revenue on the basis of the information you supply them about your individual circumstances. The Inland Revenue will issue you with a Notice of Coding, or tax code, which gives the amount of money you can earn tax free and detailing what benefits have been deducted.

It's a good idea to set money aside regularly to cover your yearly tax bill. Information about tax assessments and filing returns can be obtained from your local office of the Inland Revenue, and many local accountants offer free advice on the basics.

**ACTIVITY**

There is a helpline for those with problems relating to self-assessment: 0845 915 4515. Phone and ask if they will send you any information leaflets relating to self-employment. Keep these for reference.

## National Insurance

Most people who work are liable to pay National Insurance contributions, unless they qualify for an exemption. Self-employed people are liable for two classes of contributions, Class 2 (paid towards benefits, except unemployment) and Class 4 (paid on profits and gains). Unless you have either been excused payment because of low earnings or are a married woman or a widow with reduced liability you must pay Class 2. These can be paid either quarterly every 13 weeks, or by direct debit every month.

Employers are responsible for Class 1, earnings-related contributions to the PAYE scheme. An employee can claim for sickness, invalidity, maternity, unemployment and widow's benefit where appropriate, once enough contributions have accumulated.

### ACTIVITY

Check with your tax office or a local accountant for more information about National Insurance. Ask about small earnings exceptions, and making and deferring payments.

## VAT

Value added tax (**VAT**) is a government tax charged on most goods and services. Currently the rate is 17.5 per cent for businesses with a taxable annual turnover of £54,000 or more. As giving aromatherapy is a service, it may be liable for VAT once the turnover from the business reaches the annual amount and the business must be registered for VAT with the local office. A registration number will be issued and true and accurate records must be kept on all business transactions. Every 3 months it will be necessary to fill in a VAT return form and where output tax exceeds input tax the difference will need to be paid to Customs and Excise.

### ACTIVITY

1   Write to the Inland Revenue, Customs and Excise office and Social Security and ask for information leaflets relevant to being in business. Study the information and discuss it with your fellow students.
2   Call or write to a local accountant and ask if you can have a courtesy consultation. They are usually happy to provide free basic information. Find out whether it would be to your advantage or not to have your accounts handled by a professional.

 **Progress Check**

1   What is VAT?
2   Why is it useful to formulate a business plan?
3   What is a notice of coding?
4   What is self-assessment?

# Advertising and promotion

Planning is essential when deciding ways to advertise and promote your practice. Give some thought to what type of clients you wish to attract, then you can make decisions about such things as: the appropriate medium for advertisements, as well as the style, tone and presentation, so that you engage the audience's attention. Consider what are the five or six most vital pieces of information that should appear in any form of advertising for aromatherapy. Promotion needs to be cost-effective as well and there are usually local avenues of free advertising. There are many ways to promote yourself besides advertising. A few of these are included here.

## Suggestions for ways to promote your practice

- Offer to give one treatment free for every five treatments received.
- Offer to give half-price treatments to patients who introduce a friend to your practice.
- Offer treatments as birthday or Christmas presents, with an attractive card the giver can use, which announces the gift treatment and gives details about yourself and how to book.
- Donate introductory treatments for prize draws at school fundraisers and association meetings.
- Write letters introducing yourself to local groups such as the Women's Institute, National Women's Register, Weight Watchers and support groups for such conditions as arthritis and ME (myalgic encephalomyelitis). Offer to give talks and demonstrations.
- Participate in any local complementary medicine 'fairs', though you need to check these out first to see how suitable they are and how productive they might be. If there are no such events, think about organising one yourself or with other local holistic practitioners.
- Create a business card and letter-headed stationery.
- Create a leaflet for distribution to the public. Research the best sites where you might leave your leaflets for free distribution.
- Write to your local GP practice manager introducing yourself, explaining aromatherapy and offering to arrange a meeting to discuss with them how aromatherapy might be useful to their patients. Restrict yourself to one or two conditions, which are common and which usually respond well to aromatherapy, and offer to do a trial period giving treatments for these. Such treatments may save the practice money on their prescription bills.
- Have a special day or half-day a week in which you treat children and/or new mothers free. Have a special day for clients with a specific condition, such as asthma or pre-menstrual syndrome.
- When you open your practice, and whenever you have something substantially new of interest to the public, send a **press release** to the local papers to try and get them to cover the event. The press release should be very brief but contain essential information: your name, address and telephone number, time, date, address of the event and a brief description of its nature in such a way as to engage the interest of the editor. Try to find an interesting, new or unique angle to promote your business.

## Websites

If you have an internet service provider, it may offer you free webspace you could use for advertising your practice. Also, professional associations have websites, which should have some space dedicated to promoting their members to the public, such as a referral register. Check out your local town, village or district council to see if your practice could be included on their websites.

## Giving talks

Giving talks to local groups of interested people is a very good way of promoting your practice and increasing public awareness of aromatherapy and complementary medicine in general. There are many organisations and groups looking for speakers at their regular meetings, for example, the Women's Institute, the National Women's Register, support groups for various conditions such as fibro-myalgia, arthritis, eczema, asthma and civic groups, such as the Soroptimists, Rotary or Lions Club. More doctors, nurses and midwives are becoming aware of the benefits of complementary medicine; they want to know more and might be interested to have you as a speaker to their local associations.

### Plan ahead and organise

As with any other activity, planning ahead is important. Before you even begin to outline your ideas, think about the kind of audience you have, so you can direct the tone and level of the talk to them, to their interests and experience as far as you can. Being able to tie the information in the talk to specific aspects of their lives gives it more value.

Think about any posters or other visual material you could bring that will help you illustrate your ideas. As well as simply talking about aromatherapy, consider what activities you might also include to get the audience involved with essential oils; for example, demonstrating a facial massage, getting members of the audience to practise some massage on each other, having some scent samples of pure essential oils versus synthetic scents to pass around. Plan what equipment you would need for any activity such as towels, cushions, smell strips.

When planning the talk itself, put yourself in the position of members of the audience and think up questions they might have about aromatherapy. Then gear your talk to try to answer these questions. For example, if there are doctors in the audience, they might be very concerned to know about levels of training and professionalism, as well as about the therapeutic aspects. Be prepared to answer their concerns. Be sure to emphasise in the talk the safe handling and storage of essential oils. Remember that members of the audience are potential clients so they will want to know about costs, confidentiality, what is actually involved in a massage (including timing, type of massage), and often simply whether treatment is painful or not. Be prepared to answer such questions, and have your business cards ready.

Brainstorm and note down all the ideas that you want to cover, then think through them again and organise them. Aim to have an introduction and a conclusion to round off the talk, and decide in what order you want to discuss your ideas. If you make notes use headlines to highlight the main points, and make some notes of the information under each. It is perfectly acceptable to use notes when speaking. Before you give your first public talk, practise it on a helpful friend or family member, or at least in front of a mirror. This will take out some of the anxiety about public speaking.

## GOOD PRACTICE

Brainstorming is a technique for generating ideas on a subject. The group or individual first thinks up and lists in no particular order all the ideas that come to mind on that subject, even the most wacky ones, and not worrying about their value at this stage. Only then is each idea considered in turn and rejected or kept. Next they are placed in order of importance or priority for action.

### Gaining confidence

Giving talks to the public is daunting for many people, especially at first. It helps if you can start with small, familiar groups. The more talks you give, the easier it becomes. But there is always likely to be the odd question that comes as a surprise. The best approach is to speak from your own experience, including your life experience in general; give concrete, specific examples whenever possible, and above all don't be worried about admitting when something is outside your experience. It is perfectly acceptable to admit this, though it is helpful if you can think of someone to whom you can refer the questioner in order to obtain an answer.

## REMEMBER

When speaking in public you are representing not only yourself but aromatherapy as a whole. A positive appearance and manner helps promote confidence and reflects well on the profession.

## ACTIVITY

1 Brainstorm a list of questions you think an audience of midwives might ask about aromatherapy. What special areas would you need to concentrate on for this audience? Repeat this for a WI group. Compare your lists with those of two fellow students and make adjustments as needed.

2 With a partner, if possible, work out your answers for the following questions and then compare them:
   How would you answer the question 'How many treatments does a person usually need?'

Think of 10 ways in which aromatherapy (with or without massage) works that you might mention in a talk.

How would you answer the question 'How do I know if a practitioner is suitably qualified?'

How would you answer the question 'How do you know which oils to choose?

3   In groups, practise giving a 10-minute talk to each other.
4   Practise giving a 15-minute talk in front of the mirror at home.

## Key Terms

You need to know what these words mean. Go back through the chapter or check in the glossary to find out.

- ♦ accounts
- ♦ business plan
- ♦ cash flow forecast
- ♦ press release
- ♦ tax return
- ♦ VAT

# APPENDIX 1
# CASE HISTORIES

The following case history summaries are offered to help illustrate the points made about taking case histories and record keeping made in Chapter 3.

## Case 1

Mrs A, aged 49, married, mother of two young adult children (in further education), part-time school assistant

*Enquiry*: Mrs A presented with a history of pain in her neck, shoulders, and from the mid-back around to the chest sometimes, onset within the past year. She had had a course of six osteopathic treatments, the practitioner diagnosed the fundamental cause of her pain as tipped pelvis leading to a trapped nerve, postural imbalances. Treatments had helped but not fully relieved the problem. Mrs A reported also suffering from headaches on the left side, migraine-like and that she becomes ill with nausea and headache before, surprisingly, something nice is about to happen. She is under quite a lot of pressure due to a combination of stress at work and taking on a lot of responsibility for the home and family, including care of her husband's mother. She is trying hard to keep going but feels at her breaking point. She has been to counselling to see if that could help but has not taken the decision to really tackle the problems that came up.

She has no serious medical conditions in her history. Medication consists of HRT and use of coproxamol, especially at night, for relief of back and neck pain. She has taken antibiotics for repeated colds.

Her physique is small, slight and very slender. She feels the cold. Her constitutional type is melancholic–sanguine.

Relevant facts from her history included:

- low energy level: she felt tired and low
- she was not sleeping well
- she had had three colds since Christmas with sore throat, coughing – dry, tight chest and had lost her voice. The glands in her throat swell when she gets a cold
- she gets a slight sneezing allergy in the summer. Her skin is sensitive to perfumes; she gets blotches
- her periods had always been troublesome, heavy and painful. Somewhat less so now on HRT
- she only takes exercise when she walks into town for shopping
- her home life is stressful as she worries a lot about her family, and also does a lot for them, as well as working herself. Her job is also stressful as she is expected to deal with some very difficult pupils at playtimes and lunch
- postural examination confirmed pelvic imbalance with right hip line raised and very tight muscles across the sacral-iliac area

♦ her diet is a reasonably healthy one (e.g. brown bread, little sugar, healthy snacks). The evening meal is a cooked one of meat and vegetables. She does like her crisps though.

*Assessment*: Mrs A's immune system is weakened (repeated colds, stress). Her energy is weakened due to stress factors in her life, poor sleep and considerable pain, which is very wearing. She is coping with little support from her husband, but this is partly due to the fact that she has not communicated with him about her condition and situation, so he hasn't been aware of it. I feel, and discuss with her, that she needs to let him know that she needs more support from him and also that she needs to communicate to her children that they need to take more responsibility for themselves. She has gotten in the habit of doing so much for them and not taking time for nourishing herself.

*Therapeutic strategy*: Relaxing massage with emphasis on shoulder, neck and back areas: muscle releasing, relaxing tension, increasing circulation and healing. I will use much more carrier oil than normal as oil itself helps nourish the body, relax and calm the nervous system and muscle tension.

Weekly treatments for four weeks and then reassess.

*Essential oils*: Jasmine for stress and to induce relaxation and a euphoric feeling, and sense of being cared for; this contributes to enhanced immunity.

Basil, linalool for stress, anxiety, muscular pain, headache; stomachic; respiratory antispasmodic, and antimicrobial, relieves catarrh and sinus congestion; nervine, relaxant. Enhance immunity. Warming and clearing energy. Promotes clarity of perception, calms the mind.

Lavender for stress, anxiety, pain; antimicrobial; enhance immunity. Harmonises the blend.

*Carrier*: Almond oil to nourish the skin.

*Second consultation*: Mrs A reported feeling 'unbelievable' relief. She had had no headache for five days. The pain in her neck–shoulders–back had been relieved for several days, but had returned and felt tender again, front and back on this day. She had not had to use the coproxamol. She was still not sleeping well. She reported that her legs feel jumpy when she goes to bed at night. I feel Mrs A is underweight, even for her frame, and raise the subject with her and suggested a range of healthy foods that she could add to her diet.

*Therapeutic strategy*: Repetition of previous treatment, including use of same essential oils. I again discussed with her the importance of taking time for herself, for some relaxation in her life and of communicating her needs to her husband and children, so she is not carrying everyone's emotional load plus all housekeeping responsibilities. The aim is to enhance her self-esteem, self-confidence. I recommended she massage her legs every evening before going to bed and I gave her a home blend of the same essential oils and carrier to use.

*Third consultation*: Mrs A reported a good response. She has been massaging her legs and feet nightly and has been sleeping better. She is taking time for herself, starting to do cross-stitch, which she enjoys. She has been able to cope with the demands of her job much better. Her anxiety is less. She is more self-aware and able to stop her mind thinking about worries in an unproductive way. She has begun to talk to her husband about the situation; their relationship is basically sound. The family stresses remain. Her husband is also under a lot of stress but has acknowledged that he has been letting her take the brunt of it. Mrs A feels able to cope with them better as she is feeling better in herself.

She reported that her legs and feet feel achy. There is some pain in her right buttock, otherwise none. She reported no headaches. Her period has started.

*Therapeutic strategy*: Keep encouraging Mrs A in her positive changes. Avoid abdominal area during massage. Give more attention to legs and feet, neck, shoulders, lower back and buttocks.

*Essential oils*: Clary sage for improving circulation in the legs; improve reproductive function; euphoric, relaxing.

Rosemary: improving circulation; analgesic for pain, strengthen immunity. Warming, tonic.

Jasmine: as above for enhancing positive feelings of well-being, relaxing.

*Discussion*: Mrs A continued to improve and continued to come monthly for treatment. This has kept her feeling much better and able to cope with her circumstances; she has more energy, sleeps well and wakes feeling well, has many fewer headaches, much less or no pain; fewer colds. She noticed her nails were improved in their condition, not so brittle. She took the initiative to make a few important positive changes in her life and relationships and this also made a big difference to her health and sense of well-being. This is an example of when the holistic approach of aromatherapy probably prevented the person becoming more imbalanced. She might otherwise have become clinically depressive.

## Case 2

Ms B. Age 55, single, full-time employment. Referral from osteopath who treated her for postural imbalances and cranial-sacral balance, but also found her very tense, and thought she would benefit more from aromatherapy.

*Enquiry*: Ms B presented with symptoms of dryness in the throat, like a fur ball, though also feels mucus at back of throat; nose is very dry. Her eyes are prone to irritation, alternating with 'filming' over them. Onset was within the past year. X-rays had been taken which found no sinus blockages. She has tried nasal sprays, inhalations recommended by chemist and antibiotics. Symptoms are worse lying down, first thing in the morning and at night. Also she gets headaches, frontal and all over, and down the neck and upper back. She feels a pressure building up in her head and face; a nagging ache, lasting all day. She is not getting good sleep.

Relevant facts from her history include:

- Her skin is very sensitive, face reddens on touching. Had acne rosaceae, but took a course of antibiotics, which appears to have cleared it. Had an episode of skin rash, for which she consulted a homoeopath and treatment cleared it.
- Does not suffer otherwise in the respiratory area, no colds, bronchitis or other.
- She tends to constipation, passing stool only once in every 2–3 days.
- She had been put on HRT but had uncomfortable side-effects (weight gain, bleeding nose) so has discontinued.
- Poor sleep.
- Her diet is a factor. She eats mucous forming foods like biscuits, meat, cakes. Takes tea and coffee.
- Her workplace is very dry.
- Physical assessment showed varicose veins and some lymph stasis in legs, though no oedema around ankles.

*Assessment*: Ms B has a sensitive skin and I will have to treat accordingly. Dryness but at the same time congestion plus tension is the pattern.

This would be a combination melancholic–phlegmatic constitution. I feel her diet – and the constipation that is its result – is a significant factor. I also think the dryness of her workplace is contributing to the irritation. She can't change this, but she can minimise its effects.

*Therapeutic strategy*: Recommend a cleansing diet for three weeks, avoiding mucous, acid-forming foods (eggs, dairy, meat, bread, cakes, biscuits and flour products, and sugar, processed foods, tea and coffee). Recommend taking breaks at work in the fresh air, avoid smoking areas. Cutting out tea and coffee, which can be drying, substitute herbal teas, dandelion coffee. Give lymphatic drainage massage to the face and neck areas. Massage helps to improve lymph and blood circulation, which benefits whole body. Take care over lower leg area. Weekly treatments for four weeks then reassess.

*Essential oils*: Lavender: relax, relieve stress; gentle, circulatory stimulant to clear blockages; analgesic for headache.

*Eucalyptus citriodora*: benefits respiratory and throat conditions, and is non-irritating and calming.

*Carrier*: Almond oil with 5% avocado oil for sensitive skin, dryness.

*Second consultation*: Ms B reported an aching in her jaw, which lasted about 36 hours. She had experienced the same after the osteopathic treatment. Otherwise she felt all right, but no significant improvement.

*Therapeutic stragegy*: Massage, as before. Recommended she drink fennel tea as an aid to digestion (counter the accumulation of mucus and toxins), cleansing and weight loss.

*Essential oils*: For the face: damask rose and sandalwood; soothing, cooling, balancing, calming.

For the body: lavender and *E. citriodora* as before.

*Third consultation*: Ms B again experienced some aching in the bones of her face immediately after the treatment but this went off soon after.

She had no film over her eyes this week and no irritation. There was not the usual pressure in her nose and the throat felt a little looser, though the sense of dryness is still there. She had no pain in her neck or head during the week. She has been implementing the diet and is slimmer, feels less bloating and is feeling much better in herself. Her sleep has improved. She has more energy.

*Discussion*: Ms B continued to improve. She began to come for treatment every six weeks. The headaches occur only occasionally, and also the eye irritation and sense of pressure return occasionally, but less and less. The dryness of something in her throat receded, though it did continue. The build-up of congestion in her system has been greatly lessened by the combination of aromatherapy, massage and the diet she adopted. I believe that there is something in the atmosphere at her workplace that is irritating her mucous membranes and that since she cannot do much about this she will continue to suffer some irritation and sense of dryness in her throat. She has a new sense of well-being and is continuing on a more healthy diet. This was a very good result, though not a complete resolution of her symptoms.

# Case 3

Mrs C: aged 35, married with 2 teenage children; employed in charity fundraising.

*Enquiry*: Mrs C has had skin problems since puberty when she began to have acne and excess seborrhoea. The areas affected have been the face: forehead and chin, sometimes the cheeks; the neck and the back between the shoulder blades. Still the skin has an excess of seborrhoea all the time. In the winter the tops of the arms and legs tend to become dry and rough patches appear. Acne occurs mainly in the spring and in the following areas: across the centre of the upper back, on the neck, along the hairline and on the face; and occasionally over the neck shoulders (décolletage). The acne appears as large blind spots, which are very moist and develop pustules and burst. If the head is knocked off the skin scars, deep pits occur, which are permanent, and the area looks pitted and uneven.

Relevant factors from her history included:

- Mrs C leads a busy life, runs her household, is active socially and works full-time running a charity. She is responsible for the funding.
- Her diet is well balanced. She has no known food allergies. Fluids include plenty of water, herbal teas and red wine, a small amount taken at weekends.
- Her weight fluctuates easily. Around the time of her periods she begins to experience bloating and retains fluid. At the time of treatment she was normal weight for her age and height.
- She exercises regularly at weekends, enjoying activities with her husband.

◆ She is otherwise in good health, physically, mentally and emotionally.

*Skin examination*: Mrs C has fair, creamy white skin with no flushing or pinkness. Skin is cool to touch, soft and fine grained. There are moles on the back and tops of the arms; no freckles. The skin has a light sheen, small open pores around the base of the nose, forehead and chin.

*Assessment*: The condition is of long standing and therefore the expectation is that it will take several months before steady improvement can be seen.

The symptoms of congestion around the time of the period indicate a hormonal factor and also that the circulation is generally sluggish, which can have repercussions for the health of the skin.

There is a combination of dryness and excess moisture in the symptoms, but excess moisture is the more prominent aspect.

It is reasonable to consider that some stress, at least at times, is a factor given her busy life and commitments.

*Therapeutic strategy*: Improve circulation to the entire body and particularly to the skin; clear congestion in the skin. Ensure skin is cleansed regularly. Promote healing of skin tissues and good nourishment of the skin.

A programme of monthly treatments with applications to cleanse the skin with essential oils and hydrolats to keep skin clear of congestion and to balance pH and protect the acid mantle. Sunflower oil to be part of the cleansing agent because it is neutral, mimics sebum in its composition and so will help normalise sebum production. It also dissolves grease and make-up. Also, aloe vera gel to be included as it is anti-inflammatory, antiseptic, promotes healing and reduces puffiness and the risk of allergic reactions. Applications to include massage, exfoliation, skin brushing, warm steam towel treatments and moisturising cream.

Skin brushing helps to remove dead skin cell, lift dirt and grime and stimulate circulation. Exfoliation stimulates circulation to the skin. Warm steam towels applied to areas opens and flushes pores. Massage stretches and improves connective tissue beneath the skin, smoothes the skin and relaxes strained tissues.

Patient to continue care between treatments by self-applying a prepared low-oil moisturiser with essential oils; 50 ml of moisturiser was applied over a month and the essential oil blend was adjusted each month.

*Essential oils chosen were rotated among*: Skin healing, antibacterial: frankincense, cistus flowers, lavender, chamomile. Hormone balancing: rose, geranium.

*Treatment at consultation*:

1 Cleanse face and back with low oil cleanser. Apply hydrolat mist and blot dry.

    Aloe vera gel base 1/3 part
    Low-oil white lotion base 1/3 part
    Rosemary or sage hydrolat 1/3 part
    0.5% essential oils of citrus and geranium

2   Skin brush the back from hips to neck and the arms from hands to axilla with a large bristled body brush, using upward movements in line with lymph flow. Turn patient over gently, skin brush the face with a small facial brush using circular movements across the forehead, cheeks and down the neck to the cervical glands.

3   Exfoliate the face with a foam-cleansing base exfoliant applied by hand, using light circular movements. Rinse with warm water and spray hydrolat.

> Exfoliant ingredients: cream base $\frac{1}{2}$ part, bubble base $\frac{1}{4}$ part, hydrolat $\frac{1}{4}$ part. Mix, gradually incorporating foam-cleansing base. Finally add hydrolat until a lotion consistency is obtained.

4   Patient turns over and exfoliation is continued on the back using foam and gentle circular movements. On areas without acne a string mitt and a stronger movement are used. Pustule areas are avoided. Rinse with warm water and using a flannel mitt.

5   Apply warm steam towel to the back. Prepare with hot water to which essential oils are added. Rinse towel in water, squeeze out and apply to the back. Cover with plastic and more towels to retain heat. Leave on 1 minute, remove. Spray area with hydrolat mist and pat dry.

6   Apply moisturising cream with gentle massage movements.

> Light moisturising lotion:
>
> 30 ml cream base
>
> 15–20 ml rosemary hydrolat – enough to create a lotion consistency
>
> 5 ml *Centella asiatica* infused vegetable oil
>
> 5 ml rosehip infused vegetable oil
>
> 2% essential oils, alternating among frankincense and cistus flowers, lavender and chamomile, rose and geranium.

Treatments commenced in spring and continued monthly for 12 months. Patient also used a UV sun bed at times.

At the year's end the results were reviewed with the patient. The patient felt little had changed. The programme was changed. Treatment was to begin in the winter and was given only every two months through the spring. At the end of 8 months, the acne had reduced. There were fewer blind spots and little new scarring.

*Discussion*: This case reflects the importance of considering the holistic context of a condition. The condition was of long-standing, therefore a quick result was not expected. It took several months of treatment, over a year, before significant improvement became evident. Also the patient reported that the symptoms were season-dependent. This proved to be a very important factor. It is interesting to note that the cooler temperatures of winter can reinforce an already sluggish circulation. The ancient Greeks noted that when the weather begins to warm in the spring, often an imbalance in a humour, especially the blood/sanguine and phlegm/lymph humour, would begin to show in symptoms, or aggravation of symptoms. This seems to be what was happening in the case of this patient. Once the programme had been changed to take account of the seasons, the condition began to improve steadily.

# APPENDIX 2: CAUTIONS FOR THE USE OF ESSENTIAL OILS

The following information reflects concerns for the use of certain essential oils in certain conditions and circumstances: toxicity, skin irritation and/or skin sensitisation. They should be used with caution and within the limits of the practitioner's training and experience and willingness to take responsibility for the treatment.

## Reasons for caution

1 abortifacient, 2 carcinogenic, 3 diuretic, 4 emmenagogue, 5 parturient, 6 skin irritant, 7 potentially toxic due to high phenol or ketone content, 8 oestrogen stimulant, may affect hormone levels, 9 astringent, stops flow of secretions, 10 strongly stimulating, may affect blood pressure, nerve or brain activity (neurotoxic), 11 phototoxic, 12 mucous membrane irritant, 13 hepatotoxic

## Avoid throughout pregnancy

Certain essential oils are strongly emmenagogue or induce uterine contractions:

| | | |
|---|---|---|
| aniseed 3, 5, 8 | clove 5 | sage 3, 4, 9 |
| basil 4, 7 | hyssop 3, 4 | tarragon 1, 3, 4, 7 |
| bay 3, 4, 5 | lemongrass 3, 6 | thyme 3, 4 |
| camphor 3, 4, 6 | nutmeg 4, 5 | pennyroyal 1, 2, 5 |
| cinnamon 1, 4, 7 | parsley 3, 4, 5 | |

## Avoid in first trimester

Certain essential oils are mildly emmenagogue, or oestrogenic, meaning they may affect hormone levels and are thus best avoided in pregnancy:

| | | |
|---|---|---|
| angelica 3, 4 | coriander 8 | melissa 6 |
| cajeput 3, 6 | cumin 4 | myrrh 3, 4 |
| caraway 3, 4, 6 | fennel 3, 4, 6, 8 | peppermint 4 |
| carrot seed 3, 4 | jasmine 5 | rosemary 10 |
| cedarwood 3, 4 | juniper 3, 4, 5 | spearmint 4 |
| clary sage 4, 8 | marjoram 4 | |

**REMEMBER**

These essential oils are safe during pregnancy: mandarin, grapefruit, neroli, petitgrain, rosewood, sandalwood, tea tree, ylang ylang, benzoin, ginger.

## Avoid while breast feeding    9

| | |
|---|---|
| peppermint | sage |

## Avoid when skin will be exposed to sunlight, X-rays, radiotherapy, using a sunbed   12

Certain drugs also increase photo-toxicity of skin, so exercise caution if patient is taking the following: cardiac medication, chemotherapy, tranquillisers, garbonamptomene, Largactil, Xanthonene.

In general expressed citrus oils (not distilled) contain small quanitites of the furocoumarin bergaptene, which can render the skin more sensitive to effects of ultraviolet light, thereby increasing the chance of burning:

| | | |
|---|---|---|
| angelica | lemon | tangerine |
| bergamot | lime | verbena |
| cumin | mandarin | |
| grapefruit | orange | |

A bergamot oil that has been rendered bergaptene free is available.

## Avoid in patients with high blood pressure   10

| | | |
|---|---|---|
| eucalyptus | rosemary | thyme |
| hyssop | sage | |

## Avoid in patients with kidney disease   3

For example, nephritis:

| | | |
|---|---|---|
| juniper | parsley | black pepper |

## Avoid in patients with history of epilepsy   10

A few essential oils, which contain certain ketones, are potentially neurotoxic, i.e. because they are lipid soluble, they can pass through the blood–brain barrier and affect the central nervous system. The ketones include fenchone, pinocamphone, camphor, thujone. Not all essential oils with ketones are hazardous to these patients.

| | | |
|---|---|---|
| anise | eucalyptus | nutmeg |
| camphor | fennel | rosemary |
| cinnamon | hyssop | sage |

## Avoid in patients with sensitive skin   6

These oils are generally safe, but to be sure, conduct a patch test before using:

| | | |
|---|---|---|
| basil | caraway | clove bud |
| benzoin | cinnamon leaf | citronella |

| cumin | lemongrass | thyme |
| fennel | melissa | tea tree |
| geranium | parsley seed | verbena |
| ginger | peppermint | ylang ylang |
| jasmine | pine (*Pinus sylvestris*) | |
| lemon★ | spearmint | |

(★ Citrus oils can be an irritant if used in excess.)

## Avoid in patients with sensitive mucous membranes 13

| clove bud | spearmint | thyme |
| peppermint | | |

## Avoid in patients with history of liver damage 14

This caution applies to the oral intake of essential oils rich in phenols. Minute amounts applied to the skin, as in aromatherapy, are considered safe.

| aniseed | fennel | camphor |
| basil | cinnamon bark and leaf | |

## Patients with history of cancer

Some scientific studies have looked at the effects of essential oils, among other chemicals, on the formation or growth of cancerous cells. When instances have been found, it was only after daily application of high concentrations over many months. This is not the case with current aromatherapy practice. For the students' information, the essential oils, which contain significant quantities of safrole, beta-asorone and benzopyrene, such as cade, sassafras, calamus and yellow and brown fractions of camphor, are the ones that appear to have carcinogenic activity. Also, essential oils rich in methyl chavicol or methyleugenol, such as tropical basil, and French and Russian tarragon, should be avoided in such conditions.

## Not for general use

The following essential oils are not considered safe in general use and should be avoided unless the practitioner is specifically further trained in their use.

| almond, bitter | *Prunus amygdalus* |
| boldo leaf | *Peumus boldus* |
| calamus | *Acorus calamus* |

| | |
|---|---|
| camphor (brown) | *Cinnamomum camphora* |
| camphor (yellow) | *Cinnamomum camphora* |
| cassia | *Cinnamomum cassia* |
| cinnamon bark | *Cinnamomun zeylanicum* |
| costus | *Saussurea lappa* |
| elecampane | *Inula helenium* |
| fennel, bitter | *Foeniculum vulgare* var. *amarga* |
| horseradish | *Amoracia rusticana* |
| jaborandi | *Pilocarpus jaborandi* |
| mugwort | *Artemesia vulgaris* |
| mustard | *Brassica nigra* |
| pine, dwarf | *Pinus mugo* |
| rue | *Ruta graveolens* |
| sassafras | *Sassafras albidum* |
| sassafras, Brazilian | *Ocotea cymbarum* |
| savine | *Juniperus sabina* |
| southernwood | *Artemesia abrotanum* |
| tansy | *Tanacetum vulgare* |
| thuja, cedarleaf | *Thuja occidentalis* |
| thuja, Western red | *Thuja plicata* |
| wintergreen | *Gaultheira procumbens* |
| wormseed | *Chenopodium anthelminticum* |
| wormwood | *Artemesia absinthium* |

# APPENDIX 3: THERAPEUTIC PROPERTIES OF ESSENTIAL OILS

The following is a list of therapeutic properties and their definitions. The practitioner of aromatherapy should be familiar with these terms and their meanings. Examples of essential oils having each property are given as illustrations; they are not the only ones with such a property. The list should be extended by your own research. Check for correct species and for safety data for each oil before use.

**Abortifacient** capable of inducing an abortion *pennyroyal*

**Alterative** blood purifying, usually by acting on the liver, kidneys or lymph; *see depurative   rosemary, lemon, juniper, cedarwood, fennel, carrot seed, eucalyptus, tea tree, niaouli, cajeput*

**Anaesthetic** capable of inducing loss of sensation and of numbing pain   *clove, peppermint*

**Analgesic** relieves or reduces pain   *peppermint, bergamot, chamomile, lavender, clove, rosemary, eucalyptus, ginger*

**Anaphrodisiac** lowers sexual desire   *marjoram*

**Antacid** counters acidity, particularly excess acid in the stomach   *lemon*

**Antiallergenic** counters an allergic reaction *chamomile, melissa*

**Antibiotic** inhibits or destroys bacterial pathogens *eucalyptus, myrrh, tea tree (essential oils rich in alcohols, phenols, ketones, terpenes and aldehydes)*

**Anticoagulant** prevents formation of blood clots *geranium*

**Anticonvulsive** controls convulsions   *chamomile, clary sage, lavender*

**Antidepressant** counteracts depression, inducing positive mood   *basil, bergamot, chamomile, jasmine, lavender, melissa, neroli, rose, sandalwood, ylang ylang*

**Antiemetic** arrests vomiting, counters nausea *ginger, basil, cinnamon, fennel, peppermint*

**Antifungal** inhibits or destroys fungal infection *tea tree, lemongrass, myrrh, patchouli, thyme, geranium, coriander, cedarwood*

**Antigalactagogue** inhibits formation or flow of breast milk   *peppermint, sage*

**Antimicrobial** inhibits or destroys microscopic pathogens   *myrrh, thyme*

**Antineuralgic** reduces nerve pain   *chamomile, eucalyptus, peppermint*

**Antioxidant** inhibits oxidative damage to cell walls *benzoin, coriander, clove, cumin, lemongrass*

**Antiphlogistic** counters, reduces inflammation, fevers   *chamomile, eucalyptus, lavender, yarrow, sage, clary sage*

**Antipruritic** relieves itching   *chamomile, lavender, peppermint*

**Antirheumatic** relieves pain of osteo-arthritis, rheumatoid arthritis   *benzoin, cajeput, chamomile, eucalyptus, cypress, juniper, lavender, marjoram, rosemary, niaouli*

**Antisclerotic** prevents hardening of tissue due to chronic inflammation   *lemon, garlic, onion*

**Antiseptic** destroys or inhibits growth of microbe pathogens   *Virtually all essential oils have this property to a greater or lesser extent*

**Antispasmodic** relieves or releases muscle spasm or cramp   *chamomile, lavender, fennel, valerian, clary sage*

**Antisudorific** reduces sweating   *clary sage, sage, cypress*

**Antitussive** relieves coughing   *eucalyptus, hyssop, marjoram, pine, sage, clary sage, rose*

**Antiviral** inhibits or destroys viral pathogens *eucalyptus, hyssop, lemon, lime, camphor, tea tree, pine, niaouli, thyme*

**Aperitif** encourages appetite, promotes digestion *cardamom, ginger, bay, caraway, bergamot, black pepper*

**Aphrodisiac** excites sexual desire, promotes health of glands and reproductive organs   *jasmine, ylang ylang, clary sage, sandalwood, rose, vetivert, neroli, cardamom, patchouli*

**Astringent** having a drying and tonic effect on tissues; binding; inhibiting flow or accumulation of fluids   *sage, frankincense, cypress, geranium, lemon, immortelle*

**Bacteriacide** an agent that destroys bacteria   *tea tree, eucalyptus, niaouli, cajeput, myrrh, frankincense*

**Balsamic** soothing and healing like a resinous balm *myrrh, pine, benzoin*

**Carminative** relieves or prevents flatulence   *basil, black pepper, fennel, cardamom, chamomile, ginger, lemon, marjoram, peppermint*

**Cephalic** acting on the disorders of the head   *basil, peppermint, sage, rosemary*

**Cholagogue** promotes the flow of bile   *lemon, rosemary, peppermint, yarrow*

**Choleretic** promotes the formation of bile *peppermint*

**Cicatrisant** promotes healing of wounds by formation of scar tissue   *bergamot, chamomile, clove, cypress, frankincense, geranium, juniper, lavender, patchouli, tea tree*

**Cordial** a traditional term for general stimulant, tonic; also a heart or cardiac tonic  *melissa, marjoram, neroli, rose, lavender, benzoin*

**Counter irritant** reducing pain or irritation in an area by provoking an increase in local circulation, or a minor irritation to the skin in another, *see* rubifacient  *black pepper, ginger, eucalyptus, juniper, rosemary, pine*

**Cytophylactic** encouraging growth of leucocytes, cells which defend against infection  *eucalyptus, peppermint, tea tree.* (According to Valnet (1982), most essential oils are cytophylactic.)

**Decongestant** relieving mucous congestion in the upper respiratory tract  *peppermint, tea tree, eucalyptus, cajeput, niaouli, sage*

**Depurative** blood purifying, usually by acting on the liver; *see* alterative  *rosemary, lemon, juniper*

**Detoxicant** neutralising toxic substances  *frankincense, fennel, juniper, tea tree*

**Diaphoretic** promotes sweating, stimulates circulation to the skin, *see* sudorific  *angelica, camphor, chamomile, ginger, black pepper, hyssop, mints, myrrh, juniper, pine, rosemary, sage, thyme, yarrow*

**Digestive** promoting good digestion  *basil, marjoram, ginger, sage, rosemary, thyme, oregano, fennel, cardamom, cumin, mandarin, lemon, bergamot, cinnamon*

**Disinfectant** destroying germs  *All essential oils are disinfectant to a greater or lesser degree*

**Diuretic** promoting the flow of urine  *juniper, cedarwood, cumin, coriander, carrot seed, cypress, sandalwood, fennel*

**Emmenagogue** promoting and regulating menstrual flow  *angelica, lavender, juniper, basil, clary sage, fennel, cumin, jasmine, myrrh, rose, rosemary*

**Emollient** soothing and softening to tissues  *chamomile, geranium, lavender, rose, sandalwood, mandarin, immortelle*

**Escharotic** corrosive or caustic, used to treat warts and skin cancers  *lemon, tea tree, garlic, cinnamon*

**Expectorant** promoting discharge of mucus and phlegm from the lungs and throat  *benzoin, basil, angelica, eucalyptus, ginger, thyme, yarrow*

**Febrifuge** lowers, reduces a fever  *bergamot, melissa, peppermint, chamomile, myrrh, niaouli, palmarosa, patchouli, sandalwood, camphor*

**Galactagogue** promoting the flow of breast milk  *fennel, dill, jasmine, cubeb, coriander*

**Haemostatic** stops blood flow, haemorrhage, *see* styptic  *geranium, lemon, cinnamon, cypress, rose*

**Hepatic** strengthens the liver function  *rosemary, lemon, carrot seed, grapefruit, immortelle, peppermint*

**Hypertensive** increases blood pressure  *camphor, hyssop, pennyroyal, sage, thyme, rosemary* (note: this effect is extrapolated from the fact that these oils stimulate the circulation)

**Hypoglycaemic** low in blood sugar, hence an oil that helps lower blood sugar levels  *eucalyptus, juniper, geranium*

**Hypotensive** reduces blood pressure  *jasmine, lavender, marjoram, melissa, ylang ylang*

**Insecticide** kills or repels insects  *cypress, eucalyptus, lavender, geranium, peppermint, citronella, tea tree, thyme, may chang, patchouli*

**Laxative** promoting evacuation of bowel  *black pepper, fennel, ginger, camphor*

**Leucocytisis** increasing the activity or numbers of leucocytes, the white blood cells responsible for fighting infections. See cytophylactic

**Nervine** calming and/or restoring to the nerves or nervous system, relaxing  *basil, bergamot, marjoram, jasmine, lavender, melissa, rose, sandalwood, ylang ylang, vetiver*

**Parasiticide** kills parasites, e.g. fleas, lice,  *eucalyptus, lemon, lemongrass, peppermint, rosemary, thyme, tea tree*

**Parturient** aids parturition or labour and childbirth by stimulating uterine contractions  *lavender, clary sage, jasmine, clove bud, juniper, peppermint*

**Pectoral** a remedy acting on disorders of the chest, i.e. lungs  *cajeput, eucalyptus, niaouli, pine, benzoin, hyssop*

**Prophylactic** preventing disease, many essential oils have this property, if used  *lavender, eucalyptus, rosemary, juniper, ylang ylang, jasmine, ginger*

**Restorative** restoring vitality, health, spirits  *bergamot, basil, camphor, pine, mints*

**Rubifacient** drawing local circulation to an area of skin to produce redness  *black pepper, ginger, eucalyptus, juniper, rosemary, pine*

**Sedative** calming to the central nervous system, counters hyperactivity of function  *benzoin, chamomile, clary sage, frankincense, jasmine, lavender, rose, melissa, sandalwood, vetivert, ylang ylang*

**Splenetic** tonic or strengthening to the spleen  *angelica, black pepper, fennel, immortelle*

**Stimulant** increasing the activity of an organ or function, e.g. circulation, peristalsis, secretions, muscle contractions, kidneys  *basil, bay, cajeput, camphor, clary sage, fennel, hyssop, juniper, rosemary, sage, peppermint, myrrh*

**Stomachic** tonic or strengthening stomach functions, digestion  *bay, basil, cardamom, juniper, nutmeg, patchouli, rosemary, rosewood, sage, thyme*

**Styptic** arresting haemorrhaging, bleeding (usually astringents)  *cinnamon leaf, cypress, juniper, geranium, lemon, lime, pine (turpentine/terebinth), rose otto*

**Sudoriphic** promotes sweating, stimulates circulation to the exterior, *see* diaphoretic  *angelica, camphor, chamomile, ginger, black pepper, hyssop, mints, myrrh, juniper, pine, rosemary, sage, thyme, yarrow*

**Tonic** strengthening to an organ, tissue, function or system; choice depends on the area  *basil, clary sage, black pepper, frankincense, geranium, myrrh, juniper, sage, rosemary, yarrow*

**Vasoconstrictor** causing smooth muscles of the blood vessels to contract  *chamomile, cypress, geranium, peppermint, rose*

**Vasodilator** dilates blood vessels, which relieves strain on the heart and helps in hypertension  *carrot seed, lemongrass, marjoram*

**Vermifuge** expels worms  *carrot seed, cinnamon, clove, eucalyptus, niaouli, tarragon, thyme*

**Vulnerary** wound healing, promoting healing of skin, muscle, bone by inhibiting infection and stimulating regeneration of tissue  *benzoin, elemi, frankincense, immortelle, lavender, myrrh, rosemary, tarragon, tea tree, yarrow*

# APPENDIX 4: ESSENTIAL OIL ENERGETIC AND THERAPEUTIC CHART

The chart may be used to support constitutional treatment as well as choosing oils by therapeutic property.

For reasons of space only the main actions of essential oils are given. Most other properties can be derived from one or more of these.

**Key: W**=warming  **C**=cooling  **M**=moistening  **D**=drying or draining  **B**=balancing – i.e. amphoteric, regulating, or normalising an excess or deficient condition. **t**=top note  **m**=middle note **b**=base note.

**Notes:** Warming: a warming oil can also have an anti-inflammatory or antipyretic effect, following the principle of like curing like and synergy; assessment of the patient's energetic pattern is needed to determine its appropriateness. It can help on the emotional and mental levels, e.g. countering the coldness of depression.

Cooling: has a refreshing effect and can counter an excess heat or inflammation, whether physical (as in fever), emotional (as in anger) or mental (overactive thoughts, overworking).

Moistening: while all essential oils are drying to an extent due to their volatility, in some this is outweighed by the additional ability to promote healthy secretions and or moisture in the tissues.

Drying: this effect can be based on several properties, e.g. diuretic, astringent, diaphoretic. It includes the action of some oils that drain excess fluids or reduce fluid congestion.

Stimulating: increasing the activity of an organ or system, or of the vital force (blood, lymph circulation, bile or gastric secretion). The symbol '+' indicates a stronger effect.

Diaphoretic, diuretic and emmenagogue properties stimulate specific functions.

Nervine: acting on the nervous system by calming, relieving spasms or strengthening (toning). '+' indicates a stronger effect.

Alterative: blood and lymph purifying. The means varies with the oils, e.g. via liver decongesting, killing pathogens or stimulating the increase of leucocytes.

Digestive: promoting good digestion which helps reduce toxic accumulation; enhances nutrition.

Respiratory: Relieving congestion or expectorant.

Diaphoretic: sudorific; promoting sweating.

Diuretic: promoting excretion of urine. Helping drain excess fluids.

Emmenagogue: includes also the concept of moving blood that may have become congested or blocked; a condition that can affect men and women.

Astringent: drying and/or strengthening tissues.

Vulnerary: promoting healing of tissues.

Tonic: strengthening to an organ or function; rejuvenating.

Mental-emotional: calming, restorative, euphoric/uplifting, invigorating, refreshing, comforting, promoting clarity. See individual profile for detail.

**Method:** To hone the selection of oils based on constitutional type or energy pattern of the patient: First, check the energy of an oil, then check the therapeutic properties match the effect needed, finally refer to the details of each oil in Chapter 11. Students are encouraged to add to or revise the information in light of their experience or tutor's instruction.

| ESSENTIAL OIL (*=ABSOLUTE) | NOTE | ENERGY | THERAPEUTIC ACTION | | | | | | | | | | | Mental Emotional |
|---|---|---|---|---|---|---|---|---|---|---|---|---|---|---|
| | | | Stim. | Ner-vine | Dig. | Alt. | Resp. | Diaph | Diur. | Emm. | Ast. | Vuln. | Tonic | |
| Basil | t | W D | • | • | • | • | • | • | | • | | • | | Calming, promotes clarity |
| Benzoin* | b | W D/B | • | • | • | • | | | • | | • | • | | Calming, comforting, uplifting |
| Bergamot | t | C D | | • | • | | • | | • | | • | • | | Euphoric, refreshing, calming |
| Black pepper | b | W D | • | • | • | • | • | • | • | • | | | | Promotes clarity, calming |
| Cajeput | t | W D | • | • | • | | • | • | | | | | | Promotes clarity, invigorates |
| Cardamom | m | W D | • | • | • | | • | | | | | | • | Calming, promotes clarity |
| Carrot | m | W D/B | • | • | • | • | • | | | • | | | • | Calming |
| Cedarwood, A | b | W D | • | • | | • | • | | • | • | • | | | Calming, promotes clarity, euphoric |
| Cedarwood, T | b | W D | • | | | • | • | | • | • | • | | | Calming, restorative |
| Cedarwood, V | b | W D | • | • | | • | • | | • | • | | | | Calming, restorative |
| Chamomile, R | m | C B | • | • | • | • | • | • | • | • | • | | | Calming, uplifting |
| Chamomile, G | m | C M | • | • | • | • | • | • | | • | | | | Calming, uplifting |
| Citronella | t | C M | | • | | • | | • | • | | | | • | Uplifting, calming |
| Clove bud | b | W D | • | • | • | • | • | | | | | | • | Comforting, promotes clarity (memory) |
| Clary sage | t | W D | • | • | • | • | • | | | • | | | • | Euphoric, calming, invigorating |
| Coriander | t | W D | • | • | • | • | | | | • | | | • | Uplifting, promotes clarity |
| Cypress | b | W D | • | • | • | • | | • | • | | • | | • | Restorative, invigorating |

| ESSENTIAL OIL (*=ABSOLUTE) | NOTE | ENERGY | Stim. | Nervine | Dig. | Alt. | Resp. | Diaph | Diur. | Emm. | Ast. | Vuln. | Tonic | Mental Emotional |
|---|---|---|---|---|---|---|---|---|---|---|---|---|---|---|
| Eucalyptus | t | W D | •+ | • | • | • | • | • | • | | | • | | Promotes clarity, invigorating, refreshing |
| Fennel | m | W D | | • | • | • | | | • | • | | | • | Balancing |
| Frankincense | b | W D | | •+ | • | • | • | | • | • | | • | • | Calming, euphoric |
| Geranium | m | C M/B | | • | • | • | | | | | • | • | • | Uplifting, refreshing |
| Ginger | t | W D | • | • | • | • | • | • | | | | | • | Balancing |
| Grapefruit | t | C D | • | | • | • | | | • | | • | | • | Euphoric, restorative, calming |
| Hyssop | t | W D | •+ | • | • | • | • | • | • | | • | | | Calming, promotes clarity |
| Jasmine* | b | C D/B | | •+ | • | | • | | | | | | | Euphoric, calming |
| Juniper | b | W D | •+ | • | • | • | | • | • | • | • | • | • | Invigorating, uplifting |
| Lavender | m | W D/B | • | • | • | • | | • | • | • | | • | • | Euphoric, calming |
| Lemon | t | C D | • | | • | • | | • | • | | • | | • | Euphoric, refreshing, invigorating |
| Lemongrass | t | C M | | | • | • | | • | • | • | | | | Calming, uplifting |
| Lime | t | C D | • | • | • | • | | • | | | • | | • | Uplifting, refreshing, invigorating |
| Mandarin | t | C D | • | • | • | | | | | | • | | • | Refreshing, calming |
| Marjoram, Sweet, Spanish | m | W D/B | • | • | | | • | • | • | • | | | | Calming, comforting, restorative, promotes clarity |
| May Chang | m | W D/B | • | • | | | | | | | • | | • | Euphoric |
| Melissa | m | C D/B | • | • | • | • | • | • | | | | | • | Calming, refreshing, uplifting, euphoric |
| Myrrh | b | W D | • | • | • | • | • | | | • | • | • | • | Calming, promotes clarity |
| Myrtle | m | W D | | • | | • | • | | | | | | | Refreshing, uplifting |
| Neroli | b | C M/B | • | • | • | • | | | | | | | • | Refreshing, calming, euphoric |
| Niaouli | t | W D | •+ | | | • | • | • | | | | | • | Promotes clarity, uplifting |
| Orange, bitter/ Petigrain | t | C D/B | | • | • | • | | | | | • | | | Refreshing, calming, euphoric |
| Orange, bitter/ Bigarade | t | C D/B | | • | • | • | | | | | • | | • | Refreshing, calming euphoric |
| Palmarosa | t | C M | • | | • | • | | | | | | • | • | Calming, uplifting |
| Patchouli | b | W D/B | • | | • | | | • | • | | | | • | Calming, promotes clarity |
| Peppermint | t | C/W B | • | • | • | • | • | • | • | • | • | | • | Refreshing, uplifting, invigorating |
| Pine | m | W D | • | | | • | • | • | | | | • | • | Invigorating, promotes clarity, refreshing |
| Rose | b | C B | | •+ | • | • | | | | • | • | • | • | Euphoric, calming, comforting |

| ESSENTIAL OIL (*=ABSOLUTE) | NOTE | ENERGY | Stim. | Ner-vine | Dig. | Alt. | Resp. | Diaph | Diur. | Emm. | Ast. | Vuln. | Tonic | Mental Emotional |
|---|---|---|---|---|---|---|---|---|---|---|---|---|---|---|
| Rosemary | m | W D | •+ | • | • | • | • | • | • | | • | | • | Invigorating, promotes clarity, (concentration, memory), restorative |
| Sage, Spanish | t | W D | • | • | • | • | | | | | • | • | | Invigorating, uplifting |
| Sandalwood | b | C D/B | | •+ | • | • | • | | | • | • | | • | Calming, euphoric |
| Spearmint | t | W D | • | • | • | | • | | | | • | | | Refreshing, invigorating, uplifting |
| Tea tree | t | W D | • | | | • | • | • | | | • | • | • | Invigorating, restorative |
| Thyme | t | W D | •+ | • | • | • | • | • | | | • | | • | Invigorating, restorative, promotes clarity (concentration) |
| Valerian | b | W D | | • | • | | | | • | | | | | Calming |
| Vetiver | b | C M | • | • | • | • | | | | | | | | Calming, euphoric |
| Yarrow | m | C D | | • | • | | | • | • | | • | • | • | Promotes clarity |
| Ylang Ylang | b | C M | • | •+ | | | | | | | | | • | Calming, euphoric, restorative |

# GLOSSARY

**ABC** – it stands for Airway, Breathing, Circulation – the important aspects to check first when giving first aid to an unconscious casualty.

**Absolute** – the substance produced from a concrete, pomade or resinoid, which undergoes solvent (ethanol) extraction at room temperature followed by filtering and distillation at low temperature to remove the solvent.

**Accounts** – the full and accurate record of all business transactions. The record is backed up with evidence, such as receipts for all purchases, chequebook stubs, bank statements, etc.

**Active listening** – listening with full attention to hear the other person's message, being receptive and supportive.

**Adaptation** – the means by which the body adapts or changes in response to a new or ongoing stress by making adjustments in its functions to ensure survival. It is part of the General Adaptation Syndrome, which Hans Seyle described as the series of responses to non-specific stressors.

**After care** – the period of an aromatherapy consultation after the treatment is given in which the practitioner explains to the client the likely effects and responses to the treatment and any relevant observations he or she has made, formulates a home blend, answers any questions, makes recommendations to enhance the client's health and so forth.

**Amphoteric** – in natural medicine, capable of producing a balancing effect between two extremes.

**Anabolism** – metabolic activity in which the body builds up complex substances and tissues from simple substances.

**Anosmia** – the loss of the sense of smell.

**Aromatogram** – a test for the best essential oil to inhibit or kill a pathogen. A swab of infected material is taken, the bacteria cultured in a petrie dish and different essential oils introduced to see which one has the best efficacy for that individual's tissue.

**Business plan** – a document setting out the strategy as to how a business will be set up and funds obtained for any needed expenditure; required by banks before they will agree a loan.

**Catabolism** – metabolic activity in which the body breaks down complex substances into simpler substances.

**Carbon cycle** – the natural cycle by which carbon is taken up and released by living organisms.

**Cash flow forecast** – a prediction of how much cash a business is likely to generate in a specified period of time in the future. The cash flow itself is the difference between the outgoings and receipts over a given period.

**Charge** – the plant material placed in the extraction tank.

**Chemotype** – two or more plants of the same species, which demonstrate variation in the chemical constituents of their volatile oils.

**Chloroplast** – the chlorophyll-containing component of plant cells.

**Code of ethics or practice** – standards of conduct set by professional organisations for their members; includes such subjects as working within the limits of training, confidentiality and security of information.

**Compound** – a substance constituted of atoms or ions of two or more different elements.

**Concrete** – a semi-solid mass produced in the first stage of solvent extraction. Used for plants such as rose whose essential oils would be damaged by the high heat of distillation.

**Constitutional type** – a term indicating one's genetic predisposition to certain characteristics, be they physical, mental or emotional; to certain patterns of imbalance; and to certain responses to a given condition or situation.

**Continuing professional development** – the obligation of the practitioner to undertake, at regular intervals, further study or training to maintain high standards of competence.

**Covalent bond** – a type of molecular bond formed by the sharing of electrons between atoms.

**Dicotyledon** – a form of plant in which two seed leaves appear at germination.

**Dynamic** – characterised by vital energy, power; energised, capable of activity.

**Eliciting** – respectfully evoking all relevant information from the client to elucidate the case; bringing into the light, into awareness.

**Elimination channels** – the five routes or systems by which the body cells and systems remove waste and toxins, namely the skin, the kidneys, the lungs, the lymph, the colon.

**Endorphin/enkephalin** – a type of neuropeptide or hormone released from the pituitary gland, which binds to the opiate receptors on cells causing such things as analgesia and euphoria. 'The brain's own morphine' (C. Pert).

**Enfleurage** – extraction by macerating or soaking plant material in an oil or fat.

**Essential fatty acids (EFAs)** – lipid substances found in fats and oils that are essential for the body's functions and which are not manufactured by the body but must be obtained from foods.

**Expression** – extraction by preparation and the pressing of the peel; used for citrus fruit.

**Family** – the category of plant taxonomy below an order and above genus.

**Fixed oil** – a non-volatile oil.

**Functional group** – that part of a molecule made up of a single atom or group of atoms, which substitutes for hydrogen and significantly affects the properties and behaviour of the molecule.

**Gas chromatography** – test for ascertaining the identifiable components of a gaseous substance; used to verify an agreed standard range of components present in a sample of essential oil and rule out adulteration. The data sheet resulting is the chromatogram.

**Genus** – the category of plant taxonomy below a family and above a species.

**Healing crisis/achievement** – a naturopathic concept describing the process of healing, which the body undertakes to balance itself, e.g. when it is ready to eliminate the fundamental cause of a disease condition. Indications may include such things as headaches, a fever, increased elimination via the skin, kidneys or respiratory system. The patient feels discomfort, especially if the body is not prepared for it, but more energy and positive well-being when it has passed.

**Hepatotoxic** – capable of damaging the liver or inducing disease in the liver.

**Holistic** – an approach to health care that recognises: (a) that health is a dynamic state of balance between the three main aspects of human life, the physical, mental–emotional and spiritual. It follows that the cause of disease lies not only in the physical sphere, and that any treatment given for a disease needs to address each aspect, not only the physical one; (b) that the body itself functions in an intelligent and integrated way and a symptom of imbalance in any one part cannot be understood or treated in isolation from the other parts and aspects of the organism; (c) an organism is integrated with its surroundings and cannot be understood in isolation.

**Homeostasis** – the body's feedback mechanisms for maintaining optimum levels of gases, ions, water and nutrients, as well as pressure and temperature to ensure its health.

**Hydrocarbon** – a compound containing only hydrogen and carbon.

**Hydrophilic** – a property of a molecule, which makes it attracted to water.

**Integrity** – a word derived from the Latin for wholeness indicating a state of inner and outer honesty and high ethical standing. 'Integrity of tissues' indicates their strength and sound functioning.

**Intention** – that aspect of treatment in which the practitioner's mind and energy is directed towards the goal of working with the natural healing energy without force. It is a positive but passive state, being open to change, facilitating the body's own self-healing mechanisms.

**Intuition** – that aspect of the mental faculties, which relies on non-logical modes of understanding beyond reason or physical perception.

**Isomers** – compounds having the same molecular formula (presence of the same atoms or elements), but differing in how these are structured, which gives them different properties.

**Limbic system** – a combination of structures within the brain associated with learning, memory and emotions. It includes the hippocampus, the pituitary gland and is closely linked to the hypothalamus and the amygdala.

**Limits of training** – the responsibility a practitioner has to recognise when a client has needs that cannot be met by his or her skills; knowing when to refer a client to another practitioner; not practising in ways for which one is not trained and qualified.

**Lipids** – a group of compounds, also known as fats or oils, characterised by being insoluble in water. Fats are solid at room temperature while oils are fluid. Phospholipids are fats in which a part of the molecule carries an electrical charge, making it partly soluble in water and partly not. Phospholipids are important to the structure and behaviour of cell membranes.

**Lipophilic** – attracted to and able to dissolve in fats.

**Lipophobic** – not attracted to and not able to dissolve in fats or lipids.

**Mixture** – a substance formed by elements which blend but do not bond chemically.

**Monocotyledon** – a form of plant in which one seed leaf appears at germination.

**Neuropeptide** – *see* peptide.

**Neurotoxic** – damaging to the nervous system or tissue and causing disease.

**Nitrogen cycle** – a natural cycle in which nitrogen is taken up and released by living organisms.

**'Nose'** – a professional creator of perfumes. A nose is trained to detect several thousand individual odours.

**Osmosis** – diffusion of a fluid across a semi-permeable membrane until there is equal concentration of fluid on both sides.

**Peptide or neuropeptide** – a protein molecule secreted by neurons, lymphocytes and monocytes, and capable of conveying information to cells which stimulates certain behaviours. Also called a cytokine.

**Perfusion** – flowing or passing through a substance, layer, tissue or membrane.

**Pharmacokinetics** – the pathways through which a substance moves after entering the body, the ways it is changed during its journey and how this determines its biological activity.

**Pharmacology** – the study of the biological activity, or effect, of substances when introduced into the body.

**Photosynthesis** – the process by which plants use the energy of sunlight to synthesise carbohydrates from carbon and water.

**Polarity** – indicating a type of bond formed in a molecule. If it is polar, the molecule is more hydrophilic and reactive; if it is apolar or non-polar the molecule is more hydrophobic.

**Pomade** – the fat saturated with essential oil produced during the enfleurage method of extraction before further processing by mixing the fat with alcohol, which allows the essential oils to be separated off.

**Presence** – a state of mindfulness and inner awareness, which is – as much as possible – free of concern for either past or future and fully open to or accepting present experience without prejudging what occurs.

**Provenance** – the place of origin; in aromatherapy indicating also the series of operations the plant material's volatile oil undergoes from growing, harvesting and extraction to transportation, bottling and marketing. Lack of quality control at any stage can depreciate the resulting essential oil.

**Qualitative research** – research conducted by use of subjective experience of participants.

**Quantitative research** – research conducted by objective measurements.

**Quenching** – in aromatherapy and perfumery, the ability of one or more components in an essential oil to buffer or lessen the effect of others.

**Recovery position** – the position into which an unconscious casualty is placed when giving first aid.

**Referral** – advising and facilitating the transfer of a client's care, or part of it, to another practitioner more qualified to deal with a condition or situation.

**Rejuvenation** – the correct application of techniques, procedures and substances, which enhance the vitality, health and well-being of the whole organism and inhibit or protect against wear and tear or the ageing process.

**Risk assessment** – a process of evaluating potential risks in a workplace and providing for the means to minimise or exclude them.

**Secretory cells** – specialised cells in plants which secrete aromatic molecules.

**Sensitisation** – a process in which the body becomes more than normally sensitive to a substance and produces a reaction.

**Smell fatigue** – the loss of the awareness of an odorant; the sensory fibres lose their responsiveness as they accommodate to continuous stimulation.

**Solvent extraction** – modern method of extraction of essential oils using various solvents.

**Species** – the category ranking below a genus in taxonomy of organisms and above subspecies.

**Stages of disease** – a naturopathic concept identifying the stages through which the body's healthy functioning degrades and disease manifests. Stages include: acute, sub-acute, chronic, degenerative.

**Stress response** – the body's natural response to stress of any kind through a sequence of nervous and hormonal changes that affect the mind, emotions and physical functions.

**Synergy** – a term describing the phenomenon that the whole is greater than merely the sum of its individual parts or that when the different parts are fully present and act in concert, a greater, different energy and effect is created than can be attributed to any single part on its own.

**Taxonomy** – the classifying of organisms in an ordered way, which shows natural relationships.

**Tax return** – the form supplied by the Inland Revenue for the purposes of tax collection on which you record your earnings for the past year, any capital gains and your net profit.

**Terrain** – a French term indicating the background condition of the body that either leaves one vulnerable to disease or enables the body to withstand stressors, pathogens, disease-causing factors.

**Therapeutic space** – a period of time and/or a place in which the client enjoys comfort, security and calm so that mind and body can become deeply relaxed and thus more open to inner healing mechanisms.

**Transference** – projecting on to another person responsibility for one's happiness or for one's negative reaction to a situation. Usually used in the context of a therapeutic relationship, e.g. between a psychotherapist and client, but applicable to aromatherapy practice.

**Treatment record** – the maintenance of a record of a client's case history, and of each therapeutic encounter, and any treatment or recommendations given.

**Variety** – a subdivision of a species indicating naturally occurring or selectively bred populations or individual plants.

**VAT** – it stands for value added tax or the amount charged to most goods and services. An aromatherpist, the provider of a service, may be liable to pay VAT once the turnover of the practice reaches a specified limit, currently £54,000.

**Vital force** – the power that creates and sustains the universe and every thing and creature in it; the energy that gives and maintains life and well-being.

**Viscous** – having a high resistance to flow; a term describing the extreme thickness and adhesive quality of a fluid substance.

**Volatile** – evaporating easily at normal temperatures.

**Yield** – term referring both to the product and the quantity of essential oil on distillation.

# REFERENCES AND FURTHER READING

Ahmad, Jaimal and Qadeer, Ashhar (1998) *Unani, the Science of Graeco-Arab Medicine*, Lustre Bress Pvt. Ltd., New Delhi.

Actander, S. (1960) *Perfume and Flavour Materials of Natural Origin*, published by the author, Elizabeth, New Jersey.

Alexander, Michael (2001) *How Aromatherapy Works: Synthetic and Efficacious Pathways of Essential Oils in the Human Physiology, Vol. I. Principal Mechanisms of Olfaction*. Whole Spectrum Arts and Publications, Odessa FLA.

Armstrong, Fauvre and Heidinsfeld, Vera (2000) 'Aromatherapy for deaf and deaf/blind people living in residential accomodation', in *Complementary Therapies in Nursing and Midwifery*, **6**, 180–88.

Balch, James F. and Balch, Phyllis A. (2000) *Prescription for Nutritional Healing*, Avery Publishing, New York.

Belaiche, P. (1979) *Traite de Phytotherapie et d'Aromathique*, Maloine, Paris.

Ball, John M. D. (1990) *Understanding Disease*, C. W. Daniel, Saffron Walden.

Battaglia, Salvatore (1995) *The Complete Guide to Aromatherapy*, The Perfect Potion, Queensland, Australia.

Caddy, Rosemary (1997) *Essential Oils in Colour: Caddy Classic Profiles*, Amberwood Publishing, Guildford.

*Culpeper's Complete Herbal* (1995) Wordsworth Editions Ltd, London.

Clark, Sue (2002) *Essential Chemistry for Safe Aromatherapy*, Churchill Livingstone, London.

Davis, Patricia (1995) *Aromatherapy A–Z*, Second edition, C. W. Daniel, Saffron Walden.

Frawley, David (1991) *Ayurvedic Healing Course*, American Vedic Institute, Santa Fe.

Frawley, David and Lad, Vasant (1986) *The Yoga of Herbs*, The Lotus Press, Santa Fe.

Gattefossé, René-Maurice (1993) *Gattefossé's Aromatherapy*, edited by Robert Tisserrand, C. W. Daniel, Saffron Walden.

Gibbs, June (1997) 'Introducing Niaouli', *Aromatherapy Times*, vol. 1, no. 35, International Federation of Aromatherapy, London.

Grieves, M. (1984) *A Modern Herbal*, Savas Publishing, Adelaide/Jonathan Cape Ltd, London.

*Hippocrates*, translated in eight volumes by W. H. S. Jones, Paul Potter, Wesley Smith (1968–1994) Loeb Classical Library, William Heinemann, London.

Kenton, Leslie (1985) Ageless Ageing, Century, London.

Johnson (1985) *H & R Guide to Fragrance Ingredients,* R. Gloss and Co., London.

Kusmirek, Jan (2002) *Liquid Sunshine: Vegetable Oils for Aromatherapy*, Floramicus, Glastonbury.

Lawless, Julia (1992) *The Encyclopedia of Essential Oils*, Element Books, Shaftesbury.

Manniche, Lise (1989) *An Ancient Egyptian Herbal*, British Museum Publications, London.

Manniche, Lise (1999) *Sacred Luxuries, Fragrance, Aromatherapy and Cosmetics in Ancient Egypt*, Opus Publishing, London.

Maury, Margarite (1989) *Margarite Maury's Guide to Aromatherapy*, C. W. Daniel, Saffron Walden.

Mernagh-Ward, Dawn and Cartwright, Jennifer 1997 *Good Practice in Salon Management*, Nelson Thornes, Cheltenham.

Miller, Light and Miller, Bryan (1998) *Ayurveda and Aromatherapy*, Motilal Barnasidass, New Delhi.

Mitchell, A. and Cormak, M. (1998) *The Therapeutic Relationship in Health Care*, Churchill Livingstone, London.

Montague, Ashley (1986) *Touching: the human significance of skin*, Harper Collins, London.

Murray, Michael and Pizorno, Joseph (1990) *Encyclopedia of Natural Medicine*, Little, Brown and Company, New York and London.

Newman-Turner, Roger (1990) *Naturopathic Medicine*, Thornsons-HarperCollins, London .

Pert, Candace (1988) *Molecule of Emotions: Why You Feel the Way You Feel*, Simon & Schuster, London.

Pert, Candace (1999) *Molecules of Emotion*, Pocket Books, London.

Piesse, S. (1895) *Des Odeurs, des Parfums, et des Cosmetiques*, Paris.

Piesse, S. (1905) *Histoire des Parfums*, Paris.

Pitman, Vicki (2000) *Herbal Remedies*, Vega Publishing (Chrysalis), London.

Price, Len and Price, Shirley (1999) *Aromatherapy for Health Professionals*, Churchill Livingstone, London.

Schnaubelt, Kurt (1998) *Advanced Aromatherapy*, Healing Arts Press, Rochester, Vermont.

Seyle, Hans (1990) *The Stress of Life*, McGraw-Hill, London.

Stuart, Malcolm (1989) (ed.) *Encyclopedia of Herbs and Herbalism*, CEEPI/Dealerfield.

Susskind, Peter (1986) *Perfume: the Story of a Murder*, Penguin, London.

'The ABC Clinical Guide to Herbs' (sample chapter for German chamomile), *Herbalgram, the Journal of the American Botanical Council*, 2003, **58**, 34–46 www.herbalgram.com .

Tierra, Michael (1998) *Planetary Herbology*, The Lotus Press, Santa Fe, California.

Tisserand, Robert (1977) *The Art of Aromatherapy*, Healing Arts Press, Vermont.

Tisserand, Robert and Balacs, Tony (1995) *Essential Oil Safety: A Guide for Health Care Professionals*, Churchill Livingstone, London.

Valnet, Jean (1982) *Practical Aromatherapy* C.W. Daniel, Saffron Walden.

Worwood, Valerie Anne (2001) *Aromatherapy for the Beauty Therapist*, Thomson Learning, London.

Aromatherapy Consortium
PO Box 6522
Desborough
Kettering
Northants NN14 2YX.
info@aromatherapy-regulation.org.uk
Tel: 0870 7743477

Independent testing companies
  Traceability Ltd
  Jenny Warden
  www.traceabilityltd.co.uk

Professional associations, UK
  The International Federation of Aromatherapy
  182 Chiswick High Road
  London W4 1PP
  Tel: 0208 742 2650
  www.int-fed-aromatherapy.co.uk

  The International Federation of Professional
  Aromatherpists
  82 Ashby Road
  Hinckley, Leicestershire LE10 1 SN
  Tel: 01455 637897
  www.ifparoma.org

Essential oil suppliers, UK
  Butturber and Sage
  7 Tessa Road
  Reading RG1 8HH
  Tel: 0118 9505100
  www.butterburandsage.com

Fragrant Earth Ltd
Orchard House
Magdalen Court
Glastonbury, Somerset TA
Tel: 01458 831216
www.fragrantearth.co.uk

Rosa Medica
The Barn
Crickham
Wedmore, Somerset BS28 4JT
Tel: 01934 712848

Saffron Oils
Belmont House, Newport
Saffron Walden, Essex CB11 3RF
Tel: 01799 540622

Shirley Price Aromatherapy
Essentia House
Upper Bond Street
Hinckley, Leicestershire LE10 1RS
Tel: 01455 615466
www.shirleyprice.co.uk

The Essential Oil Company
Worting House
Basingstoke
Hampshire RG23 8PX
Tel: 01256 332737
essoil@aol.com
www.eoco.org.uk

# INDEX